FOURTH EDITION

JONG'S
COMMUNITY
DENTAL HEALTH

"As man advances in civilization and small tribes are united into larger communities, the simplest reason would tell each individual that he ought to extend his social instincts and sympathies to all members of the same nation, though personally unknown to him. . . ."

Charles Darwin, 1882

FOURTH EDITION

Jong's Community Dental Health

Edited by

George M. Gluck, DDS, MPH

Associate Professor
Division of Comprehensive Care and Applied
   Practice Administration and
   Behavioral Sciences
New York University College of Dentistry
New York, New York

Warren M. Morganstein, DDS, MPH

Senior Associate Dean
Professor, Department of Oral Health
   Care Delivery
Baltimore College of Dental Surgery
Baltimore, Maryland

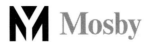

St. Louis Baltimore Boston Carlsbad Chicago Minneapolis New York Philadelphia Portland
London Milan Sydney Tokyo Toronto

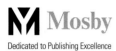
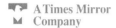

Dedicated to Publishing Excellence

A Times Mirror
Company

Publisher: Don E. Ladig
Acquisitions Editor: Penny Rudolph
Associate Developmental Editor: Angela Reiner
Project Manager: Mark Spann
Designer: Judi Lang
Manufacturing Supervisor: Karen Boehme
Editing and Production: Top Graphics
Cover Designer: David A. Scott

FOURTH EDITION

Printed in the United States of America
Composition by Top Graphics
Printing/binding by R.R. Donnelley & Sons Company

Mosby–Year Book, Inc.
11830 Westline Industrial Drive
St. Louis, Missouri 63146

International Standard Book Number 0-8151-3488-6

97 98 99 00 01 / 9 8 7 6 5 4 3 2 1

CONTRIBUTORS

Myron Allukian, Jr., DDS, MPH
Director–Community Dental Programs
Boston Department of Public Health
Boston, Massachusetts

Rima Bachiman, DDS, MPA
New York University College of Dentistry
New York, New York

Tryfon Beazoglou, PhD
Department of Pediatric Dentistry
School of Dental Medicine
University of Connecticut Health Center
Farmington, Connecticut

Muriel J. Bebeau, PhD
Professor
University of Minnesota School of Dentistry
Minneapolis, Minnesota

Helene Bednarsh, BS, RDH, MPH
Director, HIV Dental Ombudsperson Program
Boston Department of Public Health
Boston, Massachusetts

Lester E. Block, DDS, MPH
Director of Graduate Studies in Public Health
University of Minnesota School of Public
   Health
Minneapolis, Minnesota

Joseph Boffa, DDS, MPH
Associate Professor
Department of Dental Care Management
Goldman School of Graduate Dentistry
Boston University Medical Center
Boston, Massachusetts

David O. Born, PhD
Professor and Director
Division of Health Ecology
University of Minnesota School of Dentistry
Minneapolis, Minnesota

James Crall, DDS, ScD
Department of Pediatric Dentistry
School of Dental Medicine
University of Connecticut Health Center
Farmington, Connecticut

Marianne B. DeSouza, RDH, BA, MS
Director, Greater New Bedford Tobacco
   Control Program
New Bedford, Massachusetts

Eliezer Eidelman, Dr Odont, MSD
Department of Pediatric Dentistry
Hadassah School of Dental Medicine
The Hebrew University
Jerusalem, Israel

Diana L. Mercado Galvis, RDA, RDH, MS
New York University
New York, New York

Eugene Hittelman, EdD
New York University
New York, New York

Alice M. Horowitz, PhD
National Institute of Dental Research
National Institutes of Health
Bethesda, Maryland

Jeffrey P. Kahn, MPH, PhD
Director, Center for Bioethics
University of Minnesota
Minneapolis, Minnesota

Bennett Klein, Esq.
Director, AIDS Law Project
Gay & Lesbian Advocates & Defenders
Boston, Massachusetts

Nancy R. Kressin, PhD
Center for Health Quality, Outcomes and
    Economic Research
VA Medical Center
Bedford, Massachusetts

Madalyn L. Mann, MS
Associate Professor
Goldman School of Dental Medicine
Boston University
Boston, Massachusetts

David G. Pendrys, DDS, PhD
Department of Behavioral Sciences and
    Community Health
University of Connecticut Health Center
Farmington, Connecticut

Benjamin Peretz, DMD
Department of Pediatric Dentistry
Hadassah School of Dental Medicine
The Hebrew University
Jerusalem, Israel

Burton R. Pollack, DDS, MPH, JD
Dean, School of Dental Medicine Health
    Sciences Center
State University of New York at Stony Brook
Stony Brook, New York

Lynda Rose, BA
Goldman School of Dental Medicine
Boston University
Boston, Massachusetts

Terri S.I. Tilliss, RDH, MS, MA
Associate Professor, Dental Hygiene
University of Colorado Health Sciences
    Center School of Dentistry
Denver, Colorado

PREFACE

Immense changes have taken place in the delivery of dental care with consequent changes in the field of community dental health. The fourth edition focuses on the most salient issues.

In part the changes are due to the efforts and influences of new editors who have endeavored to preserve the integrity and philosophy of the Jong editions. Most of the changes relate to current data, recent initiatives, and shifts in public policy.

The most far-reaching modifications occur in the following chapters: Chapter 2, which presents an overview of dental care delivery; Chapters 4 and 17, which address transmissible diseases; Chapter 6, which focuses on the impact of emerging ethnic groups; Chapter 9, which discusses epidemiology; Chapter 15, which presents a comprehensive analysis of how to read the scientific literature and explains the elements of informatics and how to access the literature; and Chapter 16, which addresses bioethics and community dental health.

Chapter 2, from an economist's perspective, describes the impact of managed care and changes in the dental workforce. It also includes a forecast of the needs of the dental workforce for the next decade. Chapters 4 and 17 discuss the specific roles of dental team members in the treatment of patients with HIV. The historic and biologic evolution of HIV is described as taking place through legislation and legal cases involving practitioners and patients. The efforts of the Centers for Disease Control and Prevention, the Food and Drug Administration, and the Occupational Safety and Health Administration are highlighted. In addition, the implications and impact of the Americans with Disabilities Act on the practice of dentistry are discussed. Chapter 6 describes sensitivities to health care that are based on cultural differences. Chapter 7, which discusses geriatric oral diseases, analyzes important demographic changes and suggests their potential significance for dentistry. Chapter 9 succinctly defines epidemiology, provides an overview of epidemiologic strategies, and summarizes the distribution of oral diseases in the population. The diseases discussed range from dental caries and dental fluorosis through the oral manifestations of AIDS. The author suggests how knowledge of epidemiology may assist the dental team member. Chapter 15, uses clearly labeled tables to list and define the elements of acceptable research papers. It describes in practical terms how the computer can be used to access information. Chapter 16 presents concepts related to the nature of a profession and discusses "justice" as it applies to the distribution of scarce dental health resources. Six bioethics/community dental health ethical dilemmas are presented along with the author's analysis.

In other chapters sections have been added to address effective preventive programs, practical material for dental health education, and steps to be followed in the planning of community dental health programs.

George M. Gluck
Warren M. Morganstein

ACKNOWLEDGMENTS

Any book is a collaborative enterprise. Certainly a book such as this one, which integrates the works of various contributors, owes much to the work of many individuals. The co-editors are responsible for the selection of topics and contributors. At times the editors have felt like the organizers of a community dental health symposium.

This book has benefited from the inspiration, cooperation, assistance, wisdom, and generosity of many people. Our managing editor and her staff at Mosby have been especially helpful. However, most of all, the book owes its theme, its organization, and the commitment of many of the contributors to the early work of Dr. Anthony Jong, who at the time of his death was an associate dean and chairman of the department of dental public health at the Boston University dental school. Dr. Jong had forged this book out of his dual interests: providing dental care for the underserved and inspiring dental students and dental hygiene students to pursue their interest, if not their career, in the field of dental public health.

The editors are dedicated to the continuation of Dr. Jong's legacy and would be remiss without mentioning Dr. Jong's greatest inspirations: his wife, Pat Westwater Jong, and his two children, Jessica and Alex.

George M. Gluck
Warren M. Morganstein

CONTENTS

SECTION IV   RESEARCH IN DENTAL PUBLIC HEALTH

SECTION V   ETHICS AND THE LAW IN COMMUNITY DENTAL HEALTH

PERSPECTIVE

When we think about community dental health, the significance of the individual members of the dental team cannot be underestimated. The following historical perspective provides an overview of the evolution of the dental team.

Evolution of the Dental Team: An Historical Perspective

Maxine Peck, CDA, MS

The Dental Assistant

As far as is known, the first dental assistant was hired in 1865 by Dr. C. Edmund Kells of New Orleans. This first assistant, a woman, was employed for the purpose of lending an air of "respectability" when the dentist was treating a female patient. Dr. Kells discovered that an assistant could perform routine office functions in the operatory as well as at the front desk. Assistants continued to perform nonclinical functions until World War II, when efforts were made to increase the efficiency and productivity in the provision of services to the uniformed services. Assistants were trained to work chairside. Soon thereafter chairside assistants were employed in private practice.

In the 1960s efforts were made to train dental assistants and dentists to provide services in the practice of four-handed sit-down dentistry. Experimental operatory designs and work simplification techniques were applied to the delivery of dental care. To a large degree the role of the dental assistant had become institutionalized and vital to the practice of dentistry.

The first organization of dental assistants was established in 1921 in New York City. This organization was called the Education and Efficiency Society. By 1924 several groups of dental assistants had formed throughout the United States, and the first national meeting occurred in conjunction with the meeting of the American Dental Association. Since then the three related professions—dentists, dental hygienists, and dental assistants—have met together on a regular basis.

In the early 1930s the dental assistant associations recognized the need to establish a formal curriculum requirement. In 1948 a certification board was established to determine the competence of dental assistants. The certification board was designed as a separate body from the national dental assistant organization. In 1957 the American Dental Association approved a set of standards for the certification of dental assistants. These regulations established that dental assistants needed to attend a 1-year course offered by an educational institution. Currently there are approximately 231 accredited dental assistant programs varying in length from 1 to 2 years. Graduates of these programs are eligible for the national dental assisting examination.

The Dental Hygienist

The "invention" of the dental hygienist is attributed to Dr. Albert Fones, who trained his dental assistant to provide preventive services for his patients in 1906. The role of the hygienist included educating the patient in oral health care and cleaning the patient's teeth. Fones also developed the first curriculum for the dental hygienist. He emphasized health care for children and advocated dental health education courses in the public schools. Although Fones is generally credited with the development of the first curriculum, it was the Ohio College of Dental Surgery that developed a program for hygienists and dental assistants in 1910. However, strong pressure from local dentists forced the program to close.

In 1915 the Connecticut Dental Practice Act required licensure for dental hygienists. Thus began the legal recognition of the progression of dental hygiene. Thereafter the number of dental hygiene programs began to proliferate gradually. In the 1940s all dental hygiene programs were required to implement a curriculum that spanned 2 to 4 years. According to the American Dental Association's Annual Report on Allied Dental Education in 1951, there were 26 programs throughout the United States, and by 1994 there were 212 programs. In 1951 there were 632 dental hygiene graduates, and in 1994 there were 4553. The number of graduates has remained relatively stable during the early 1990s.

A profile of a current dental hygienist would describe an operator who spends approximately 78% of his or her workday providing direct care in a private dental office. Approximately 95% of hygienists are employed by private practice. The remaining 5% work in diverse settings such as state and local governments, health centers, hospitals, dental and allied dental education schools, research facilities, and business and industry.

Expanded Functions

The 1960s were dominated by the notion that there was a shortage of dental care providers in the United States. One approach to increasing productivity was to better use auxiliaries in the delivery of services. The federal government established a manpower center in Louisville, Kentucky, where the expanded use of auxiliaries in the delivery of services was to be investigated. Studies concluded that auxiliaries (assistants and hygienists), when used in an innovative fashion (including expanded functions) could dramatically increase the productivity of the dental team.

This use of expanded function for auxiliaries continued into the 1970s. When the economy began to worsen, however, dentists complained of lack of busyness, and in 1973 the American Dental Association's House of Delegates passed a resolution stating clear opposition to programs that permitted expanded function research. In 1975 the American Dental Association passed a resolution that stressed "the termination of research in expanded functions and a return to traditional roles and responsibilities of dental auxiliaries."

The politics of dental allied health personnel has hovered between the need for more efficient and less expensive dental health services to the public and the perceived needs of the dental profession as articulated by the American Dental Association. When the economy is expanding and the public's buying power is sufficiently strong, the dental profession has supported increased integration of allied health personnel into the delivery process. When the economy has lagged, dentists have resisted an increased role for assistants and hygienists.

The Practice Acts

In 1915 the state of Connecticut defined the profession of dental hygiene in its state practice act. Since this action was taken, every state has described the qualifications and the licensing mechanisms for dental hygienists. Despite areas of similarity, state practice acts and state provisions describing the dental hygienist are remarkably varied. Dental assisting is not universally defined. State practice acts may range from the simple mention of the dental assistant profession to a series of processes including different levels of skills required, state examinations, and educational requirements.

Supervision of state dental practice acts is undertaken by boards of dental examiners or boards of dentistry. For the most part, members of these boards have traditionally been dentists. Over the past 30 years, however, increasing numbers of representatives of dental allied health personnel and of the lay public have been included. Most observers would agree that the inclusion of nondentists on these boards has had a liberalizing effect and has fostered innovation in the enforcement of the dental practice act.

SECTION I

Dental care delivery

CHAPTER 1

Dental public health: an overview

Lester E. Block

The dental profession has primary responsibility for the oral health care of the public and, through the state dental practice acts, virtually has exclusive jurisdiction over the provision of this care. Although the public might not think of the major dental diseases—dental caries and periodontal disease—as particularly serious ones, the magnitude of the problem, as evidenced by the universality of the diseases and the extensive levels of untreated pathologic conditions, results in a public health problem of major proportions.

Each dentist, dental hygienist, dental assistant, and dental laboratory technician is, in fact, a health care worker combating diseases that jeopardize the health of the public.

Dental public health is simultaneously a field of study within the broader field of public health and one of dentistry's eight specialties. Although dental public health evolved from organized dentistry, its philosophy and substance have been more reflective of public health. This difference arose in part because the focus of the dental practitioner is the individual patient, whereas the focus of the dental public health practitioner is the community. In

today's complex society, however, dental health issues cannot be the exclusive concern of any one sector of dentistry. In view of current economic, political, and social factors, which are increasingly influencing the health services delivery system in the United States, dental public health and organized dentistry will of necessity find it mutually beneficial to work together more closely because the goals of both are the same: optimal dental health for all Americans and universal access to comprehensive care.

In the dental public health field the current emphasis on the total dental care delivery system and its impact on oral health status has been increasing. This increasing focus on the delivery of dental care has been primarily related to the development of alternative delivery systems (e.g., dental health maintenance organizations, independent practice associations, preferred provider organizations), the increased role of third-party payers (e.g., insurance companies), the increasing role of government in the payment for care (e.g., Medicare and Medicaid), an overall increasing emphasis on cost control, and an increased concern about the quality of care.

3

What is public health?

The reader must be wondering why a book titled *Community Dental Health* would have as the title of its first chapter "Dental Public Health: An Overview"? Why not "Community Dental Health: An Overview"? Unfortunately, the answer to that question is not simple, and the debate as to what to call the field described in this chapter has been ongoing for more than 80 years. What, if anything, is the difference between public health and community health? Actually, the question should be what is the difference between *community* and *public* because health is common to both terms.

Public is defined as the community or the people as a whole—public equals people. It is a group of people living in the same locality and under the same government (i.e., society as a whole) or a group of people having common interests or characteristics.

Community is defined as a group of people who live in one area and have common interests—an interacting population of various kinds of individuals living together—the public, or society, a social group of any size who share government and reside in a specific locality.[1-4]

After comparing the above definitions, it may be difficult to discern a difference between the two words, yet a difference does exist for a significant number of people. Part of the reason for this perception of difference can be explained by the science of semantics (the study of meaning), in which the difference between the *connotation* (the suggestion of a meaning by a word apart from the thing it explicitly describes or names) and the *denotation* (a direct specific meaning of a word as distinct from an implied or an associated idea) of words is explored.[1,5]

In the case of the words *community* and *public*, although the denotation of both words is essentially the same, the connotation for some people is not. It may initially appear that the issue of connotation versus denotation is su-perfluous, but it should be emphasized that one of the major problems in the development of sound public policy is the use of ambiguous words. This issue is especially true in regard to the debate over health care reform, the major public health policy issue of the 1990s.

Writing or speaking about reform is like writing about integrity. Nearly everyone is interested in it, but hardly anybody stops to explain what it means. "The trouble with integrity," said Steven Carter, "is that everyone is expected to have it, but everyone who uses the word means something different."[6] Currently the term health care *reform* is being used by legislators or policy pundits to describe any proposal that they make to change the health care system, regardless of the consequences of that change. Reform is not simply change—it is change that leads to improvement in form, structure, and quality, in other words, beneficial change.[1] Legislators often use the word *reform* to imply that what they are proposing is in the public interest.

When hearing a word or term used in a political debate or discussion, it is worth remembering what Humpty Dumpty said after being asked by Alice what was meant by a word he had just used: "When I use a word," he said, "it means just what I choose it to mean. Neither more, nor less."[7]

Many think that the term *community health* is associated with the 1960s and early 1970s, a time when America's social consciousness was raised and a "war on poverty" was declared by "The Great Society," a war intended to raise the social, economic, and health status of the less affluent members of our society and provide every U.S. citizen with a decent standard of living and comprehensive medical and dental care. Federal government funding was made available for the development of "community health centers" and for dental and medical schools to create or expand departments that would focus on public health issues. In a sense this was a new beginning that led to a large expansion of community health care facilities and community health departments and programs at dental and dental hygiene schools.

Because the term *public health,* in the minds of certain segments of the public and a number of the administrators who would be developing these departments and health centers, was often associated with the poor and with low-quality care, the decision commonly was made to substitute the word *community* for *public* because *community* did not have the negative connotation of the word *public.*

In reality, the term community health was not born in the 1960s and 1970s. It was commonly used during and before the 1920s. Community health centers were organized before World War I and increased in number during the war largely because of an effort to overcome the shortage of health care providers, who were then serving in the military. During the 1920s it was acknowledged that the "public health problem of today is a community problem" and that the health of the individual cannot be separated from the health of the community at large (meaning the location in which people reside).[8]

It would be misleading, however, to suggest that the community health centers of the 1960s and 1970s were an outgrowth of those in the 1920s.[9] The earlier centers primarily focused on prevention, social welfare services, and nutrition; they provided little, if any, treatment. This was often the result of a bargain struck between provider organizations and the public health authorities. A blatant example is the following published promise of the George White Health Unit located in Boston from the 1920s to 1940s: "No prescriptions given; no sickness treated." The concept of community health centers of the 1960s and 1970s was derived from European models such as the Peckham Health Center in England. U.S. health workers who had studied and trained in these international models and who later participated in the civil rights movement in the South were in-

strumental in promoting the concept of the community health center, which provided total care.[10]

Although some still view the concerns of community health as focusing on personal health care provided in the local community, others use the term *community health* to mean environmental health activity; still others have in mind the totality of personal health services for the community. Cecil Sheps[11] suggests that the term *community health* is comparable to and synonymous with public health and "encompasses the full range of health services, environmental and personal, including other major activities such as health education of the public and the social context of life as it affects the community, the latter referring to a total population. And this is not limited to governmental efforts." Thus both public health and community health could be seen as "the effort that is organized by society to protect, promote, and restore the health and quality of life of the people." Specific activities within public health change as the "needs and demands of the society which they are serving undergo change."[11]

The word *community* is currently used to refer to a particular kind of population for which a hospital or a health network is responsible, typically a geographic area smaller than a state but possibly as large as a county or major city.

DEFINING PUBLIC HEALTH

In defining *public health,* it is helpful to define *health* first. The traditional dictionary definition of health is being free from disease or pain.[4] This limited definition has proved insufficient to address issues of public health concern, and the World Health Organization (WHO) created a more encompassing definition in its constitution. WHO defines *health* as "a state of complete physical, mental and social well-being and not merely the absence of disease or infirmity."[12] A problem with the WHO definition is that it is impossible to quantify, and the criteria of freedom from disease, stress, frustration, and disability are actually incompatible with the process of living and aging. As Dubos has stated, "Complete and lasting freedom from disease is but a dream remembered from imaginings of a Garden of Eden designed for the welfare of man." Thus Pickett and Hanlon[12] suggest considering health as a continuum under which a disease or injury may lead to an impairment, which may lead to a disability, which may lead to a dependency requiring external resources or aids to carry out activities of daily living. Health in this continuum then can be defined as "the absence of a disability."

Knutson[13] defined *public* as "of or pertaining to the people of a community, state, or a nation," and he offered a simple yet comprehensive definition of public health:

Public health is people's health. It is concerned with the aggregate health of a group, a community, a state, or a nation. Public health in accordance with this broad definition is not limited to the health of the poor, or to rendering health services or to the nature of the health problems. Nor is it defined by the method of payment for health services, or by the type of agency responsible for supplying those services. It is simply a concern for and activity directed toward the improvement and protection of the health of a population group in the aggregate.

A more widely used definition of public health was developed by Winslow[14] in 1920:

The science and art of preventing disease, prolonging life, and promoting physical and mental efficiency through organized community effort for the sanitation of the environment, the control of communicable infections, the education of the individual in personal hygiene, the organization of medical and nursing services for the early diagnosis and preventive treatment of disease, and the development of the social machinery to insure everyone a standard of living adequate for the maintenance of health, so organizing these benefits as to enable every citizen to realize his birthright of health and longevity.

This definition shows great understanding in that Winslow, more than 70 years ago, recognized the impact of social, educational, and economic factors on health. Winslow, however, did not include either health care or mental health in his definitions, two areas that have more recently come to be of significant public health concern.

Public health work has expanded from its original focus on asepsis to, in sequence, sanitary engineering, preventive physical medical science, preventive mental medical science, the positive or promotive as well as social behavioral aspects of personal and community medicine, and more recently the promotion and ensurance of comprehensive health services for all.

In general, public health is concerned with four broad areas: (1) lifestyle and behavior, (2) the environment, (3) human biology, and (4) the organization of health programs and systems. Thus public health is concerned with keeping people as healthy as possible and controlling or limiting factors that impede health and is the organization and application of public resources to prevent dependency that would otherwise result from disease or injury.

Regardless of the definition of public health, there will continue to be a lack of the crispness, instant recognition, and understanding associated with the definitions of other specialties. The average citizen has difficulty identifying public health, let alone defining it. In a nonrandomized street survey of the public's understanding of public health, it was found that when a member of the public was told that the surveyor's profession was public health, the surveyor was met in most cases with a blank stare. It was only after the surveyor mentioned well-known public health institutions (e.g., the Centers for Disease Control and Prevention), health departments, specific programs (e.g., tobacco control, immunizations, school health education), and activities such as disease surveillance, outbreak investigation, and occupational health that the confused expression on the face of the interlocutor gave way to a nod of semirecognition.[15]

POPULATION HEALTH

To complicate the confusing semantic state of affairs, another substitute term for public health has appeared recently in the literature: *population health*. Again, the dictionary definition of *population* is similar to that of *public*, and one could correctly equate the terms *public health* and *population health*.[4,16] However, the word *population* is also being used in the phrase "population-based health services." In this context it describes services that are focused on improving the health status of the public, rather than on the actual treatment of that population. These services include "health promotion, community health protection, personal prevention and assistance in gaining access to care."[17]

The best advice I have heard regarding the clearest way to explain public health is this: instead of trying to define it, describe its mission and purpose by giving specific examples, such as public health is safe food, healthier teeth from fluoridated water, installation of seatbelts and airbags in all cars resulting in decreased mortality and injuries, a decline in cigarette smoking, a healthier American diet, a decline in the rate of coronary heart disease, declines in infant and maternal mortality, immunizations against childhood diseases, clean water and air, a reduction in cervical and breast cancer deaths, a reduction in tooth loss as a result of wearing mouthguards, and so on.[15]

FOCUS ON HEALTH CARE AT EXPENSE OF PUBLIC HEALTH

In 1977 Dever[18] proposed a model for developing health policy that incorporated a broader concept of health that included, in addition to the system of health care organization, lifestyle (self-created risks), environmental risk, and human biology. Dever was concerned with the apparent mismatch of pub-

lic resources expended on health care–related activities and factors contributing most prominently to morbidity and mortality. He noted that the United States focused most of its health resources on health care despite the extensive role that these other factors played in the level of health of its population. Although nearly two decades have passed since Dever's observations were made, they remain valid.[19]

In a 1990 analysis of causes of death in the United States, it was found that the role of lifestyle in mortality had changed little since 1977. Half of all deaths could still be attributed to tobacco, diet and activity patterns, alcohol, microbial agents, toxic agents, firearms, sexual behavior, motor vehicles, and illicit drug use. With health resources continuing to be focused on personal health care, it is clear that the mismatch between resources and health determinants continues. When it is noted that less than 1% of the aggregate amount for all health care in the United States was spent on population-based public health activities, it becomes clear that the mismatch is even more extensive than many may realize.[19] It is worth noting that public health receives only 3% of the total health dollar.[20]

FUTURE OF PUBLIC HEALTH REPORT

The most recent and major influential review of public health is the 1988 report by the Institute of Medicine's (IOM), *The Future of Public Health*.[21] The report details the findings of a blue-ribbon committee appointed by the IOM to study the public health field. Among the areas addressed is the previously mentioned issue of the definition of public health. The report defines the mission of public health as the fulfillment of society's interest in ensuring the conditions in which people can be healthy; it states that the substance of public health–organized community efforts should be aimed at the prevention of disease and promotion of health. In addition, the report states that public health links many disciplines and rests on the scientific core of epidemiology.[21] Public health practitioners share the belief that the public's health "can be improved by altering conditions—behavior, the environment, biological interactions, and the organization of services—that might otherwise, at a future time have an adverse impact on health."[12]

The organizational framework of public health encompasses "both activities undertaken within the formal structure of government and the associated efforts of private and voluntary organizations." The history of dental public health as well as of public health has been one of "identifying health problems, developing knowledge and expertise to solve problems, and rallying political and social support around solutions."[21]

The report indicated that the primary concern of public health is health promotion and disease prevention because society relies on the public health system to ensure clean air and water, safe food, healthy lifestyles, and epidemic-free communities. During past years the thrilling advances in technology and science have led to a major health-related focus of society on diagnosis and cure and as a result, the public health infrastructure has deteriorated "like a two-lane highway in the shadow of an interstate." The landmark report declared the current system to be fragmented and rudderless to the point of "disarray." The report, which has been called one of the most important reports in the annals of American health care, exposed a litany of weaknesses, gaps, and challenges that threatened to overwhelm "this nation that has lost sight of its public health goals."[22]

The major problems cited in the report include the acquired immunodeficiency syndrome (AIDS) epidemic, pollution-related diseases, the surge in chronic diseases characteristic of an aging population, inadequate funding of public health agencies, and the growing health care needs of the indigent. Since the publication of the report, several other threats have emerged. Among these are:

- New and reemerging infectious diseases (e.g., a resurgence of tuberculosis), which have been identified as an urgent public health problem demanding a response that may be beyond the financial means of public health agencies. A number of these diseases have become resistant to antibiotics, threatening to reverse hard-won gains.
- The rising tide of violence that has come to be viewed as a major public health problem.
- An antiregulatory movement that has swept through Washington, threatening government's ability to enforce standards and regulations, especially in the areas of environmental and occupational health and health safety.
- Food-borne and water-borne microbes going undetected and environmental hazards unaddressed.[22]

These more recent trends have been the focus of a 1996 IOM Round Table to assess whether the 1988 IOM report's conclusions are still current enough to remain valid into the next millennium as the year 2000 is fast approaching.[22-24]

The IOM report identified three core public health functions: assessment, policy development, and assurance.[21] The American Public Health Association,[25] the national organization that addresses issues of public health concern, delineated these three core functions as follows:

- *Assessment* can be best understood as a process whereby factors that threaten the health of a population are identified, followed by a determination as to whether resources are available to effectively deal with the identified health problems. Public health agencies must assess personal health, environmental health, community concerns and resources, and data on the quality, range and use of public and private medical and dental services.

- *Policy development* is the development of policy by public health agencies in response to specific community and national health needs. Public health agencies must develop comprehensive public health policies to improve health conditions, ensure that policies are politically and organizationally feasible and respect community values; devise measurable objectives and implementation strategies; and identify resources needed to implement the health policies developed.
- *Assurance* means that public health agencies are responsible for seeing that conditions contributing to good health, including high-quality services, are available to all. These agencies also must provide essential public health and environmental health services; respond to personal and environmental health emergencies; administer quality assurance programs and guarantee care for those unserved in the current health care marketplace, including recruiting and retaining health care practitioners to provide appropriate services.[25,26]

Alfred Sommer, dean of the School of Hygiene and Public Health, Johns Hopkins University, in an address to a group of public health professionals describing the future of public health, stated that its viability lies in "developing a data system for measuring and tracking the health of the public more effectively; integrating curative and preventive services at both individual and societal levels; and evaluating success and modifying the system when needed to achieve it."[27]

WHAT IS DENTAL PUBLIC HEALTH?

The American Board of Dental Public Health[28] modified the Winslow definition of public health and defined *dental public health* as

. . . the science and art of preventing and controlling dental disease and promoting dental health

through organized community efforts. It is that form of dental practice which serves the community as a patient rather than the individual. It is concerned with the dental health education of the public, with research and the application of the findings of research, with the administration of programs of dental care for groups, and with the prevention and control of dental disease through a community approach.

A problem with the presently accepted definitions is that they imply that dental public health is concerned only with organized community efforts and only with the dental health of aggregate populations. Now is a good time to reevaluate these definitions and to amend them so that they more accurately reflect current public health activities and interests. A suggested modification of Knutson's definition of public health is: Dental public health is a concern for and activity directed toward the improvement and promotion of the dental health of the population as a whole, as well as of individuals within that population.

COMMUNITY DENTAL HEALTH AND DENTAL PUBLIC HEALTH

In addition to the use of the terms *community dentistry* and *community dental health* (used by schools of dentistry to avoid using *dental public health* or *public health dentistry*), the terms *health ecology, dental ecology,* and *social dentistry* also came into use in the 1960s and 1970s. With so many names used to represent the same field, it is no wonder that both the public and the dental and dental hygiene professions were confused about what these departments did or represented.

During this period of name confusion, a leading dental public health practitioner in 1973 called on the American Board of Dental Public Health to hold an election to vote on a new name for the specialty to avoid being thought of as "those federal and state employees who couldn't make it in private practice" and to "better identify with the changing world of dentistry."[29] At that time I pointed out that a rose by any other name is still a rose and that, as Shakespeare wrote, "The fault, dear Brutus, is not in our stars, but in ourselves. . . ."[30]

Given the confusion in regard to the meaning of the terms *dental public health,* previously called *public health dentistry,* and *community dentistry* or *community dental health* (the term used in the title of this book), for all practical purposes *dental public health* and *community dental health* can be considered equivalent terms. For the remainder of this chapter the term *dental public health* will be used.

DENTAL PUBLIC HEALTH PRACTITIONERS

It is generally agreed that those people who are interested in careers and leadership roles in dental public health should be knowledgeable in both oral health practice and dental public health. Most dental public health practitioners are initially educated as dentists or as dental hygienists and then pursue graduate-level training in dental public health. Dental public health training programs are offered primarily at schools of public health and schools of dentistry. Competency objectives for dental public health specialists have been developed by a committee established by the American Board of Dental Public Health. Although these objectives will be specifically applied to the education and qualifications of dentists desiring to become dental public health specialists (at this time there are no specialties in dental hygiene), they certainly can be applied to all dental public health educational programs. The objectives fall within four overall categories: (1) health policy and program management and administration, (2) research methods in dental public health, (3) oral health promotion and disease, and (4) oral health services delivery system.[31-33]

The specific areas of knowledge and expertise, aside from those in oral health, include planning, implementation, operation, and evaluation of dental public health programs; policy process; regulation; management information systems; human resources management; financial management; marketing; communications; quality assurance; and risk management.[31,33]

DIFFERENCES BETWEEN DENTAL PRACTITIONERS AND DENTAL PUBLIC HEALTH PRACTITIONERS

The question is often asked: What are the differences between the practice of clinical dentistry and dental public health? Box 1-1 indicates the major conceptual differences.

At a forum held in 1994 on the occasion of World Health Day—The Year of Oral Health, Richard L. Wittenberg, the president and chief executive officer of the American Association for World Health, stated that "for too long oral health has been a topic overlooked or dismissed as a secondary health issue." He called for raising the awareness of critical and oral health issues and motivating change in communities across the United States. He cited the following facts that he said "were staring us in the face."[35]

- More than 20 million U.S. workdays are lost annually because of oral disease or the need for dental care.
- Each year, 8600 people die as a result of oral cancer, much of which should be preventable.
- Baby-bottle tooth decay is preventable but still affects thousands of young children because of lack of awareness of proper infant feeding.
- The elderly have special oral health needs and are vulnerable to periodontal disease and oral cancers.
- Many populations in the United States do not have access to fluoridated water, a highly effective means of preventing tooth decay.
- Dental sealants can be nearly 100% effective in preventing dental decay but are woefully underused.

BOX 1-1

CONTRASTING ASPECTS OF DENTAL AND DENTAL PUBLIC HEALTH MODELS OF PRACTICE

Dental Model	*Dental Public Health Model*
Purpose: to maximize the dental interests of individual patients	Purpose: to maximize the dental health status of a population, community, public
Work content: to provide personal dental health	Work content: to develop, implement, and evaluate programs to improve dental health education; creation of health services systems
Practitioner is concerned with risk-benefit calculus for individual patients	Practitioner is concerned with relative cost benefits of different community interventions or strategies
Practitioner's primary moral obligation is to individual patients	Practitioner is obliged to think in terms of how best to allocate community resources
The ideal is the provision of state-of-the-art services	The use of appropriate technology, which may not be state-of-the art
Patient-specific needs are relevant for decision making	Population-based measures of need are of primary importance
Outcomes are measured in terms of changes in individual patients	Outcomes are measured in terms of community change

Modified from Gray BH: *Milbank Q* 70:535-556, 1992.

Following these comments, Carlyle Guerra de Macedo, then the director of the Pan American Health Organization (PAHO), pointed out that:

Oral health's role as an integral part of general wellness has long been overlooked by the citizens of the world. . . . Since health encompasses more than just the absence of disease, it is crucial that we stress the maintenance of good oral health in relation to the entire healthy self. . . . Yet in the case of oral health, preventive measures have not been implemented to their fullest potential, even though relatively small investments would yield lifelong benefits.[35]

The reality is that millions of Americans are still at risk for oral health problems because of the following factors:

- They are unaware of simple and practical oral health practices, underlying oral and medical conditions, compromised immune systems.
- A failure on the part of society to promote and provide community preventive measures and, for many people, a lack of access to oral health care. About 150 million Americans lack dental insurance, an important factor in seeking care, 40% of Americans do not visit the dentist each year, and a much larger percentage does not receive what the readers of this book would call comprehensive care. It is the field of dental public health that has as one of its primary missions the redressing of the above inequities in our society.[35]

The multidisciplinary character of dental public health is important to appreciate. Many professional disciplines, which are discussed in later chapters, are involved in the field of dental public health. The more important of the disciplines are epidemiology and biostatistics; health economics; political and other social and behavioral sciences; biologic and physical sciences; and health education, health administration, and nutrition.

The dental profession has recently been focusing more on dental public health–related interests in its attempt to increase the strength and effectiveness of the profession and to improve the oral health of the population.

The major reason for this increased interest is the perception on the part of organized dentistry that it is facing critical issues, such as the rising cost of dental education, the increased indebtedness of students, the perceived oversupply of dental personnel, the increasing number of alternative forms of developing services, deregulation, and a highly competitive marketplace.[36]

To address the projected future problems confronting the dental profession, in the early 1980s the American Dental Association (ADA) established the Special Committee on the Future of Dentistry,[36] which produced a report in which a series of issues and their implications were raised and discussed.

Although this document is more than a decade old, its concern that the future would bring to the dental profession a more complex and more challenging set of problems that will need to be addressed using the knowledge and skills of the dental public health field, while not as prescient as it was in the 1980s, is still relevant.

The closer alignment of public health and organized dentistry also applies to organized medicine. A visitor to an American Medical Association's House of Delegates meeting thought he was at a public health meeting. He suggested that medicine needs the association with public health because a concern for public health makes medicine more complete. Public health practitioners should welcome this interest by both organized medicine and dentistry in that public health alone does not have the resources to accomplish its goals and it requires the help of others. Public health is the health of all people and therefore is everyone's business.[37]

PLANNING, IMPLEMENTATION, AND EVALUATION OF DENTAL PUBLIC HEALTH PROGRAMS
Planning and implementation

The definition of dental public health leaves the specific objectives of a dental public health program to be developed. Dunning[38] has raised a number of important questions that should be addressed if a program is to be planned effectively:

1. What are the dental needs of the community or population?
2. How extensive is the demand for dental treatment in the population?
3. What dental personnel are available to serve the population, and what is the political climate in regard to the type of staffing that can be used?
4. What is the prevailing philosophy of the people regarding the extent of health care they expect to receive and the manner in which they are willing to receive it?
5. To what extent will the prevention of disease obviate the need for treatment? If in fact preventive measures could accomplish this goal, would they be acceptable for a particular society or segment of society?
6. What scope of service will be offered in a public program, who will receive the service, and in what manner will the service be delivered?
7. How can the service be adjusted to the mores of the population?

Implementation and evaluation of programs

In its stated recommendations regarding the implementation of dental public health programs, the WHO Expert Committee on Dental Health [39,40] suggested that it is important to view a perceived dental health problem within the context of the prevailing health problems and the overall situation of the respective country, region, or community.

Six phases of planning have been identified and should be followed in this sequence: (1) collection of preliminary information, (2) establishment of priorities, (3) selection of targets and objectives, (4) consultation and coordination, (5) drafting of the plan, and (6) periodic assessment and readjustment.

Evaluation and quality

Program evaluation is required if one is to know what, if anything, the program has accomplished, whether the objectives have been achieved, and to what extent has the program contributed to the improvement of the dental health of the community (see Chapter 13). Without information regarding conditions that existed before a program has begun (baseline information), it is not possible to determine the program's impact.[41]

The main criteria for evaluation of dental health programs include:

1. *Effectiveness:* Has the stated objective been attained?
2. *Efficiency:* How much has the attainment of the stated objective cost, and how did that cost compare with the anticipated costs?
3. *Appropriateness:* Has priority been given to the most useful strategy for the attainment of the stated objectives, and is the strategy acceptable?
4. *Adequacy:* Has the program addressed the overall health problem or was it directed at only part of it? Did the program equitably address the needs of all segments of the population?

From a public health perspective it is important to understand that quality of care is not just the quality of individual services. Schonfeld[42] has suggested that four levels be used to evaluate the quality of dental care programs: the first would evaluate the provided individual restoration, procedure, or service; the second would evaluate the impact of that procedure or service on the overall health of the mouth; the third would consider the patient's total oral health and the influence that dental care has had on the attitude toward dentistry and on dental-related behavior; and the fourth would look at the family and the community, evaluate the level of dental care provided for groups and communities, and determine the number and social distribution of persons receiving adequate dental care.

A continuing system of evaluation can indicate:

1. Whether the prevalence of dental disease is changing
2. Whether existing disease is being treated at a greater or lesser rate than new disease is occurring
3. If any groups in the community are not receiving the appropriate level of care that is needed
4. If providers of services are performing at acceptable levels
5. Whether the provided preventive or educational measures being conducted are effective in reducing needs or promoting demands for treatment.[43]

Dental disease

For better understanding of the public health impact of dental disease, one should keep in mind that dental diseases are not reversible and are not self-curing (see Chapter 9). Although preventive procedures are highly successful in reducing the prevalence and incidence of the major dental diseases, prevention has not been able to eliminate them. Therefore, in addition to a preventive component, a treatment component is an essential element of any dental public health program.[44]

At least three unique characteristics of the two most common dental diseases of the mouth—dental caries and periodontal disease—are important to consider: (1) they are of universal prevalence; (2) they do not undergo remission or termination if left untreated but accumulate a backlog of unmet needs; and (3) they usually require technically demanding, expensive, and time-consuming professional treatment. The importance of these characteristics is frequently underestimated by both clinicians and nondental public health practitioners.[44]

Almost all individuals are subject to continually recurring attacks of dental disease. For this reason most people experience a periodic need for services from the time their teeth erupt. Especially in childhood, failure to detect and treat infectious diseases has a more significant impact on total physician labor requirements than the failure to detect and treat dental diseases has on dentistry because most children affected by infectious diseases (e.g., the flu) either die or recover with no treatment. Dental disease, however, if left untreated, continues to develop and accumulates a backlog of needs almost always requiring surgical excising of hard or soft tissues and the replacement of diseased, defective, or missing tissues.[44]

Role of federal and state government in public health

Although the focus in this chapter is on government-related activities, it should be clear from the previous discussion of the meaning of public and community health that neither is exclusively in the domain of government. However, the more formal public health programs and activities are generally under the aegis of government.

Although there is no constitutionally defined role for the federal government in the maintenance of public health, and such activities have traditionally been the province of the states under their police power, nonetheless, over the years there has been a continuing gradual development of a federal presence in the health field. This has come about primarily because of the (1) responsibility for special population groups, such as merchant seamen, members of the armed forces, veterans, and Native Americans; (2) constitutional power to regulate interstate commerce, from which most of the regulatory power of the federal government in health is derived; (3) grants-in-aid to states and institutions for a wide variety of activities; and (4) sponsorship and financial participation in the payment for health services (for example, Medicaid and Medicare).[45,46]

See Appendix A for a description of the departments of the federal government.

Federal government dental activities

The federal government's role in focusing on dental health–related concerns is primarily within the jurisdiction of the Department of Health and Human Services (DHHS). This role has been significantly reduced in recent years from what formerly was an identifiable organizational presence to one that was found by the Interim Study Group on dental activities in the late 1980s to be fragmented, lacking, and uncoordinated, preventing the Department of Health and Human Services from effectively carrying out its responsibilities. Most important, the study group was unable to identify within the department either a discernible oral health policy or a mechanism whereby oral health perspectives are assured of receiving appropriate consideration in the development of health policies.[47]

The most recent inventory of resources and activities devoted to dental and oral health, completed in 1988, revealed that the oral health activities of the DHHS, as well as the resources devoted to those activities, "have been disaggregated, dispersed, reduced drastically, or altogether eliminated since 1972." The inventory also found that the emphasis on decentralization over the past years caused the various department programs that share the same goal of improving oral health to be severely fragmented, leading to decreased interagency communication, limited collaboration, duplication of efforts, and uncoordinated programs lacking direction or purpose. In addition, the communication lines between federal and nonfederal sectors of the oral health care community, including state and local programs and other oral health organizations, have decreased.[47,48]

The inventory pointed out that it was difficult to find any central unit in DHHS that has dental health policy as its mission and that there was no discernible oral health policy. This current situation is a far cry from department activities in the 1960s and 1970s, when there was a strong, coordinated oral health focus.[48]

No study of this kind has been conducted since then. However, little appears to have changed and the critical comments made by the study group are currently applicable.

ORAL HEALTH COORDINATING COMMITTEE OF U.S. PUBLIC HEALTH SERVICE

One of the positive outcomes of the Interim Study Group's report was the formation of the U.S. Public Health Service Oral Health Coordinating Committee.[49] The committee is chaired by the Chief Dental Officer of the Public Health Service (PHS) and its membership is composed of a dentist from each of the following agencies: National Institute of Dental Research, Agency for Health Care Policy and Research, Centers for Disease Control and Prevention, Food and Drug Administration, Health Resources and Services Administration, and the Indian Health Service. The coordinating committee has served as a forum for keeping its members informed about dental activities in each others' agencies. It has also published several monographs on issues of importance to dental public health.

With the Assistant Secretary of Health no longer the head of the Public Health Service

and in a position to encourage communication and cooperation between the eight agencies within the PHS, it is still too early to determine whether the recent reorganization will result in more or less fragmentation of federal dental activities (see Appendix A).

DENTISTRY IN PUBLIC HEALTH SERVICE AND U.S. PUBLIC HEALTH SERVICE COMMISSIONED CORPS

In 1994 the seventy-fifth anniversary of dentistry in the U.S. Public Health Service was celebrated. Before 1919 the most notable dental public health activity began in 1901 when Dr. Frederick McKay surveyed the presence of mottled enamel, also known as "Colorado Brown Stain," which he linked to the water supply. In 1908 Dr. McKay joined with the father of modern dentistry, G.V. Black, to continue his field observations. In 1912 the Army Dental Corps was established, and in 1913 the Navy Dental Corps was created. Also in 1913 the Department of the Interior initiated contractual arrangements with itinerant dentists to provide care on Indian reservations. The PHS involvement in public health was then limited to research at its Hygiene Laboratory (predecessor of the National Institutes of Health), a small number of field epidemiologic studies, and direct care to primarily merchant seamen through a network of hospitals and relief stations.[50]

In March 1919, after the end of World War I, veterans of that war were made a new category of federal beneficiary and were eligible to receive dental services from the PHS. In June 1919 Dr. Ernest E. Buell, who had served as a major in the Army Dental Corps, became the first commissioned dentist in the PHS and later the first Chief of the Dental Section.[50]

The U.S. Public Health Service Commissioned Corps should be distinguished from the PHS—an umbrella agency composed of eight constituent agencies. The U.S. Public Health Service Commissioned Corps is one of the six or seven uniformed services and is primarily composed of commissioned corps officers. Dentistry is one of 11 categories of health professionals in the PHS, and dentists have been commissioned since 1919. Clinical positions available to entry-level dental officers are currently found in the Federal Bureau of Prisons (FBoP), the Indian Health Service (IHS), the National Health Service Corps (NHSC), and the U.S. Coast Guard (USCG).[51]

In 1994 there were approximately 130 dental officers assigned to the FBoP, 410 assigned to the IHS, 45 assigned to the NHSC, and 65 assigned to the USCG. Through the Commissioned Officer Student Training and Extern Program (COSTEP), the PHS allows dental students to serve in assignments for periods of 31 to 120 days.[52] Most dentists employed in the PHS become commissioned officers, although civil service employment is an option.

A sign of progress since the previous edition of this book is that dental hygienists can now be commissioned in the U.S. Public Health Service with either a focus on public health planning and evaluation activities or on the clinical treatment of patients and the implementation of community prevention and promotion programs. Dental hygienists in the PHS come under the category of Health Service Officers, one of the 11 PHS professional categories. Although a graduate degree is not required for the commissioning of a dental hygienist (the minimum academic requirement is a bachelor's degree), a master's degree is preferred for hygienists interested in working in a public health position.

Not all officers in the NHSC are assigned to PHS agencies. Dentists and dental hygienists can be employed in clinical programs or research, regulatory, and administrative programs.[51]

Clinical programs are found in the IHS, the FBoP, NHSC, and the USCG.[51] Research, regulatory, and administrative programs are found in the National Institute of Dental Research (NIDR), the Centers for Disease Control and Prevention (CDC), the Food and Drug Administration (FDA), and the Agency for Health Care Policy and Research (AHCPR).[51]

FEDERALLY FUNDED DENTAL ACTIVITIES

No detailed fiscal analysis of expenditures for federal dental activities has been compiled since 1988. In fiscal year 1988, the total expenditures for federally funded dental activities was $579,824,835, of which $256,573,835 was for programs of the PHS. Approximate allocations by type of PHS program are 52% or $135 million for activities related to dental research, 42% for direct provision of dental services, 4% for activities related to education and training, and 2% for technical assistance and support activities. For a detailed analysis of federal expenditures, see Ginsburg and Schmidt.[48]

Dental activities undertaken by the federal government can be placed in two categories and are distributed among the several agencies of the department, which has been allocating approximately 1.25% of its budget for these activities.[53]

The first group of dental activities consists of programs that seek to improve the nation's capability to provide better oral health protection. They include biologic research, disease prevention and control, planning and development programs in dental labor, education and services research, and regulation and compliance functions such as quality assessment. These programs account for about 40% of the department's dental budget. The other 60% is assigned to the second group, which includes those programs concerned with the provision of dental services.[53]

HEALTHY PEOPLE 2000— ORAL HEALTH 2000
Healthy people 2000

Healthy People 2000 is a publication of the DHHS. It lists 297 different health objectives to be achieved by the year 2000. Among these are

16 oral health objectives that address reductions in dental caries, periodontal disease, oral cancer, and dental trauma from accidents, as well as improvement in use of oral health services, dental sealants, and fluorides.[54]

Healthy People 2000 follows the previously published (1979) *Healthy People,* which established goals and objectives for 1990. *Healthy People 2000* has been developed hand in hand with the revision of *Healthy Communities 2000: Model Standards,* the workbook for applying the objectives in *Healthy People* to individual community needs.[55]

Oral Health 2000 is a nationwide program that unites private, public, and voluntary sectors in a prevention-based education and service initiative that is based on the 16 oral health objectives of *Healthy People 2000,* the federally led national agenda for improved public health. Major attention is to be focused on the use of fluorides, mouth guards, tobacco use cessation, periodontal disease and the health of special target groups such as diabetics, the elderly, the disabled, and minority populations at highest risk for oral diseases. The program is sponsored by the American Fund for Dental Health.[35]

Dental activities of state public health agencies

Unfortunately, there are few national data on current activities of either the dental or medical activities of the state health departments. The reason is that funding formerly available from the PHS for collection of this information has been withdrawn. As of 1990, however, of the 50 state health departments, plus the District of Columbia, American Samoa, Guam, Puerto Rico, Trust Territory, and the Virgin Islands, the following states or locations had no reported dental budget: Alaska, Connecticut, Maryland, Mississippi, Nevada, North Dakota, South Dakota, Wisconsin, Trust Territory, and the Virgin Islands. The remainder of the states

reported a total of $54,390,000 expended on dentally related activities. Twenty-five states and the District of Columbia reported having spent a portion of the Maternal and Child Health Services block grant on dentally related services. Twenty-five states reported expending a portion of their prevention block grant on dentally related services. Few state health agencies reported expending more than a limited portion of their budget on dentally related services.[56]

STATUS OF STATE DENTAL PUBLIC HEALTH PROGRAMS

From observing the status of dental public health programs at the state level, it is evident that the status of these programs has been on the decline in regard to staffing, organizational status, and financial and organizational support.

A 1991 survey of state dental health programs by the Association of State and Territorial Dental Directors indicated that only 39 of the 50 states had an oral health program. Eight states had recently lost a dental director position. Where programs existed, two thirds had conducted oral health assessments. Many fewer had surveyed other oral diseases, and only about one fourth provided screenings for oral cancer. Only one state had a mouthguard program, and fewer than half the states were directly involved in the provision of oral health care to low-income persons.[57]

A 1993 follow-up survey clearly documented the continuing problems. Ten states reported no state dental director, only 38 had dental directors, and of those only 33 were full-time.[57]

The 1991 survey found strong evidence to suggest that the states in which a statutory basis for a dental public health program existed had more stable programs. In 93% of those states with the statutorily supported programs, the level of services remained stable or had increased in the past 2 years, whereas only 28%

of programs in states without such authority had not declined. The report proposed the development of a model statute that state or local dental public health groups could propose to their legislatures.[57]

In regard to funding of and expenditures by state dental programs, it is clear that most programs have experienced sharp reductions in resources with several experiencing sharp reductions in both personnel and program dollars.[57]

A survey of budget trends for state and territorial oral health programs showed that from 1984 to 1989, public oral health expenditures increased at a much slower rate (46%) than did overall public health expenditures (68%). During that period the number of states with no categorical oral health expenditures increased from 3 to 8 and the number of states with no block grant expenditures for oral health also increased from 9 in 1984 to 17 in 1989.[57]

Evidence unquestionably suggests that "state dental public health programs have been weakened by ever tightening budgets, poorly articulated oral health needs and priorities, and the failure to modify and integrate traditional dental program activities into more broadly based health programs." The *Year 2000 Oral Health Objectives for the Nation* cannot be achieved, especially among high-risk populations, without state oral health programs.[57]

At one time virtually all state health departments had a dentist directing their dental health programs. More recently, in addition to the downsizing of these state dental programs, there has been a trend toward nondentist administration, primarily dental hygienists with master's degrees.

In 1996 the states of Colorado, Idaho, Maine, Michigan, Minnesota, Montana, North Dakota, Oregon, Utah, and Washington had dental hygienists directing their state health department's dental program. New Jersey's dental program is currently directed by a nurse.[58]

LOCAL DENTAL PUBLIC HEALTH PROGRAMS

The "Future of Dental Public Health Report" indicated that "little information has been gathered about these programs."[58] Local programs vary widely across the nation, but a lack of data about them makes generalization about differences, clientele served, population density, organizational structure, and funding difficult. During the past 25 years, however, it is clear that the overall number of local dental public health programs has decreased significantly. A study of 150 local dental programs published in 1988 found that 20% reported that their dental program ranked "low" or "lowest" in the organizational structure in which they operated and only 34% believed that their programs had a high priority in their organizations.[59]

FEDERALLY FUNDED HEALTH CENTERS

Dental health care programs that are part of neighborhood, rural, migrant, and homeless health centers—founded largely through federal dollars—have experienced extreme difficulties in recent years. Approximately half of these centers lack a dental program, and no standards have been established for preventative dental care for children. Between 1984 and 1989, the dental personnel at these centers declined by 11%, and about 60 centers previously offering dental services no longer provided them.[57]

FUTURE OF DENTAL PUBLIC HEALTH

In response to the previously described IOM 1988 landmark report, *The Future of Public Health,* leaders in the dental public health community, recognizing that the important pronouncements contained in that report also applied to dental public health[21] (public oral health), conducted an in-depth review of dental public health's origins, scope of responsibilities, and its future challenges and roles. The findings from this review were published in *The Future of Dental Public Health Report.* In response to the question "Where does dental public health stand today?" the report acknowledges that the current environment in which federal, state, and local level dental health programs exist is conflicting, inconsistent, and infused with ambiguous policies. Although the oral health needs are documented with persistent and emerging oral health problems, oral health is given a low priority by health planners. The report states that the contributions of dental public health professionals are not well understood by either the dental profession or the broad field of public health. The report suggests that dental public health leadership "must strive to articulate the public's oral health needs more clearly to dental, public health and health policy makers." The following six interrelated goals are recommended for dental public health as a pathway to improved effectiveness:

1. Earn support from the public.
2. Earn support from policy makers.
3. Earn support from program administrators.
4. Earn support from the dental community.
5. Ensure recruitment and profession development of dental public health personnel.
6. Ensure collaboration with colleagues.[57]

Use and delivery of dental services

Several important distinctions, especially concerning dental care, exist in regard to the need for care, the demand for care, and the actual use of services. A dental need is considered to exist when an individual has dental disease, although the individual may not perceive this need. A demand for care exists when an individual believes there is a need for care and is able to translate that need into actively obtaining care. Sheiham,[60] however, believes that a demand for care exists when the individual perceives a need for and wishes to receive care, even though that person may not actually obtain treatment. Use occurs only when the individual actually receives care.[60] Sheiham's concept considers that one may perceive a need, may desire that the need be treated, and then, in an attempt to make a demand on the delivery system, find the system unable or unwilling to provide treatment. For example, the individual may not be able to afford care, there may not be an available source of care, or the provider might not accept the individual for treatment.

As stated previously, a major concern of public health is the issue of access to care and the fact that access to health services is not equitably distributed among population groups in this country. This has been especially true in regard to the delivery of dental services. Access to even basic medical and dental care for all our citizens is still not a reality. The uneven distribution of health services hits the poor and minorities hardest, with substantial numbers of underserved people "who are different ethnically from the controlling group." The United States, along with South Africa, is still the only developed country with no national policy ensuring that all citizens have access to health care.

The term *rationing* has been used in regard to limiting the distribution and allocation of health services. What has been seen in this country in regard to rationing is that millions of Americans do not get the care that they need. Aside from the Oregon Health Program, there is currently no official governmental policy to ration care. The term *de facto rationing,* however, is being used to describe situations in which care is denied or not provided because of economic or social factors that are brought about by the nature of society and its health care system.[61] Whereas the term *rationing* has to date been applied primarily to medical services, it should not be long before it begins appearing in the dental literature.[62]

FORMS OF DENTAL HEALTH SERVICES

Historically, dental health services in the United States have been classified into three groups:

1. Services provided by dentists and dental auxiliaries and financed by the patient or a source other than the government
2. Services provided by nongovernment dentists and dental auxiliaries partly or entirely remunerated by the government
3. Services provided by dentists and dental auxiliaries employed by the government, such as military personnel

The prevailing philosophy in the United States continues to place the primary responsibility for health and the acquisition of health services on the individual and not on society, even though there has been increased involvement for payment by the federal, state, and local governments. In the 1940s the ADA established the Council on Dental Health. One of the fundamental principles formulated by a council subcommittee was that the responsibility for the health of the people of the United States is first that of the individual, then the community, then the state, and last the nation.[63] This attitude that the individual has the first responsibility contrasts with an attitude in European countries that suggests that society as a whole is responsible. By the 1970s national state-operated social programs were the norm in Europe. It has been suggested that the catastrophic events that befell Europe, primarily the effects of two wars in the first half of the twentieth century, hastened the development of social welfare programs in European countries. The United States, it must be remembered, largely escaped the physical and social devastation of those wars.[64,65]

IMPACT OF HEALTH CARE REFORM AND MANAGED CARE ON PUBLIC HEALTH

During the past 10 years there has been an evolving revolution in the financing and delivery of health care services. Although this revolution to date has affected medicine and public health significantly more than it has dentistry and dental public health, it is unlikely to remain that way.

The revolution has involved the increasing movement toward a health care system driven by market forces and the projection that the majority of Americans will be enrolled in one of the merging integrated health systems that will manage the care of their subscribers primarily under a capitated payment system. Under such a payment system, unlike that of a fee-for-service system, a predetermined payment is made to the integrated health system, which essentially agrees to provide all needed health services. Under the fee-for-service system, payment is made only for those services that have been provided.

One could say that organizations providing care under a capitated system become accountable for the health and wellness of their subscribers. Theoretically, the healthier their subscribers, the fewer services these subscribers require and the less it costs the health care plan. If these plans are to be accountable for the health and financial risks associated with the community of the individuals they enroll, the plans will be required to manage the care of their "communities" or population of subscribers.

The concept of health care providers managing the health and health care of a population is a relatively new one for providers but a traditional one for public health. The management of a population's health will require the skills and competencies encompassed within the public health disciplines such as epidemiology, administration, environmental health, biostatistics, health services research, and health education. In fact, the skills and competencies of the public health disciplines are the basic tools for assessing the health needs of populations, developing programs of intervention, and evaluating their costs, efficacy, and outcomes.[66]

However, at the same time that health care plans are employing public health–trained personnel and focusing more on the health status of their subscribers, there is a developing concern that this focus will be directed only at those aspects of health that have an impact on the bottom line of the plan's financial statement, rather than as is public health's focus, on a concern for all aspects of a population's health and environment.[67]

The question that is most asked in regard to the role of public health in a managed care environment is: Who will be responsible for maintaining the public's health? (Will it still be public health agencies, will it be integrated health care systems, or a combination of both?) It was stated earlier that the capitation system for paying for health care gives managed care organizations (e.g., health maintenance organizations [HMOs], the prototype of prepaid managed care plans), a potential interest to actively improve their enrollees' health status because the plans' expenses should be lower and their profits higher if the enrollees use fewer services. An HMO interested in truly taking responsibility in meeting its enrolled populations' health needs could take a public health approach and address these needs as if they occurred in a community of enrollees, and focus on overall prevention. However, although prevention may pay in the longer run, it is an investment in the future; it may only be in a plan's interest to expend resources on keeping an enrollee healthy, if that enrollee remains with the plan long enough to allow the plan to realize savings from the reduced use of more expensive services as a result of those prevention measures. Prevention measures such as exercising, developing healthful eating habits, and dental health education require up-front investments that may not "pay off" until years later. Efforts to control more general public health problems such as community violence and reducing environmental hazards require complex and expensive programs that would benefit the entire community as well as the plan's subscribers in a given community. In this type of situation there could well be the incentive for cooperative agreements between plans and public health agencies. Although the potential exists for public health agencies and managed care organizations to develop closer working relationships, agencies that operate in the name of public health should be wary of delegating core functions and responsibilities to managed care organizations.[68]

The challenge facing the dental care delivery system will be no different from the one now facing the rest of the health care delivery system. The mandate in health care today is to realign economic incentives to produce fair prices, real value, reasonable profits, and predictable cost growth while improving or maintaining access to care, reducing inappropriate care, improving quality, and promoting optimal health. The challenge from a public health perspective is to ensure that in the effort to control costs, access, and quality are not sacrificed.[69]

• • •

Harold Hillenbrand,[70] former executive director of the ADA, stated in 1977:

The United States is the only industrially developed country in the world without a coherent, identifiable national health program and has only now reached the stage of making a statement of intent. . . . The delivery of dental health care is not now, if it ever was, solely a problem for the dental profession. Real solutions must be found in the unselfish collaboration of dentists, the other health professions, the dental auxiliaries, social and behavioral scientists, epidemiologists, educators, statisticians, government and public health officials, consumers, and a whole host of others. There are enough problems to challenge and plague us all.

Since then little has changed, and Hillenbrand's words are as appropriate in the late 1990s as they were in 1977. There is still much for dental professionals and dental public health to accomplish to meet the dental needs of the people in the United States and "enough problems to challenge and plague us all."

Waldman and Niessen[71,72] point out that since the 1980s much of the public media reporting about dentistry has focused on the improvement in oral health status, the increase in access to care, and the improved ratio of dentists to patients. As a result of this "positive" coverage, the perception on the part of state and national policymakers has been that all is well with dental health and there is no longer a need to expend public dollars on dentally related programs. Although the dental and dental hygiene professions can be proud of the progress that has been made, there is still a long way to go before the oral health status of U.S. citizens is at an acceptable level. As an analogy to the overreaction to improving dental health indicators, one could compare the example of someone who has just received a 50% increase in salary from $4 to $6 per hour. That would certainly be a significant percentage-wise increase, but trying to support a family in the United States in 1997 on $6 per hour is virtually impossible.

In regard to dental disease, in spite of the improvements in the status of dental health, more than 50% of the population is not caries-free.[71] To help ensure that dental health receives a fair share of third-party and public funds, a continued emphasis on "the rest of the story," as newscaster Paul Harvey says, is necessary. Once a perception becomes planted in the public mind, it is difficult to change it. One of the problems faced by public health practitioners is effectively communicating their "message" to the public and public policy makers. The fact that there appears to be a numerically significant improvement in dental health status can be misleading to the less informed. Thus, despite continuing improvements in a number of dental public health indicators, there is still much to be accomplished before the goals of universal access to dental care and optimal dental health for all can be achieved.[72,73]

There is little doubt that public health and social welfare programs have been under attack since the 1994 elections. As the philosophy of individual responsibility has been increasing along with the belief that the federal government should no longer be actively involved in efforts to protect and promote the public's health, there has been a rising concern among public health practitioners that the health status gains that have been achieved in past years are in danger of being reversed. This challenge will call for increasing vigilance on the part of dental and dental public health practitioners to ensure that the improvement in oral health status is not reversed.

REFERENCES

1. *Merriam-Webster's collegiate dictionary,* ed 10, Springfield, Mass, 1993, Merriam-Webster.
2. *American Heritage dictionary of the English language,* ed 3, Boston, 1992, Houghton Mifflin.
3. *Saunders encyclopedia and dictionary of medicine, nursing, and allied health,* ed 6, Philadelphia, 1992, WB Saunders.
4. Urdang L, editor: *The Random House college dictionary,* rev ed, New York, 1988, Random House.
5. Hayakawa SI: *Language in thought and action,* ed 2, New York, 1964, Harcourt, Brace & World.
6. Carter SL: *Integrity,* New York, 1996, Basic Books.
7. Carroll L: *Through the looking glass,* New York, 1982, Julian Messner.
8. Burnham AC: *The community health problem,* New York, 1920, Macmillan.
9. Kovner AR, Martin SP: *Community health and medical care,* New York, 1978, Grune & Stratton.
10. Sidel VW, Sidel R: *Reforming medicine: lessons of the last quarter century,* New York, 1984, Pantheon Books.

11. Sheps CG: *Higher education for public health: progress and potential,* New Orleans, Oct 22, 1974, Delta Omega lecture, American Public Health Association.
12. Pickett G, Hanlon JJ: Philosophy and purpose of public health. In *Public health administration and practice,* ed 9, St Louis, 1990, Mosby.
13. Knutson JW: What is public health? In Pelton WJ, Wisan JM, editors: *Dentistry in public health,* ed 2, Philadelphia, 1955, WB Saunders.
14. Winslow CEA: The untilled field of public health, *Mod Med* 2:183, 1920.
15. Koplan JP: Defining public health, *Curr Iss Public Health,* 1:241, 1995.
16. Nerenz DR: Who has responsibility for a population's health? *Milbank Q* 74:43, 1996.
17. Washington Department of Health: *Core public health functions: a progress report from the Washington state core government public health functions task force,* Olympia, Wash, 1993.
18. Dever GEA: Epidemiological model for health policy analysis, *Social indicators research,* 2(4):451-466, 1976, Dordrecht, The Netherlands, D Reidel.
19. Salman ME: Public health policy: creating a healthy future for the American public, *Fam Commun Health* 18: 1995.
20. Gordon L: Public health is more important than health care, *J Public Health Policy,* 14(3):261-264, 1993.
21. Institute of Medicine Committee for the Study of the Future of Public Health, Division of Health Care Services: A vision of public health in America: an attainable ideal. In *The future of public health,* Washington, DC, 1988, National Academy Press.
22. Public health system under siege, *American Medical News,* p 2, Jan 8, 1996.
23. Siege relief, *American Medical News,* p 17, Jan 8, 1996 (editorial).
24. Kent C: A long-neglected system strains to respond to a rising threat, *American Medical News,* p 7, Jan 8, 1996.
25. American Public Health Association: *Public health in a reformed health care system: a vision for the future,* Washington, DC, 1993.
26. Keppel KG, Freedman MA: What is assessment? *J Public Health Manage Pract* 1:1, 1995.
27. Sommer A: Viewpoint on public health's future, *Public Health Rep* 110:657, 1995.
28. American Board of Dental Public Health: *Guidelines for graduate education in dental public health,* Ann Arbor, Mich, 1970, American Board of Dental Public Health.
29. Waldman HB. *J Public Health Dent* 37(1):95, Winter 1977 (letter to editor).
30. Shakespeare W, *Julius Caesar,* act 1, scene 2, line 134.
31. American Board of Dental Public Health: Competency objectives for dental public health, *J Public Health Dent* 50:338, 1990.
32. Rozier GR: New opportunities for dental public health, American Association of Public Health Dentistry's *Communique* [newsletter] 9:1, 1990.
33. Rozier GR: Proceedings: workshop to develop competency objectives in dental public health, *J Public Health Dent* 50:330, 1990.
34. Gray BH: World blunders and the medical profession: conflicting medical cultures and the ethical dilemmas of helping, *Milbank Q* 70:535, 1992.
35. American Association for World Health: *Oral health for a happy life,* Washington, DC, 1994.
36. American Dental Association: *Strategic plan report of the American Dental Association's special committee on the future of dentistry: issue papers on dental research, manpower education, practice and public and professional concerns,* Chicago, 1983, American Dental Association.
37. Foege W: On AMA's interest in public health, *Am Med News* 29:4, 1986.
38. Dunning JM: Dental needs, resources, and objectives. In Dunning JM, editor: *Principles of dental public health,* ed 2, Cambridge, Mass, 1970, Harvard University Press.
39. World Health Organization Expert Committee on Dental Health: *Organization of dental public health services report,* WHO technical report series no 298, Geneva, 1965, World Health Organization.
40. World Health Organization Expert Committee on Dental Health: *Planning and evaluation of public dental health services report,* WHO technical report series no 589, Geneva, 1976, World Health Organization.
41. Dunning JM: A word of warning in incremental dental care, *NYJ Dent* 38:56, 1968.
42. Schonfeld HK: Peer review of quality of dental care, *J Am Dent Assoc* 79:1376, 1969.
43. Burt BA: Administration of public dental treatment programs. In Slack GL, editor: *Dental public health,* Bristol, United Kingdom, 1974, John Wright and Sons.
44. Young WO: Dentistry looks toward the twenty-first century. In Brown WE, editor: *Oral health dentistry and the American public,* Norman, Okla, 1974, University of Oklahoma Press.
45. Wilson FA, Neuhauser D: *Health services in the United States,* ed 2, Cambridge, Mass, 1985, Ballinger.
46. Brandt E: The federal contribution to public health. In Scutchfield FD, Keck CW, editors: *Principles of public health practice,* Albany, NY, 1997, Delmar Publishers.
47. Interim Study Group on Dental Activities: *Improving the oral health of the American people opportunity for action: a study of the oral health activities of the Department of Health and Human Services,* Rockville, Md, 1989, Department of Health and Human Services.

48. Ginsburg S, Schmidt RE: *An inventory of resources and activities devoted to dental and oral health in the Department of Health and Human Services,* Bethesda, Md, 1989, Richard Schmidt Associated Ltd.

49. Public Health Service Oral Health Coordinating Committee: Membership list, Bethesda, Md, Oct 1995.

50. Snyder LP: Seventy-five years of dentistry in the Public Health Service and the Commissioned Corps: Public health through service, research and prevention. In *PHS dental notes special edition,* Bethesda, Md, 1994, US Public Health Service.

51. Furman LJ, Arnold M: Final draft—U.S. Public Health Service dental programs, March 25, 1996, Homepage, DePAC.

52. US Public Health Service: *U.S. Public Health Service Commissioned Corps—standard dental recruitment concepts,* Bethesda, Md, May 1995.

53. Greene JC: Federal programs and the profession, *J Am Dent Assoc* 92:689, 1976.

54. American Public Health Association, Professional Affairs Division: *Summary of healthy people 2000,* Washington, DC, 1991, American Public Health Association.

55. McGinnis MJ: *Healthy people: public health macroview* 3:4, Washington, DC, 1990, Public Health Foundation.

56. Public Health Foundation: *Public health agencies 1990: an inventory of programs and block grant expenditures,* Washington DC, 1990, Public Health Foundation.

57. Corbin SB, Martin FR: The future of dental public health report—preparing dental public health to meet the challenges: opportunities of the 21st century, *J Public Health Dent* 54:80, 1994.

58. Association of State and Territorial Dental Directors, *State dental directors,* 1995, The Association.

59. Kuthy R, Odum JG: Local dental programs: a descriptive assessment of funding and activities, *J Public Health Dent* 48:36, 1988.

60. Sheiham A: Planning for manpower requirements in dental public health. In Slack GL, editor: *Dental public health,* Bristol, United Kingdom, 1974, John Wright and Sons.

61. Lundberg GD: National health care reform: an aura of inevitability is upon us, *JAMA* 265:2566, 1991.

62. Block LE, Freed JR. A new paradigm for increasing access to care—the Oregon health plan, *J Am Coll Dent* 63:30, 1996.

63. Wilson WA: The future role of government in dental practice and education, *J Am Coll Dent* 40:111, 1973.

64. Burt BA: Financing for dental care services. In Striffler DF, Young WO, Burt BA, editors: *Dentistry, dental practice and the community,* ed 3, Philadelphia, 1983, WB Saunders.

65. Willcocks AJ: Dental health and the changing society. In Slack GL, editor: *Dental public health,* Bristol, United Kingdom, 1981, John Wright and Sons.

66. Lamm RD: Critical challenge, *Public Health Rep* 111:224, 1996.

67. Pew Health Professions Commission: *Critical challenges: revitalizing the health professions for the twenty-first century, the third report of the Pew Health Professions Commission,* San Francisco, December 1995.

68. Brown RE: With managed care, what role for public health? *Nation's Health* 26:2, 1996.

69. Sumaya CV: Oral health for all: the HRSA perspective, *J Public Health Dent* 56:35, 1996.

70. Ingle J, Blair P, editors: *International dental care delivery systems,* Cambridge, Mass, 1978, Ballinger.

71. Niessen L: Some myths in dentistry and their implications for public health, American Association of Public Health Dentistry's *Communique* [newsletter] 8:1, 1989.

72. Waldman HB: The future of dentistry: we need to tell the whole story, *J Am Coll Dent* 57:46, 1990.

73. Alluhian M Jr: Oral diseases: the neglected epidemic. In Scutchfield FD, Keck CW: *Principles of public health practice,* Albany, NY, 1997, Delmar Publishers.

CHAPTER 2

An overview of the U.S. dental care delivery system

Tryfon Beazoglou

This chapter provides an overview of the U.S. dental care delivery system. It is not intended to be a thorough review of the system but rather a brief description of its main components.

A dental care delivery system is efficient when its structure, organization, and performance satisfy the dental needs of the population it serves in the best way possible. This requires efficiency in the education and training of its dental manpower as well as in the production, distribution, consumption, and financing of dental services. Furthermore, to remain efficient over time, a dental care delivery system must adapt promptly to the changing needs of the population it serves.

Dental education

An important component of a dental care delivery system is the production of dental manpower, which includes dentists and auxiliary personnel. The appropriate education, training, type, and number of dentists and auxiliary personnel contribute to the effective satisfaction of the dental needs of a population.

In short, typical education and training of dentists in the United States is extensive and consists of (1) a college degree (4-year predental program) and (2) an undergraduate dental education (4-year program with emphasis in basic sciences during the first 2 years and clinical sciences in the last 2 years).[1] Graduates of such a program, once they pass a license examination, are permitted to practice dentistry in a geographically restricted area.

In the last 70 years dental education and training has changed substantially in structure, intensity, and duration. Predental education today has reached, and often has surpassed, the 4-year post–high school education.

Progress in biomedical sciences and the desire to effectively meet the ever-changing dental needs of the American people has led to the division of labor in the dental care delivery system. This division of labor, on one hand, has led to the creation of allied professions (e.g., dental hygienist, dental assistant, laboratory technician) that require fewer years of education and training and, on the other hand, to postgraduate dental training and specialization. More specifically, today only about 42% of dental school graduates practice dentistry immediately (general practitioners); the next 29% receive postgraduate training (Advanced Education in General Dentistry [AEGD], General Practice Residency [GPR]); and the remaining 29% enter one of the eight recognized dental specialties.[1]

Recent evaluations regarding the effectiveness of dental education and training underline some obvious weaknesses in this component of the dental care delivery system. They include the (1) need for more effective integration between predental and dental education, (2) need for more effective integration between basic and clinical sciences, (3) lack of periodic certification of practicing dentists, and (4) need for more effective use of auxiliary personnel. Proposals for the correction of these and other alleged shortcomings of the dental education system are contained in the Pew Commission report,[2] the Institute of Medicine (IOM)[3] report, and more recently in the advocacy of the "oral physician."[4] A consequence of the above proposals would be an increase in dental education for at least 1 year.

Currently the broader dental education system produces about 3900 dentists, 4500 dental hygienists, an equal number of dental assistants, and about 600 laboratory technicians a year, although these numbers have fluctuated significantly over the years (Table 2-1).

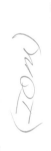

Structure and organization of the dental care delivery system
CHARACTERISTICS OF DENTISTS

The trends in dental education and increases in population and income over time have led to an increase in dental manpower. The most recent available data indicate (Table 2-2) that the total number of dentists in the United States was 174,777, whereas the number of active private practitioners was 138,094 (less than 80% of the total). Table 2-2 indicates that the number of people per active private practitioners was 1,826. This equals approximately 60 dentists per 100,000 population. It is estimated that the dentist/population ratio, which has already started declining, will be about 58 per 100,000 in year 2000 and 47 per 100,000 by 2020. It should be noted that these estimates also predict that the absolute number of active dentists will start to decline after the year 2000.[5]

It is worth noting, following recent trends of enrollment in dental schools, that the number of female dentists is increasing rapidly and accounted for almost 9% of the total number of active private practitioners in 1991.[6]

Table 2-3 shows the distribution of active dentists in private practice by specialty. Obviously, general practitioners account for the ma-

Table 2-1. Number of graduates from dental schools and allied dental education programs—selected years 1960-1994

Year	Dentists	Hygienists	Dental assistants	Laboratory technicians
1960	3,253	—	—	—
1970	3,749	2,465	2,955	359
1975	4,959	4,568	5,972	836
1980	5,256	5,184	5,958	1,068
1985	5,353	4,024	5,855	986
1990	4,233	3,953	3,940	596
1994	3,875	4,553	4,490	608

Data from American Association of Dental Schools: *Deans' briefing book, 1994-95,* Washington, DC.

jority of practitioners. This split between general practitioners and specialists is almost the opposite of that in medicine.

Table 2-4 presents the distribution of active practitioners across the nine regions of the country. Clearly, there are many dentists in every area, although there is significant variation in the number of people per dentist. However, there are other important sociodemographic factors, besides the number of people in an area, that influence the location of dentists and the dentist/population ratio (e.g., income per capita).[7]

Table 2-5 shows the age distribution of active private practitioners. This demographic characteristic may usually be another interesting feature of dental manpower. However, in lieu of the trends previously discussed, this table carries a very important message regarding the future supply of dental manpower. It reveals

Table 2-2. Number of dentists and population and population/dentists ratio in the United States, 1991

Category of dentist	%	No.
Total number of dentists	100.00	174,777
Professionally active dentists	86.26	150,762
Active private practitioners	79.01	138,094
Male	91.23	125,988
Female	8.77	12,106
Population		252,160,000
Population/active private practitioners		1,826

Data from American Dental Association: *Distribution of dentists in the United States by region and state,* 1991, Chicago, 1993, The Association.

Table 2-3. Distribution of active private practitioners by specialty in the United States, 1991

Dental specialty	%	No.
General practitioner	81.51	112,564
Specialist	18.49	25,530
Oral and maxillofacial surgeon	3.76	5,188
Endodontist	1.86	2,567
Orthodontist	6.04	8.342
Oral pathologist	0.08	108
Public health dentist	0.18	244
Prosthodontist	1.68	2,323
Periodontist	2.76	3,810
Pediatric dentist	2.13	2,948
TOTAL	100.00	138,094

Data from American Dental Association: *Distribution of dentists in the United States by region and state, 1991,* Chicago, 1993, The Association.

Table 2-4. Distribution of active private practitioners in the United States by region, 1991

Geographic region	No. of active private practitioners	Population (thousands)	Population/dentist ratio
New England	8,626	13,195	1,530
Middle Atlantic	25,984	37,766	1,453
South Atlantic	20,724	44,403	2,143
East South Central	6,682	15,350	2,297
East North Central	23,626	42,427	1,796
West North Central	9,289	17,812	1,918
West South Central	11,692	27,151	2,322
Mountain	7,423	14,036	1,891
Pacific	24,047	40,020	1,664
TOTAL	138,094	252,160	1,826

Data from American Dental Association: *Distribution of dentists in the United States by region and state, 1991,* Chicago, 1993, The Association.

Table 2-5. Age distribution of active private practitioners in the United States, 1991

Age of dentist	No. of dentists	%
<35	20,714	15.0
35-44	48,471	35.1
45-54	34,247	24.8
55-64	22,095	16.0
65+	12,567	9.1
TOTAL	138,094	100.0

Data from American Dental Association: *Distribution of dentists in the United States by region and state, 1991,* Chicago, 1993, The Association.

that in the next 10 to 20 years the number of retiring dentists will outpace the new entrants in the profession.

CHARACTERISTICS OF DENTAL PRACTICES

The organization and characteristics of dental practices play an important role in determining the efficiency of a dental care delivery system. First, the size of a dental practice may have significant consequences on access to dental care, as well as the unit cost or fees of dental services. The presence of economies or diseconomies of scale and the extent of dental markets are the main determinants of the dental practice size.

Table 2-6 indicates that dentists are organized in small-size practices. In fact, more than 96% of all dental practices in the United States consist of one-dentist (84%) or two-dentist practices. It is estimated that less than 4% of all dental practices can be considered group practices with three or more dentists. If this pattern of dental practice size persists with little change for many years, it strongly suggests lack of significant economies of scale. This and

Table 2-6. Distribution of active private practitioners and dental practices by size

Size of practice	All dentists (%)	All practices* (%)
One dentist	68.1	84.0
Two dentists	20.0	12.3
Three or more dentists	11.9	3.7
TOTAL	100.0	100.0

Data from American Dental Association: *The 1995 survey of dental practice,* Chicago, March 1996, The Association.
*Total number of practices (111,959) was estimated with the assumption that the mean number of dentists in the category "three or more dentists" is four.

Table 2-7. Office space, operatories, auxiliaries, and dental office equipment—all active private practitioners, 1994

Office space (sq. ft., mean)	1,687
Operatories (no., mean)	4.0
Auxiliaries (no., mean)	4.0*
Dental office equipment (% use)	
Composing light-curing unit	92.6
High-speed air handpiece with fiber optics	71.2
Panoramic x-ray unit	54.1
Ultrasonic scaling unit	86.8
Electrosurgical unit	45.1
Nitrous oxide analgesic equipment	57.4
Automatic x-ray film processor	78.8
Sterilizable handpiece	97.9
Intraoral video camera	19.1
Surgical laser	1.7
Biologic indicator	71.2
Silver recovery unit	13.7
Amalgam separator	16.8
Computer processing services	62.3

Data from American Dental Association: *The 1994 survey of dental practice,* Chicago, August 1995, The Association.
*Independent dentists.

additional evidence[8] seem to run contrary to the prevailing conventional wisdom that claims that larger practices are more efficient than smaller practices.

Additional evidence of the relative small size of dental practices is offered by Table 2-7. This table shows the square feet of office space, number of operatories, and auxiliary staff in an average dental practice. Furthermore, it indicates the frequency by which specific units of dental equipment are used in dental practices. Table 2-8 provides further details regarding the frequency and number of specific type of auxiliary staff employed by dental practices. It should be noted that although a dental practice employs, on the average, four auxiliaries, the

Table 2-8. Auxiliary personnel in dental practices—independent dentists, 1994

Type of auxiliary personnel	% Practices	Mean no.
Dental hygienist	63.2	1.0
Chairside assistant	91.6	1.5
Secretary/receptionist	90.7	1.1
Dental laboratory technician	5.9	0.1*
Bookkeeper/business personnel	32.6	0.2*
Sterilization assistant	9.4	0.1*

Data from American Dental Association: *The 1995 survey of dental practice,* Chicago, May 1996, The Association.
*Estimated.

number varies from none to more than seven auxiliary staff (Table 2-9).

Dentists, auxiliary staff, equipment, and dental office space are contributing factors in the production process of a dental practice. Table 2-10 provides estimates of the specific contribution of each of three major inputs (i.e., dentists, auxiliary staff, and equipment) in the production of dental services. Conventional measures of dental output are number of visits and gross billings in a year. When visits are used as an output measure of a dental practice, Table 2-10 shows that the contribution of dentists is about 46%, whereas that of auxiliary staff and equipment is about 37% and 17%, respectively. In contrast, when gross billings are used as an output measure of a dental practice, the contribution of dentists decreases to about 33% and that of auxiliary staff increases to about 51%; equipment contributes about 16%. Clearly, the contribution of auxiliary staff in the gross billings of a dental practice is not only significant but exceeds that of the dentist(s).

In itself, the preference of most dentists to organize their practices in small units would be relatively unimportant. However, this preference does assume importance, given the fact that studies have indicated that constant returns to scale characterize the production of dental services (i.e., cost per unit involved in the production of dental services does not de-

Table 2-9. Percent of all independent dentists employing auxiliary personnel (part-time or full-time)

No. of employees	%
None	8.6
One	5.8
Two	10.2
Three	15.3
Four	14.8
Five	13.4
Six	9.1
Seven or more	22.9

Data from American Dental Association: *The 1994 survey of dental practice,* Chicago, August 1995, The Association.

cline with size of the practice).[8] Stated another way, employers and other buyers have relatively less economic incentive to promote larger, more organized dental practices. Dentists, on the other hand, have valid reasons to wish to retain the current practice structure. For example, patients select dentists on the bases of proximity and referrals by other patients (Table 2-11). As a result, dental practices tend to draw from a limited geographic area. This in turn imposes several limitations on the number of dentists a viable practice can support. In addition, the relatively small size of

Table 2-10. Relative contribution of major inputs in production of dental services

Production inputs	Dental output	
	No. of visits (%)	Gross billings (%)
Dentist(s)	45.63	32.71
Auxiliary staff	36.89	51.40
Equipment	17.48	15.89
TOTAL	100.00	100.00

Data from Crakes G: *An economic estimation of dental practice production process,* University of Connecticut, Storrs, Conn, 1984 (doctoral dissertation).

Table 2-11. Percentage distribution of sources of new patients—all dentists, 1994

Source of new patients	% New patients
Patients	61.9
Other dentists	16.5
Other professionals	3.6
Advertising	6.3
Capitation/close panel contracts	4.4
All other	7.3

Data from American Dental Association: *The 1994 survey of dental practice,* Chicago, August 1995, The Association.

dental practices is a significant advantage in terms of access to dental care. In other words, for a given number of active dentists, the smaller the size of a dental practice, the larger the number of dental practices operating in a community. Consequently, more dental practices implies better access, lower indirect costs (travel expenses, travel time), and increased use of dental services, other things being equal.[9]

Financing of dental care services

Health care expenditures in the United States reached $949.4 billion in 1994, represent-ing more than 14% of the gross national product, the value of all goods and services produced in the United States (Table 2-12). The absolute, relative, and per capita amount of health care expenditures is the highest in the industrialized world. As a result, much of the impetus for the development of means to control health care expenditures can be attributed to corporate and public concern over both the absolute level of expenditures involved and the rate of increase in these expenditures over time. This push emanates from two major characteristics of the health care system: (1) health care expenditures are paid mostly indirectly (81.6%), and (2) the government (federal, state, and local) is a major payer (44.3% of total expenses). In addition, both of these dimensions are increasing over time (Table 2-13).

Aggregate expenditures for dental care services amounted to almost $44 billion in 1994, yielding an average per capita expense of about $169 (Table 2-14). In contrast to medical care, dental care is almost exclusively financed by private sources (95.7%). The share of the government (local, state, and federal) in financing dental care is less than 5% and is not increasing over time. More specifically, although dentistry recently has tried to have dental benefits included under Medicare, the huge federal deficits with which the government is faced make it implausible that the gov-

Table 2-12. Gross national product (GNP), national health care expenditures (NHCE) and their share to GNP—selected years 1960-1994

Year	GNP (billion $)	NHCE		
		Aggregate (billion $)	Per capita ($)	NHCE/GNP (%)
1960	506.5	26.9	141.50	5.31
1970	992.7	73.2	340.78	7.37
1975	1,598.4	130.7	582.18	8.18
1980	2,742.1	247.2	1,051.47	9.01
1985	4,053.6	428.2	1,720.37	10.56
1990	5,567.8	697.5	2,687.86	12.53
1994	6,726.9	949.4	3,309.81	14.11

Data from Bureau of Economic Analysis and Health Care Financing Administration, Washington, DC, 1997.

Table 2-13. National health care expenditures (NHCE) and sources of payment—selected years 1960-1994

Year	NHCE (billion $)	Source of payment		
		Private direct (%)	Private insurance (%)	Public funds (%)
1960	26.9	48.7	21.9	24.5
1970	73.2	34.4	22.4	37.2
1975	130.7	29.0	24.8	41.5
1980	247.2	24.4	28.2	42.4
1985	428.2	21.8	31.9	41.6
1990	697.5	21.3	33.3	40.8
1994	949.4	18.4	33.0	44.3

Data from Bureau of Economic Analysis and Health Care Financing Administration, Washington, DC, 1997.

Table 2-14. Aggregate and per capita expenditures for dental services and their sources of payment—selected years 1960-1994

Year	Expenditures for dental services		Source of payment		
	Aggregate (billion $)	Per capita ($)	Direct (%)	Private insurance (%)	Public funds (%)
1960	2.03	11.38	97.1	1.9	1.0
1970	4.87	24.13	90.8	4.5	4.7
1975	8.22	38.44	82.1	11.8	6.0
1980	13.73	60.85	66.4	28.6	4.8
1985	22.57	95.40	56.6	40.2	2.9
1990	32.88	132.51	48.9	47.9	2.8
1994	43.76	169.01	47.3	48.1	4.2

Data from Bureau of Economic Analysis and Health Care Financing Administration, Washington, DC, 1997.

ernment's role will be increased. In comparison, government financing of physician and hospital services amounted to 32% and 59%, respectively, and is growing. Out-of-pocket payments for dental care by consumers amounted to 48.6% of total dental care expenditures in 1994, whereas private third-party payments amounted to 46.9%.

Table 2-14 suggests substantial continuous growth in dental benefit plans in the last 30 years. However, several obstacles seem to be developing to prevent further expansion of the proportion of the population covered. Specifically, the bulk of dental insurance, both indemnity and capitation, is employer sponsored. However, employers are resisting efforts to expand coverage and are, in fact, actively attempting to reduce or eliminate their contribution. More recently, these efforts have been accelerated as changes in the tax code reduced the indirect subsidies of dental insurance premiums previously enjoyed by businesses. In any event, the period of rapid expansion of dental benefit plans seems to be drawing to a close.

Clearly, dental expenditures grew substantially between 1960 and 1994. This growth re-

flects the combined effects of changes in dental prices, population, and per capita use. In the following discussion, an attempt is made to assess the individual effects of these three factors. Fig. 2-1 shows the trend over time of three price indexes: the Consumer Price Index (CPI), the price index for medical care services, and the price index for dental care services. Obviously, the price index for dental services has risen faster than the CPI, but at a rate lower than the price index for medical care services. The price effects on dental expenditures are shown in Fig. 2-2. This figure indicates the aggregate nominal expenditures for dental services, which are rising at an increasing rate, and the aggregate real expenditures (deflated by the price index of dental services), which have increased at a decreasing rate since the early 1970s. Fig. 2-3 provides the per capita nominal and real dental expenditures (per capita use). Clearly, this figure shows that the per capita use of dental services has been remarkably stable in the last 15 years in spite of the significant improvement in the oral health of the U.S. population.

It is worth noting that the share of dental

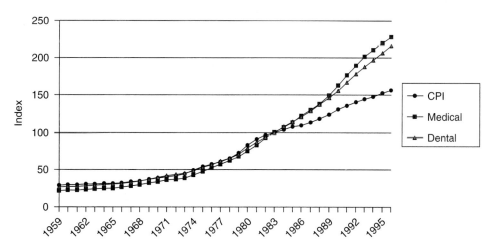

Fig. 2-1. Price indexes for all items (CPI), medical care, and dental care, 1959-1995.

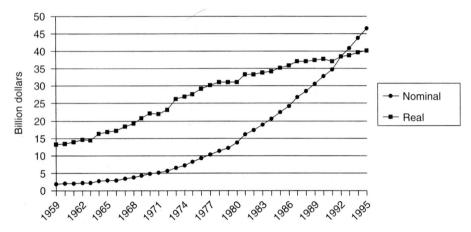

Fig. 2-2. Aggregate nominal and real dental expenditures, 1959-1995.

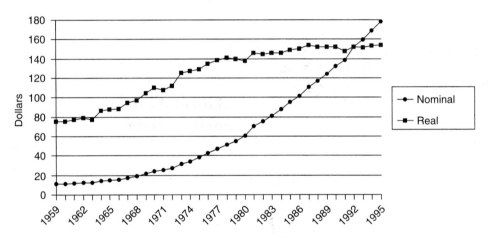

Fig. 2-3. Per capita nominal and real dental expenditures, 1959-1995.

care expenditures in the total health care budget is falling constantly. For example, it has fallen from 7.55% in 1960 to 4.61% in 1994.

Performance of the dental care delivery system

Dentistry in the United States is considered the finest in the world and has been since World War II.[10] The following discussion is a brief assessment of the performance of dentistry in the United States, with the use of structural (education/training), process (services, access), and outcome (oral health status) measures.

STRUCTURAL MEASURES

The education and training of practicing dentists in the United States is the most extensive in the world. A typical program lasts almost 10 years and consists of predental, dental, and postdental education and training.

PROCESS MEASURES

The dental sector provides primary care services and increasingly effective diagnostic, preventive, and cosmetic services. Per capita use of dental services has been relatively stable for the last 10 to15 years, and dental price inflation has been lower than that of hospital and physician services. It should be noted that more than 60% of the U.S. population visit dental practices at least once per year. The average number of visits per person per year is 2.1.[11]

OUTCOME MEASURES

The most important measure of performance of the dental care delivery system is the oral health status of the American population, which is among the best in the world. The oral health of the U.S. population has been characterized by a marked reduction in (1) the incidence of caries, (2) the amount and severity of periodontal disease, and (3) the percentage of the adult population that is edentulous.[12-15] Similar improvements can be found in a variety of other oral health conditions. This does not suggest that there does not exist a substantial amount of dental need, particularly in lower socioeconomic class groups, but it does reflect the improved oral health status combined with the development of more effective therapies and the impact of fluorides and other preventive measures that will significantly reduce the potential for substantial increases in the demand for dental care services, the level of dental care expenditures, or both.

OVERUTILIZATION OF DENTAL CARE SERVICES

Despite claims that significant variations in procedure rates between dentists suggest both overuse by patients and overtreatment by dentists, relatively few hard facts exist.[16] Moreover, much of the evidence that does exist is mixed. For example, it has been argued that truly excessive treatment or use is relatively rare and that the use of expensive services that may have only a marginal impact on oral health is a much greater problem.[17] Others have argued that the purported excess variations could in fact reflect inappropriate undertreatment in some cases or be an artifact of the study methodology.

Two important implications flow from these conclusions. First, the current lack of adequate research on the clinical cost-effectiveness of different dental treatments provides ample room for even competent dentists of goodwill to disagree on the need for treatment. Second, if this is true, the imposition of more stringent managed care programs would be unlikely, in the absence of improved data, to reduce the practice variation. In any case, the potential argument that major changes in current patterns of utilization review are necessary because of the existence of significant excessive utilization/treatment would appear to rest on a less than firm foundation.

Managed care and dental care[18,19]

The increased willingness to question the efficiency and effectiveness of the health care system is most obvious in the considerable interest among individuals, employer groups, and government in supporting the development and growth of alternative systems, arrangements, and organizations. These methods have included reimbursement incentives (e.g., the diagnosis-related group [DRG] reimbursement system used by Medicare) to reduce use of services; the imposition of rate and capital construction review processes; the development of a resource based relative value scale to establish "appropriate" physician payment levels; the creation of a variety of utilization, precertification, and concurrent review processes to limit the amount of specific services delivered or to modify where and by whom services are delivered; and the promotion of managed care systems or patient cost sharing as means of controlling the demand for health care.

The development of these new arrangements has transformed the former predominantly solo fee-for-service system into a sophisticated market-oriented and third-party–dominated health care system. In this system consumer and provider personal preferences and practices are subordinated to group ethical, moral, and financial norms. As a result, the roles of both the patient and the physician in exclusively deciding the course of diagnosis and treatment of an illness have been diminished.

Managed care plans are systems of financing and delivering comprehensive care with few exclusions and limitations and low deductibles and coinsurance. They include, among others, health maintenance organizations (HMOs), preferred provider organizations (PPOs), and exclusive provider organizations. Managed care is believed to address several prevalent problems embedded in the medical care sector. Prominent among them is the control of the high and ever-increasing cost of medical care, the promotion of primary and preventive care, and the control of inpatient care. Group practice, comprehensive coverage, capitation (instead of fee-for-service payment), and continuity of care are additional features of managed care.

Today managed care is the dominant system in the medical care sector; almost two thirds of the insured population in the United States subscribe to managed care programs.[20,21] The participation of physicians in managed care is also high; as of 1993, 75% of all physicians had a managed care contract.[22] The characteristics and performance of the medical sector and the level of participation by physicians and consumers make managed care in medicine a reality.

There is considerable common ground between medicine and dental medicine. After all, the oral cavity is part of the human body. However, there are significant differences between dental and medical care with respect to the nature of disease and services, as well as the organization, financing, and performance of their corresponding delivery systems.

What is offered by managed care in dentistry that would improve the dental care delivery system? Is it improvements in productivity or administrative bureaucracy in the dental office? Is it more comprehensive insurance coverage, more preventive and less restorative care? Is it improvements in access, quality, and continuity of care? Or is its main thrust cost containment? The reality is that the basic ingredients and problems present in the medical sector that managed care seeks to address are absent in the dental sector. Some of the reasons are discussed here.

EFFICIENCY

There are no potential productivity gains to be made by integrating the financing and delivery of dental care in group practices (e.g., dental maintenance organizations). First, a group dental practice, contrary to popular belief, is not economically more efficient than a solo practice.[23] Dental practices remain small because of a lack of scale economies. Second, existing evidence indicates that administrative costs of capitated systems are relatively high (some as high as 45% of the premium).

DISEASE AND SERVICES

Dental diseases affect most of the population throughout their lives. Dental diseases are preventable and, for the most part, not life-threatening. In addition, diagnosis and treatment of dental disease is usually accurate, effective, and relatively inexpensive. There is very little inpatient dental care. In contrast, specific medical diseases do not affect most of the population and most of them are not preventable. In addition, the diagnosis of medical diseases is more difficult, whereas treatment is often less effective and much more expensive. Furthermore, an important component of medical care services consists of inpatient care provided in hospitals.

PREVENTIVE AND COMPREHENSIVE CARE

The opportunity to shift patient treatment away from inpatient care and into ambulatory care is lacking in the dental sector. Yet this is the shift that has generated major savings in the medical care sector. Dental care is outpatient (primary) and increasingly diagnostic and preventive in nature. For example, between 1981 and 1994, the percent of dentists' time spent in diagnostic and preventive services increased from 18.2% to 23.4%, whereas the corresponding percent of time devoted to restorative services was reduced from 37.5% to 30.7%.[12,24] Indemnity dental insurance has an excellent record in providing coverage for primary and preventive dental care.[25] The structure of coverage of dental services has been more primary care oriented and efficient than that of medical services. Specifically, indemnity plans have provided comprehensive coverage for diagnostic, preventive, and basic restorative services and less coverage for endodontic, periodontic, prosthodontic, and orthodontic services. Most dental managed care plans, in contrast to medical ones, do not offer comprehensive coverage with low copayments and few exclusions and limitations. Contractually they tend to offer better coverage for the diagnostic, preventive, and restorative services and less coverage for the other services compared with that of indemnity plans. In fact, however, fee-for-service indemnity insurance plans appear to provide double the amount of preventive and more diagnostic (22%) and restorative (47%) care than capitation plans.[25]

ACCESS AND QUALITY

There are fewer potential gains in access, quality, or continuity of care in dentistry than in the medical care sector. Dental managed care systems are commonly subsets of the fee-for-service system. Managed care systems limit the number of providers and the sites where dental care can be sought by their subscribers. This, in turn, limits the choice of quality (provider, service) and restricts geographic access. To the extent that managed care systems use more group than solo practices, they further reduce access by increasing the indirect cost of dental care to their subscribers (travel time, travel expenses). Finally, continuity of care, which is a problem in the medical sector because of the extensive type and number of specialists, is not present in dental care; the overwhelming majority of dental services are rendered in general practices.

COST CONTAINMENT

Rising costs have not been a major problem in the dental sector. For many years the dental component of the consumer price index CPI fluctuated around the general CPI. In the last 10 years or so, dental prices have increased more rapidly than the CPI but significantly less than the price indexes for hospital or physician services. Excessive utilization or overutilization of dental services has not been a problem either. In fact, per capita use of dental services has been remarkably stable since the late 1970s.[26] In addition, the funding of dental services is basically private (the role of government is very small), coinsurance rates are high, and new technology, a major problem in escalating medical costs, is not an issue in the dental sector.

PARTICIPATION

The level of participation by consumers and providers in managed care plans has been a highly contested and often exaggerated issue, even within the same insurance companies. As Bailit stated, "There is a paucity of data on managed care and available information is often questionable."[20] With this caution he estimates that 14 to 17 million Americans subscribed to managed care plans in 1994. Marcus et al.[27] estimated 13 million subscribers in 1992. These numbers seem to be consistent with those reported by the American Dental Association (ADA) (4.3% of new patients came from capitation and closed panel contracts).[24] They also suggest that, on average, only a small fraction of the population subscribes to managed care plans. Despite this information, a late 1994 survey by the ADA indicates that almost 30% of dentists participated in managed care plans.[28]

Predicting future participation in managed care plans is not only difficult but can be self-serving and unreliable. Existing estimates regarding the percent of future participation of the population in managed care plans range from 20%[20,29] to 75%.[30] If one considers that recent gains in managed care participation came mostly at the expense of existing indemnity plans, these predictions seem to be very optimistic, if not implausible.[27]

PREMIUMS AND PROVIDER REIMBURSEMENT

The average per capita expense for dental care services was about $153 in 1993. In addition, individuals with dental insurance (about 40% of the population) spend on average 46% more than those with no insurance. If the same dental utilization rate is assumed between those with and without insurance, the average per capita expense for the former is $189 and for the latter $129.

The annual premium per subscriber in 1993, for four large managed care plans (1.5 million members), ranged between $83 and $122.20.[27] The corresponding payments to participating dentists were $54 and $80. Adding 25% copayments (out-of-pocket expenses), as in Marcus et al.,[27] converts these numbers to $68 and $100, respectively. Clearly, these reimbursement rates are significantly lower than both the average expenses per person with ($189) and without ($129) dental insurance. Dental managed care plans are basically cheap insurance

plans. These reimbursement rates may become attractive to dentists only when there is excess capacity in the dental office, the utilization rates of managed care subscribers are lower than average, or both.

Adapting to change

The health care environment has changed significantly in recent years in response to a variety of demographic, economic, and professional forces. For example, advances in biomedical technology have increased the ability to diagnose and treat disease, have expanded the potential population likely to benefit from these services, and have increased the demand for facilities, equipment, and personnel consistent with this new knowledge base. Changes have occurred in the racial and ethnic composition of the U.S. population. A growing proportion of the population is older than 65 years. Additional changes in the environment include the declining significance of manufacturing in the U.S. economy, the emerging dominance of the service sector, and the increasing participation of women in the labor force. These changes, among others, have altered the prevailing patterns of morbidity and mortality as well as the modalities of treatment.

An even more significant change affecting the health care environment during this period has been the growth of third-party payment mechanisms, both public and private, as a major influence. For example, governmental provision of health care coverage for the poor (Medicaid) and the elderly (Medicare) resulted in a tremendous expansion in the demand for medical care services. Other governmental programs supported a significant growth in numbers and types of health manpower, health care facilities, and research in both basic and applied sciences.

These efforts to increase the availability of care, improve access to care, and make medical care more equitable have produced ever-increasing levels of health care utilization, prices, and expenditures. Not surprisingly, this led to other efforts to stem the growth in health care expenditures, particularly given concerns about perceived overutilization and with overall efficiency, effectiveness, and equity of these expenditures.

In short, most individuals, providers, and health care organizations face an increasingly complex and dynamic environment—one characterized by a scarcity of resources, increased competition, and an increase in the number and variety of regulatory and planning bodies, consumer-interest groups, and business coalitions, all of whom now have more influence over the quantity and quality of care available and the conditions under which it will be provided. In this environment, managed care (including HMOs and PPOs) has become the dominant system of coverage; the share of the traditional fee-for-service health care coverage, without preadmission certification, has been reduced to 18%.

Dentistry has also experienced and weathered a number of changes. Among them were the growth and decline in the number and size of dental schools, the emergence and proliferation of third-party payment mechanisms (indemnity insurance and alternative payment plans), the decline in the incidence of dental caries, the introduction of new technologies, professional advertising and, more recently, infection control regulations. Perhaps the most important continuous change with the greatest impact on dentistry is the cyclical fluctuation in economic activity at the national, regional, and local levels. The down side (troughs) of these fluctuations seems to coincide with the periodic reemergence of alternative payment plans. The latter has been a troubling issue for a number of dentists despite the fact that its economic impact seems to have been very small.

As a result of these changes, a number of opinions and beliefs among dentists, educa-tors, insurers, and policy makers have been formed during this period; many of these lack a factual foundation. Some of these beliefs are related to dentistry and its main features, and others are associated with the various forms of third-party payment mechanisms. The latter, through marketing techniques and rhetoric, have generated much confusion as to what they represent, how big they are (market share), and the nature of their contribution, if any, to improvements in the dental care delivery system. A major part of the misunderstanding arises from the notion that what is effective and applicable in the medical care sector also is effective and applicable in the dental sector.

The notion that managed dental care has become a powerful force and is poised to take over the dental sector is more myth than reality. The dental sector is largely devoid of the features and conditions that have fostered managed care in the medical sector. Performance measures suggest that dental care has been "managed" well by independent fee-for-service providers receiving payments directly from patients and indemnity insurance plans.

It is noteworthy to state that the mix of dental services has changed and will continue to change. Diagnostic, preventive, and aesthetic services will continue to grow, and an effective recall system will become a necessity rather than a luxury. As a result, the trend to employ and manage more auxiliary personnel will also continue.

Dentistry faces two major challenges. The first major challenge is to learn to adapt to the changing environment. The oral health status of the U.S. population has improved and will continue to improve. Despite that fact, per capita utilization of dental care services has been roughly constant in the last 15 years. The total population is growing and the number of dentists per capita is declining. Soon the total number of dentists also will be declining. In addition, the long-term prospects for the state of the economy are good. On the basis of these trends, it is safe to say that use of dental services per dentist will continue to grow in the next 10 to 15 years. Remember, however, that although the long-term trend appears good, there is nothing to protect dentists from fluctuations in the state of the national or regional economy around this trend. Every time we are on the down side of economic fluctuations, utilization will be less, excess capacity will emerge, and the promotion of managed care plans will increase.

The second challenge to dentistry is to find a way to address the lingering problems of substandard oral health and limited access for the poor and the elderly in inner cities and rural areas. Hopefully, the present dental care delivery system, coupled with targeted private and public programs, is capable of meeting this challenge.

Conclusion

In conclusion, the U.S. dental care delivery system seems to be effective and efficient overall, and the future looks brighter. Claims that dentistry is on the decline as a viable and rewarding profession are not supported by available evidence. Furthermore, given current trends on both the supply and demand sides of dental markets, it seems probable that dentists and dental auxiliary staff will have ample opportunities to practice their profession and will be well rewarded for their care.

REFERENCES

1. Kennedy JE, Crall JJ: A model for dental education in the year 2005, *Forum* 13:S1, 1992.
2. *Healthy America: practitioners for 2005—an agenda for action for U.S. health professional schools,* Durham, NC, 1991, Pew Health Professions Commission.
3. Institute of Medicine: *Dental education at the crossroads: challenges and change,* Washington, DC, 1995, National Academy Press.
4. Nash DA: The oral physician . . . creating a new oral health professional for a new century, *J Dent Educ* 59:586, 1995.
5. American Association of Dental Schools: *Deans' briefing book, academic year, 1993-1994,* Washington, DC, 1995, The Association.
6. American Dental Association: *Distribution of dentists in the United States by region and state, 1991,* Chicago, 1993, The Association.
7. Beazoglou TJ, Crakes GM, Doherty NJ. Determinants of dentists' geographic distribution, *J Dent Educ* 56:735, 1992.
8. Crakes GM: An economic estimation of the dental practice production process, University of Connecticut, 1984 (dissertation).
9. House DR: A full-price approach to the dental market: implications for price determination, *J Health Polits, Policy Law* 5:593, 1981.
10. Eggleston FK: Reactor paper, *J Dent Educ* 60:908, 1996.
11. US Department of Health and Human Services: Vital and health statistics, *Dental services and oral health: United States, 1989,* Series 10, No 183, Hyattsville, Md, DHHS, 1992.
12. Brown LJ, Beazoglou T, Heffley D: Estimated savings in U.S. dental expenditures, 1979-89, *Public Health Rep* 109:195, 1994.
13. Brown LJ, Oliver RC, Loe H: Evaluating periodontal status of U.S. employed adults, *J Am Dental Assoc* 121:226, 1990.
14. Graves RC, Stamm JW: Oral health status in the United States, *J Dent Educ* 49:341, 1985.
15. Meskin LH, Brown LJ: Prevalence and patterns of tooth loss in U.S. employed adult and senior populations, 1985-86, *J Dent Educ* 52:686, 1988.
16. Grembowski D, Milgrom P, Fiset L: Variation in dentist service rate in a homogeneous patient population, *J Public Health Dent* 50:235, 1990.
17. Bailit HL: Is overutilization the major reason for increasing dental expenditures? Reflections on a complex issue, *J Dent Pract Admin* 5:112, 1988.
18. Glasgow JM, Beazoglou T, Mark H: Is managed care the future dental care delivery system? *Conn State Dent Assoc J* 67:23, 1991.
19. Beazoglou TJ, Heffley D, Mark H: Managed care and dentistry: reality and myth, *Conn State Dent Assoc J* 71:49-55, 1995.
20. Bailit H: Managed medical and dental care: current status and future directions, *J Am Coll Dent* 62:7, 1995.
21. Health Insurance Association of America: *Source book of health insurance data 1994,* Washington DC, 1995, The Association.
22. American Medical Association: *Socioeconomic characteristics of medical practice 1993,* Center for Health Policy Research, Chicago, 1994, The Association.

23. Crakes GM, Beazoglou TJ: A re-examination of the returns to scale of dental practices. Paper presented at Eastern Economic Association Annual Meeting, Pittsburgh, Pa, March 1988.

24. American Dental Association: *The 1994 survey of dental practice,* Chicago, 1995, The Association.

25. Beazoglou T, Guay AH, Heffley D: Capitation and fee-for-service dental benefit plans: economic incentives, utilization, and service-mix, *J Am Dent Assoc* 116:483, 1988.

26. Beazoglou T, Brown LJ, Heffley D: Dental care utilization over time, *Soc Sci Med* 37:1461, 1993.

27. Marcus M, Coulter ID, Freed JR, et al. Managed care and dentistry: promises and problems, *J Am Dent Assoc* 126:439, 1995.

28. Spaeth D: Managed care survey reveals low numbers, *ADA News* 26(19):3, Oct 1995.

29. Zatz M: Dental capitation programs—key decision factors. *J Am ColL Dent* 62:17, 1995.

30. Brown LJ, DePaola DP, Dugoni AA, et al. Spotlight on today's major issues; five share their views, *J Am Dent Assoc* 125:1459, 1994.

CHAPTER 3

The dental workforce

James Crall

The U.S. health care system is undergoing rapid and profound change. Unlike previous transitions of this magnitude, which generally have been the result of major federal initiatives, recent changes in the organization, financing, and delivery of health care are being instigated and shaped by market forces. Consolidation of providers and payors and the growth of managed care arrangements are only two examples of prominent structural transformations occurring within the health care system. The consequences of these fundamental alterations are uncertain and are likely to influence the medical sector sooner, and to a larger extent, than dentistry. Nevertheless, experts believe that all components of the health care workforce will be affected.[1]

Questions regarding the adequacy of the current and future dental workforce have received considerable attention recently as part of a major Institute of Medicine (IOM) study.[2] The IOM report dealt with four global issues concerning the dental workforce: (1) What are the current and projected supplies of dentists and allied dental professionals? (2) What will be the demand and need for services in the future, and how certain are the projections? (3) Are the composition and distribution of the dental workforce satisfactory? (4) Should enrollments in dental schools be increased, decreased, or held steady? This chapter reviews the IOM panel's findings regarding these issues and examines the implications of emerging environmental factors for the future dental workforce.

Workforce trends and projections

NUMBERS AND GEOGRAPHIC DISTRIBUTION OF DENTISTS

Government figures indicate that there were slightly more than 140,000 actively practicing dentists in the United States in 1991.[3] This translates to a dentist/population ratio of 56:100,000 or roughly 1 dentist per 1800 people. The number of dentists is expected to peak at a slightly higher level around the year 2000 and then gradually decline until at least 2020. The dentist/population ratio will drop earlier and more sharply; the ratio is expected to be <50:100,000 by 2010, or roughly 1 dentist per 2000 people.[3-5] Dentistry is unique in that it is the only health care profession that will experience an actual decline in the ratio of professionals to population during the next two decades.[6]

Significant increases in dental school enrollment occurred during the 1970s in response to federal initiatives to expand the health care workforce. New facilities were constructed, and class sizes were enlarged in anticipation of a growing demand for services. However, limited expansion of third-party coverage for dental services, particularly in public programs, and a downturn in the nation's economy in the early 1980s created pressures to constrict dental workforce production. Six dental schools ceased operation in the 1980s. These closures combined with reductions in class size at most institutions resulted in the equivalent of 20 average-sized dental schools being closed during the past 10 to 15 years.[7] As a result, the production of dental school graduates, which had reached a high of more than 5700 per year in 1982, declined and eventually plateaued at approximately 3900 per year in 1991.[8]

Although the number of dental school graduates has decreased considerably, the aggregate number of specialty training positions has remained relatively constant for the past quarter century. Consequently the number of specialists, who comprised 15% of all dentists in 1985, is projected to increase to 25% by the year 2010.[2] The relative stability in the aggregate number of training positions masks changes that have occurred within some specialties. For example, enrollments in endodontics and prosthodontics programs increased by roughly 50 positions (45% and 38%, respectively) between 1971 and 1994. Enrollments in oral surgery and orthodontics programs declined by roughly 40 and 60 positions during the same period (15% and 18%, respectively).[9] Enrollment in postdoctoral general dentistry training programs also has grown significantly, particularly since 1980. As a result, the ratio of first-year positions in advanced education (postdoctoral general dentistry and specialty) programs to U.S. dental school graduates now exceeds 60%.

The distribution of dentists across states and regions varies considerably and is projected to remain dynamic. New England and the Mid-Atlantic regions are expected to average 10 to 15 more dentists per 100,000 than the national average through 2020.[4] The ratio for the South Atlantic region is expected to increase to the national average by 2010, whereas the Pacific region is expected to experience a decrease from higher-than-average to below the national average. Nationwide, there were 1069 designated dental health professional shortage areas (defined as a ratio of 5000 or more people per dentist) in 1993. Government data suggest that an estimated 2100 additional dentists are needed to fill workforce needs in both urban and rural areas.[2]

CHARACTERISTICS AND CAPACITY OF THE DENTAL WORKFORCE

The demographic characteristics of the dental workforce have changed significantly during the latter half of the twentieth century. The proportion of women dentists has grown dramatically since the 1970s.[8] Women constituted 38% of the first-year enrollment in U.S. dental schools in 1990 and 48% of dental school graduates in 1995.[10] Women currently comprise 20% of dentists younger than age 40.[11]

The proportion of racial and ethnic minorities has grown over the past two decades, with Asians accounting for most of the increase. However, little has changed in terms of dental school enrollment by underrepresented racial and ethnic minorities (African-Americans, Hispanics, and Native Americans).[2] Preferred strategies for dealing with underrepresentation of certain minorities in the dental workforce and attrition after enrollment include stronger mentoring and outreach programs within dental schools.

ADA survey data suggest that less than two thirds of the available production capacity in dentistry has been used in recent years.[2] On average, dentists work fewer hours than primary care and specialty physicians, attorneys, and business executives. Thus there appears to be potential reserve capacity in the current system. However, it is not clear to what extent the observed lower workloads reflect lifestyle choices or whether the perceived "excess capacity" would accommodate increased demands for services.

ALLIED DENTAL PERSONNEL

There were roughly 98,000 licensed dental hygienists in the United States in 1989, with 71,540 practicing actively.[12] Dental hygienist enrollment grew during the 1960s and 1970s and declined in the 1980s, but not as sharply as for dentists. The Bureau of Health Professions has projected that dental hygienist jobs will grow at twice the growth rate for dentist jobs in the near term.[13] An estimated 201,400 dental assistants and 70,000 dental laboratory technicians comprised the other two major categories of allied dental personnel in 1990.[3]

The dental care delivery system has been relatively conservative in its use of allied personnel. Given changing disease patterns and manpower projections, increased attention is likely to be focused on issues regarding the optimal use of various types of health care personnel to deliver oral health services in more diverse settings.[6,14]

Policy considerations
SUPPLY, DEMAND, AND NEEDS ESTIMATES

None of the models developed by private or public organizations has been particularly accurate or useful for predicting the supply, demand, or need for dental manpower.[2,15] Inadequacies in current forecasting approaches relate to the subjectivity of dental diagnoses, lack of evidence on outcomes, lack of agreement on appropriate interventions, lack of data sources, and difficulty projecting the magnitude and direction of the effect of scientific and technologic advances. Despite the limitations of current approaches, the IOM Committee on the Future of Dental Education encouraged

continued efforts to strengthen programs that monitor trends in the supply of dental personnel and forecast the need and demand for oral health care.[2]

Public policies, economic conditions, and scientific or technologic advances also are recognized as powerful modifiers of supply and demand for dental services. After examining the available evidence, the IOM panel concluded that there is no compelling case for predicting either an oversupply or undersupply of dental practitioners in the next quarter century.[2] Accordingly, the committee recommended that policies to increase or decrease overall dental school enrollments should be avoided.

OPTIONS FOR DEALING WITH AN UNDERSUPPLY OF DENTAL SERVICES

The IOM committee noted that some factors point to a possible overall shortage of dental personnel or services but believed that future shortages could be dealt with by using the reserve capacity in the existing workforce or by increasing the productivity of "the dental team."[2] For example, dentists could work more hours; dental hygienists might assume expanded educational, periodontal, and outreach duties; dental assistants might perform expanded restorative duties; and laboratory technicians might provide complete denture services. However, state practice acts, which are heavily shaped by the economic interests of dentists, are seen as significant deterrents to such changes.[2] Other problems with the enhanced team productivity strategy include the attrition rate of dental hygienists from practice (which may be tied to their limited role at present) and variability in the educational backgrounds of dental hygienists and dental assistants. Indications are that more (rather than less) education will be needed to deal with more complex patients and responsibilities in the future. The IOM committee indicated that the role of physicians and nurse practitioners in supplying oral health services will be limited.[2]

An undersupply of services also could be addressed by reducing the use of dental care through modification of dental benefits packages and/or changing provider behaviors to eliminate possible incentives for overtreatment of insured patients. In the end the IOM committee urged caution in implementing any of these strategies so as not to discriminate against the poorer and less sophisticated patients and members of the population.[2]

OPTIONS FOR ADDRESSING WORKFORCE DISTRIBUTION AND COMPOSITION

Previous initiatives aimed at increasing the overall number of providers to deal with maldistribution problems have largely been abandoned because there is little evidence that this particular procompetitive strategy has worked. More targeted strategies (e.g., placing National Health Services Corps dentists in designated shortage areas) have been developed, but they have not demonstrated significant impact in rural and inner-city underserved areas, largely because of chronic program underfunding.

Desirable attributes for the future dental workforce

ABILITY TO FUNCTION AS PART OF AN INTEGRATED TEAM

Three recurring environmental themes seem worthy of consideration with respect to a future dental workforce. One characteristic of the emerging environment that seems likely to affect the future workforce is a move to larger and more integrated health care delivery sites and systems. A move away from solo practice has already begun in dentistry. Demographic trends, rising educational indebtedness, more costly office-based technologies, a relative increase in specialists, and the impact of managed care arrangements are likely to bolster the trend

toward greater consolidation. Thus it appears that greater emphasis on preparing practitioners to function effectively as clinicians and/or managers in larger and more integrated health care delivery settings is desirable.

ABILITY TO CARE FOR MORE DIVERSE PATIENT POPULATIONS

A second attribute that the future dental workforce will need is flexibility. More options will be available in terms of delivery system arrangements and practice options. New technologies are expected to be developed at an accelerated rate. Changes in the epidemiology of dental diseases and variations across regions and population groups will alter the focus of dental care delivery over time and demand a broader range of expertise. These factors seem to argue for developing a mechanism to provide a broader range of professional exposures and training for future practitioners on an ongoing basis, while also ensuring that they acquire a basic set of competencies to serve as a useful foundation throughout their professional careers. To achieve these goals, the education of future practitioners will most likely include the following core areas: population/environmental sciences (demography, epidemiology, health care delivery systems); biologic/biomedical sciences; behavioral/social sciences (psychology, sociology, economics); clinical dental sciences; managerial sciences (information systems, personnel management, accounting, practice and health care financing); decision sciences (clinical decision making, cost-benefit/cost-effectiveness analysis, outcomes assessment).

ABILITY TO RESPOND TO DEMANDS FOR GREATER ACCOUNTABILITY

A third characteristic of the emerging environment that merits consideration relates to increasing demands for professional accountability. Whether this demand is prompted by external organizations, such as managed care

---

BOX 3-1

IOM RECOMMENDATIONS CONCERNING THE DENTAL WORKFORCE OF THE FUTURE

1. Because the prospects for a future oversupply or undersupply of dental personnel are uncertain and subject to unpredictable scientific, public policy and other developments, the committee recommends that public and private agencies:
   a. Avoid policies to increase or decrease overall dental school enrollments.
   b. Maintain and strengthen programs to forecast and monitor trends in the supply of dental personnel and to analyze information on factors affecting the need and demand for oral health care.
2. To respond to any future shortage of dental services and to improve the effectiveness, efficiency, and availability of dental care generally, educators and policy makers should:
   a. Continue efforts to increase the productivity of the dental workforce, including appropriately credentialed and trained allied dental personnel.
   b. Support research to identify and eliminate unnecessary or inappropriate dental services.
   c. Exercise restraint in increasing dental school enrollments unless other less costly strategies fail to meet demands for oral health care.
3. To improve the availability of dental care in underserved areas and to limit the negative effects of high student debt, Congress and the states should act to increase the number of dentists serving in the National Health Service Corps and other federal or state programs that link financial assistance to work in underserved areas.
4. To build a dental workforce that reflects the nation's diversity, dental schools should initiate or participate in efforts to expand the recruitment of underrepresented minority students, faculty and staff, including:
   a. Broad-based efforts to enlarge the pool of candidates through information, counseling, financial aid, and other supportive programs for precollegiate, collegiate, predoctoral, and advanced students.
   b. National and community programs to improve precollegiate education in science and mathematics, especially for underserved minorities.

From Institute of Medicine Committee on the Future of Dental Education. Field MJ, editor: *A dental work force for the future: dental education at the crossroads*, Washington, DC, 1996, National Academy Press.

organizations, or a self-motivated desire to assess and improve the effectiveness and efficiency of treatment approaches, practitioners of the future will have powerful and affordable tools available for examining the outcomes and costs of care that they provide. In an environment where data and analyses will be viewed as basic necessities for assessing risk and determining preferred preventive and treatment strategies, computer skills are certain to be valued as basic requirements for effective case and practice management. Box 3-1 describes the IOM recommendations concerning the dental workforce of the future.

Summary

The U.S. health care system is undergoing rapid and profound change. In light of reservations about changing the current production of dental school graduates, consideration should be given to preparing future practitioners who will be able to function effectively in settings that are more integrated, diverse, and demanding in terms of accountability than those that currently exist. The ability to acquire new knowledge and skills on an ongoing basis and to adapt to changing environmental conditions will be highly valued attributes for members of the future dental workforce.

REFERENCES

1. Institute of Medicine Committee on the U.S. Physician Supply. Lohr KN, Vanselow NA, Detmer DE, editors: *The nation's physician work force: options for balancing supply and requirements: summary,* Washington, DC, 1996, National Academy Press.
2. Institute of Medicine Committee on the Future of Dental Education. Field MJ, editor: *A dental work force for the future: dental education at the crossroads,* Washington, DC, 1996, National Academy Press.
3. US Department of Health and Human Services, Public Health Service: *Health personnel in the United States: eighth report to Congress, 1991,* Rockville, Md, 1992.
4. American Association of Dental Schools Manpower Committee: *Manpower project report no. 2,* Washington, DC, 1989, American Association of Dental Schools.
5. American Dental Association, Bureau of Economic and Behavioral Research: *Annual report to the American Dental Association house of delegates,* Chicago, 1991, The Association.
6. Pew Health Professions Commission: *Critical challenges: revitalizing the health professions for the twenty-first century,* San Francisco, 1995, UCSF Center for the Health Professions.
7. Consani JW: Presentation at a meeting of the Institute of Medicine Committee on the Future of Dental Education, Washington, DC, Sept 1993.
8. American Association of Dental Schools: *Deans' briefing book: academic year 1992-93,* Washington, DC, 1993, The Association.
9. American Association of Dental Schools: *Deans' briefing book: academic year 1994-95,* Washington, DC, 1995.
10. American Dental Association, Commission on the Young Professional: *A portrait of minority and women dentists,* Washington, DC, 1992, Decision Demographics.
11. American Dental Association, Survey Center: Graduating trends, *ADA News,* Aug 5, 1996.
12. American Dental Hygienists' Association: Testimony presented at a public hearing of the Institute of Medicine Committee on the Future of Dental Education, Washington, DC, Sept 1993.
13. Institute of Medicine: *Avoiding crises,* Washington, DC, 1989, National Academy Press.
14. Kennedy JE, Crall JJ: A model for dental education in 2005, *Forum* 13:S1-8, 1992.
15. Capilouto E, Ohsfeldt R: *Health work force modeling: lessons from dentistry.* In Osterweis M et al, editors: *The U.S. health work force: power, politics, and policy,* Washington, DC, 1996, Association of Academic Health Centers.

CHAPTER 4

HIV and the role of the dental team

Terri S.I. Tilliss

The advent of the human immunodeficiency virus (HIV) and the resultant acquired immunodeficiency syndrome (AIDS) has greatly affected the practice of dentistry. The effects of this disease have had far-reaching implications, including infection control practices, ethical considerations, treatment planning approaches, and treatment modalities. It is incumbent on all members of the dental team to be knowledgeable about this disease and its prevention. A working knowledge of general and oral maxillofacial pathology, immunology, microbiology, sociology, psychology, and pharmacology is essential to a complete understanding of HIV/AIDS and to providing patient care. (For an in-depth description of the impact of infectious disease on the practice of dentistry, see Chapter 17.)

Epidemiology

The Centers for Disease Control and Prevention (CDC) reported the first cases of AIDS in the United States in 1981, although the virus was active before then in the late 1970s. The disease was first seen in homosexual men, but it since has affected the heterosexual population and has crossed all ethnic, age, socioeconomic, and gender boundaries.

As of the beginning of 1996, the cumulative number of AIDS cases in the United States reported to the CDC was slightly more than one half million nationwide, although the total number of infected people in the United States is estimated at 1 million, or 1 in every 250 persons. Worldwide, the World Health Organization estimates that 18 million adults and 1.5 million children have been infected with HIV and that by the end of the century 30 to 40 million men, women, and children will have been infected.[1] These statistics emphasize the magnitude of the HIV epidemic and make it clear that the far-reaching effects of this disease will not soon diminish.

The virus

HIV is considered a "retrovirus" in that viral ribonucleic acid (RNA) is reverse transcribed to deoxyribonucleic acid (DNA) for replication within the host. The predominant cell affected is the CD4-bearing T-helper lymphocyte. The destruction of these cells affects the body's immune response to bacteria, fungi,

48

and viruses; it is the inability of the body to fight these invaders and the resultant opportunistic infections that usually lead to the demise of the host. In this process many tissues and organs of the body can be affected.

Transmission of the virus is by three known routes: blood, sexual contact, and during the birth process. After initial infection, which may be evidenced by a nonspecific, short-lived viral illness or not evident at all, a long latency period (average 9.8 years[2]) usually ensues. This period is distinguished by a lack of clinical symptoms, yet the virus is highly communicable.

Oral health care personnel must be prepared to recognize the signs and symptoms of HIV/AIDS. It has been reported that 80% of HIV-infected individuals experience oral lesions.[3] Additionally, oral lesions may be the first recognized manifestation of the disease. There are other primary symptoms that dental team members must be alert to throughout the assessment phase, including the medical history, head and neck and intraoral examinations, and periodontal examination.

Serologic HIV testing

The dental team member with initial responsibility for examining patients in the dental setting must be alert during the assessment phase to detect or rule out HIV infection. If HIV infection is suspected, a blood test called the enzyme-linked immunosorbent assay (ELISA) is recommended to determine antibody to HIV. Two of three positive ELISA test results on the same serum specimen are followed by a more precise confirmatory test, often the Western blot, although there are others. The test should be conducted 6 months after possible infection because the virus may not be detectable sooner.

Although HIV serum testing is available to anyone wishing to be tested, it is especially critical for those whose clinical status or history suggest this need. Although a compre-

hensive sexual and drug history is recommended, in many dental settings this is not common practice.

A convenient lead-in for addressing the issues of HIV/AIDS can be inclusion of an entry on the medical history form that poses the question, "How knowledgeable are you about HIV/AIDS?—very much; some; very little; none." Another helpful introductory statement may be: "In order to provide you with the best health care possible, I need to ask you some specific questions about your lifestyle and health-related behaviors."

It can be difficult for dental personnel to suggest HIV testing for their patients. If done in a professional, caring manner, while the necessary information is being imparted, the suggestion of HIV testing can be relatively atraumatic for both parties.

The guidelines of the U.S. Public Health Service and the Presidential Commission on the HIV Epidemic[4,5] have recommended counseling and voluntary blood testing for certain persons. These relevant factors are listed in Box 4-1.

Assessment phase

Additional findings during the assessment phase may suggest a need for testing. A detailed medical history form is critical. Indeed, an array of positive responses provided by a patient can lead the alert interviewer to a concern about immune status before the patient has this awareness. Such positive responses may include extreme fatigue, frequent or chronic diarrhea, unexplained weight loss, unexplained fevers, or night sweats. Certainly there are other explanations for these conditions, but medical history findings combined with signs or symptoms evident during the examination should be addressed. Effective communication with the patient is essential to explore plausible causes for findings.

Although the dentist or dental hygienist will conduct the formal head and neck and intraoral examinations, other personnel should be alert during general appraisal of patient appearance. Extreme thinness (wasting syndrome), pallor, energy deficit, lesions of the extremities or head and neck area (possible Kaposi's sarcoma), limitations in the use or mobility of legs (possibly related to neuropathy), or a serious-sounding cough (pneumonia and tuberculosis concerns) can be noted by all personnel, including the receptionist or the dental assistant who seats the patient. Depression, memory loss, and signs of dementia may be noted by the dental team.

As the extraoral examination is conducted, the presence of lymphadenopathy, perioral lesions, or both is noted. The intraoral examination can reveal a variety of HIV/AIDS–associated conditions. These may include, but are not limited to, candidal infection of the oral mucosa, tongue, or pharyngeal area, angular cheilitis, oral hairy leukoplakia, slow-healing herpetic lesions, red/purple/blue lesions of Kaposi's sarcoma, and human papillomavirus.

The gingival or periodontal examination may reveal areas of spontaneous or nocturnal bleeding, linear gingival erythema (which may be fiery red), necrotizing ulcerative periodontitis accompanied by petechia-like patches, mild to severe periodontal destruction (including ulceration), and severe pain.

Such findings and concerns should be summarized and shared with the individual, with a special effort made not to exhibit or elicit undue alarm.

If testing is recommended, voluntariness, confidentiality, and state or federal laws impacting privacy of test results must be carefully considered. There should be a clear understanding of the difference between confidential testing and anonymous testing.

Pretest and posttest counseling

In urban settings a compassionate referral may be the extent of the role of the dental team. However, in rural or very isolated locales, dental personnel could be more involved in pretest or posttest counseling. Dental personnel are not expected to be experienced counselors, but certain skills and expertise can be helpful when this role becomes necessary in the dental setting. The following characteristics are important: emotional warmth, empathy, and restraint (neither challenging nor pushing the patient)[6]; also essential are crisis intervention skills, knowledge of HIV programs, value clarification skills, comfort in discussing issues related to sexual practices and preferences, stress management skills, and comfort with issues of death, dying, and drug abuse.[7] Certainly not all members of the dental team will possess all of these skills, but their development is an ongoing process.

When AIDS testing is being suggested, the patient should be informed about the HIV antibody test and what positive, negative, and equivocal results indicate. Prognosis issues can be mentioned briefly at this time when individuals are neither so overwhelmed by positive results nor so relieved by negative results that they fail to hear this information. Risk reduction during the interval between testing and results should be stressed, and, if indicated, information about safe sex can be provided.[8] Patients should also be made aware of the anxiety that can ensue while awaiting test results; coping mechanisms and support systems can be explored.

Dental personnel should be prepared to be supportive toward those receiving positive test results. Feelings of numbness, disbelief, panic, fear, despair, anxiety, and anger are not uncommon reactions among those with newly diagnosed disease.[9,10]

Considerations in the dental setting

In treating clients who have HIV or AIDS, it is most important that an atmosphere of honesty and trust exist in the dental setting. Patients must perceive an acceptance that encourages them to be open. In this way they can discuss current health status and medications, information that provides essential information for the practitioner. It is important for dental team members to maintain a current working knowledge about the disease and its treatment and to provide the listening ear and comforting touch that are often important to those living with the disease. Team members should have a sensitivity to lifestyle behaviors, including sexual preference and drug usage.

Personnel also should be sensitive to psychosocial issues affecting those living with HIV. Dementia, a common and sometimes early sequela of the disease, can be mistaken as a negative personality trait. Patients may also experience anger and emotional lability, which can pose a challenge for the staff. The manifestations of these behavior patterns are somewhat dependent on the patients' stage of acceptance, state of illness, and coping mechanisms.

Physical ramifications of HIV/AIDS can have an impact on dental treatment. Allowing for frequent restroom breaks is important for those experiencing chronic or severe diarrhea. The need to visit a restroom 10 to 12 times during the course of an appointment can be necessary. In addition, neuropathies, particularly in the lower extremities, can require frequent positioning changes, particularly for long appointments. Positioning also becomes critical for patients who have become extremely thin. Pillows and blankets can be provided for comfort, since protruding bones with very little body fat can lead to discomfort during long appointments. Very thin patients may be sensitive to temperature changes. Air-conditioned offices can be very uncomfortable for those with little to no body fat for insulation. Similarly, in cold climates, there may be high cancellation rates during cold, wet, or snowy weather because negotiating such conditions can seem formidable.

When intraoral dental work is being done, xerostomia can be a concern because of medications and salivary gland disease. Frequent rinsing should be provided. The need for salivary supplementation, fluorides, and diet counseling should be addressed. In addition, patients may be eating soft or high-sugar diets because of nausea, oral pain, lack of appetite, or digestion difficulties. All these factors may contribute to increased caries patterns.

Soft tissue discomfort can present a challenge because of the presence of lesions or HIV-associated gingival or periodontal inflammation or ulceration. Liberal availability of topical anesthetics, nitrous oxide, and chlorhexidine should be supported. Prescription of antibiotic or antifungal medications should be coordinated with a physician to minimize the risk of drug interaction.

Emphasis on meticulous oral hygiene is critical because the altered immune status allows bacteria to have an exaggerated effect. Acute and painful ulcerative conditions may preclude effective oral hygiene, which may need gradual introduction along with chlorhexidine to decrease bacterial load and discomfort.

Once plaque control has been achieved and the gingival/periodontal tissues have responded favorably, more complex treatment planning can begin. Some dentists and hygienists may believe that it is appropriate to offer only a compromised treatment plan to individuals with a terminal disease. Despite the illness, treatment plan options should be presented and patients should be allowed to make educated decisions. These decisions may be discussed with support staff as patients weigh their options. These treatment decisions should be supported and accepted by the staff. Aesthetics and comfort are still important with terminal illness, sometimes even more important with a disease that can so affect appearance and nutrition—a functional and attractive dentition can be critical.

It is important for dental personnel to be able to vent and share their feelings and concerns when working with the HIV/AIDS population. Emotional issues and apprehension about transmission are real for those working in this arena, even though history has shown that universal precautions have essentially prevented transmission to dental health care professionals. Personnel still need a safe forum for discussing work issues.

There are many considerations to be addressed in dealing with HIV/AIDS in the dental setting. Familiarity and experience can lead to increased comfort, confidence, and competence for dental team members when caring for those infected with HIV.

Unquestionably, HIV has had great impact on the provision of dental care and will continue to do so for the foreseeable future.

REFERENCES

1. Centers for Disease Control and Prevention: AIDS information international project/statistics. Document no 320001, April 1996.
2. Van de Waal I, Schulten EA, Pindborg J: Oral manifestations of AIDS: an overview, *Int Dent J* 43:3-8, 1991.
3. Greenspan D and others: *AIDS and the mouth,* Copenhagen, 1990, Munksgaard.
4. Centers for Disease Control: Public Health Service guidelines for counseling and antibody testing to prevent HIV infection and AIDS, *MMWR* 36:509-515, 1987.
5. Kerr DL: Presidential Commission releases report on the HIV epidemic, *J School Health* 58:306, 1988.
6. Bor R: ABC of AIDS counselling, *Nurs Times* 87:32-35, 1991.
7. Leukfeld CG: AIDS counseling and testing, *Health Soc Work* 13:167-169, 1988.
8. Tilliss TSI: Recommending serologic HIV testing for the dental patient, *Am J Dent* 8:263-266, 1995.
9. Perry SW, Markowitz JC: Counseling for HIV testing, *Hosp Comm Psych* 39:731-738, 1988.
10. McMahon KM: The integration of HIV testing and counseling into nursing practice, *Nurs Clin North Am* 23:803-821, 1988.

CHAPTER 5

Paying for dental care

Joseph Boffa

The dental care delivery sector of the U.S. economy is currently in the process of diversification and organizational restructuring. The market forces affecting dentistry in today's economy reflect trends that are shaping all health care delivery in the United States. One such development is the change of payment from a purely private out-of-pocket transaction between dentist and patient into a layered group financing of dental care through various types of third parties. This segmentation of payment is a relatively recent phenomenon, recent at least when compared with the growth of hospitalization insurance that has its roots in the 1920s and 1930s. The economic consequences of this trend are just beginning to be felt in dentistry, but they have been at work in medical care for the past three decades.

Other trends with economic consequences are unique to dentistry. One is the dramatic decline in dental caries in the United States, which has implications for the future of dental care delivery in terms of both the demand and the supply of dental services in the marketplace.

Market forces: the demand side

The major forces today in dental care demand can be summarized by two words: *insurance* and *caries,* more specifically, the increase of insurance and the decline of dental caries. Note that the 1970s can be characterized as the decade of dental insurance. In fact, one review reports that during one 6-year period (1970-1976) private-sector dental insurance grew 500%, from 4.8 to 23.1 million persons covered. Dental insurance payments by all insurers in 1981 were approximately $5.81 billion or 34% of all dental health care expenses. The latest figures for total enrollment provided by Delta Dental Plans is that in 1991 more than 100 million Americans were covered by dental insurance plans. In the period from 1991 to 1994, a recent survey indicates that the number grew to 124 million Americans covered.

Dental insurance is currently considered one of the most desirable employee benefits available. It is estimated that approximately one of every three Americans is covered by some type of dental insurance plan. In the past 10 years there has been a tremendous growth of such programs. In 1965, 2 million Americans were covered by dental insurance, whereas 148 million had medical insurance coverage. Since then, dental plan offerings by U.S. firms has steadily increased to such a point that a 1990 survey of 944 major employers indicated that 92% offered dental plans.

The influx of third-party dollars in the marketplace can act as a stimulus to increase the consumption of dental care. With dental care insurance subsidizing the market price for dental services, the consumer demand function tends to seek a new equilibrium with the market supply function. This is based on the assumption that a reduction in price to the consumer increases the demand for services.

The more dramatic result of growth of dental insurance is that payment for dental care is consolidating through control by administrators of employee benefit packages. Private industry—including both management and labor—will play a multidimensional, complex role in health care. As a consumer of health care whose potential influence derives in part from the massive numbers of workers, industry will become more intimately involved in finding equitable ways to allocate limited resources and improve the quality of the dental care delivery system.

A dramatic decrease in the incidence of dental caries is a countervailing force in the marketplace that might result in a reduction in the use of dental services.

Although most studies before 1977 showed an average incidence rate of two new cavities per child per year, recent investigations no longer support these data. The 1983 National Preventive Dentistry Demonstration Program, funded by the Robert Wood Johnson Foundation, indicated significant findings of less decay than previously reported. This 4-year national study evaluated preventive dental procedures throughout the United States, starting in the fall of 1977. Results showed that the long-standing pattern of two new cavities per child per year was no longer true.

In December 1981 the National Institute for Dental Research for the first time noted this dramatically lower caries incidence rate. Their study showed that tooth decay in children ages 5 to 17 had dropped about 33% from rates reported in Health Examination Surveys of 1963-

1965 and 1966-1970. In the early 1970s only 28% of children ages 5 to 17 were caries-free, yet by 1981 the number had increased to 37%. Over the last 30 years caries reduction as great as 60% has been observed.

More recent comparisons of decayed, missing, and filled surfaces (DMFS) data from several national surveys in the United States also indicate a substantial decrease in prevalence of dental caries and an increase in the number of caries-free children ages 5 to 17 during the last decade. In fact, a substantial proportion of children have no caries at all, although 20% of children account for 60% of all decay. Available literature indicates that this overall decline in dental caries is most likely the result of the increased use of fluoride supplements and fluoridated water supplies.

However, a reduction in dental caries has also been observed in nonfluoridated areas. A countrywide survey that was conducted in 1970 showed a definite improvement in the dental health of patients regardless of fluoride in their water supply. A study reported a 17.5% reduction in decay in Columbus, Ohio, which has a nonfluoridated water system. This statistic can most likely be attributed to the use of fluoridated water in processed foods and beverages.

The trend of caries reduction in nonfluoridated areas has also been noted in Massachusetts. Data for a 20-year period in some Dedham and Norwood neighborhood schools seem to follow national patterns, although community and school water fluoridation was not a factor during this study period. Both towns showed a marked reduction in the number of decayed and filled surfaces, as well as surfaces both decayed and filled.

In 1951 the average 16-year-old in the United States had 15 teeth affected by decay with two extractions. In 1981 the average was eight affected teeth with virtually no extractions. By the mid-1990s, 55% of school-aged children (age 5 to 17 years) exhibited no caries.

The issue, then, is: How does the reduction of dental caries translate into changes in demand for dental services? This type of data is usually difficult to obtain and often must be inferred. Dental practice revenue has traditionally been generated by treating the effects of dental caries.

A 1977 review of dental care expenditures is presented in Table 5-1. Data for 1977 are shown as a reflection of the income distribution for the typical general dental practice just before the observation by epidemiologists of a pronounced decrease in dental caries among children. As Table 5-1 points out, in 1977 operative and endodontic procedures, services to treat the effect of dental caries, accounted for 34.3% of general practice revenue.

Generally, fixed prosthetic services are also rendered to treat the effect of dental caries. Therefore a very conservative conclusion is that more than 50% of the income of a general dental practice in 1977 was earned from the treatment of dental caries.

Table 5-1. Expenditures by dental service type for U.S. general practice in 1977

Service	Expenditure (%)	$ millions
Fixed prosthetics	34.51	3,458
Operative	27.85	2,791
Removable prosthetics	9.63	965
Diagnostic	8.25	826
Preventive	7.67	769
Endodontics	6.35	636
Surgery	3.89	390
Orthodontics	1.07	107
Periodontics	.78	78
TOTALS	100.00	10,020

From Douglass CW, Day JM: Cost and payment of dental services in the U.S., *J Dent Educ* 43:7, 1979.

INTERPLAY OF MARKET FORCES

In the dental care delivery sector of the U.S. economy there are two trends: one in the direction of increased use of dental services and the other toward a net reduction in use. Although the trends seem to be polar opposites, in reality future demand for services is not easy to predict. The trend in dental caries reduction indicates that in another 10 to 20 years the present population of relatively caries-free children will be adult consumers of dental care. Traditional dental practices centering on the treatment of disease will need to face adjustments in finances and focus.

Changes in dental materials technology has led to the ability to offer an increased range of preventive and cosmetic services. As private practitioners adjust to falling volume in their main service line, they will tend to compensate by raising fees, extending the service line, increasing patient volume, or a combination of these trends.

These trends point in the direction of an expanding revenue base. However, there are also forces that are increasing costs. The Occupational Safety and Health Administration (OSHA) Standard on Occupational Exposure to Blood-borne Pathogens has had a major impact on dental practice in the United States. The standard, introduced in 1992, has been responsible for an additional cost burden placed on dental offices. These costs have placed dental practitioners in a position to contend with expenses beyond those associated with earlier, basic infection control activities. In 1991 the American Dental Association initiated a project aimed at assessing the financial impact of compliance with federal and state regulations on dental practices.

In both input from dental insurers and the Association's Bureau of Economic and Behavioral Research, it is estimated that dentists have raised their fees 8%, twice the inflation rate, to contend with these cost increases. To tease out the cost of infection control in this increase, the

ADA mailed a questionnaire to 6336 dental practitioners across the U.S., including 5059 general practitioners (79.9%) and 1277 specialists (20.1%). The response rate for this survey was 35%.

The total estimated per practice expense for all infection control was $45,718 annually. This cost represents the direct cost of supplies, equipment and employee training. This does not include the more difficult issue of the impact of more stringent procedures on labor costs.

The ADA study of 1994 indicates that the cost of compliance exceeds the direct measurable cost of supplies but also the additional workload to implement all standard requirements. Nearly all dental offices surveyed (94%) indicated devoting extra time to comply with federal regulations. In addition, half (56%) reported increased work hours for existing staff, whereas nearly a third (31%) reported the hiring of additional staff to meet OSHA requirements.

The requirements are necessary to ensure public health and worker safety. However, they involve a cost. Most larger dental offices can contend with this new burden by shifting responsibilities of current staff. Most smaller practices need to increase staff hours or hire new staff. This all occurs while the purchasers of dental care plans are seeking to keep their cost increases to a minimum.

The dental care marketplace is affected by several contending forces—including changing dental disease (need) patterns, increasing consumer purchasing power, regulated cost increases, and demand by third-party purchasers for more cost-effective care. All of these factors will influence the dental office of the future.

The office of the future may require a different mix of personnel. The dominant providers may be hygienists and other auxiliaries providing preventive and educational services rather than dentists offering highly skilled restorative services. The primary role of the dentist will be as diagnostician, coordinator of care, and provider of the more complex procedures involving both the hard and soft tissues of the oral cavity.

Does this mean less of a demand for dentists in the future? A decrease will depend primarily on overall shifts in consumer demand for dental services. At present most surveys indicate that only 55% of the U.S. population will visit a dentist in any given year, with approximately 30% seeking regular care. If the overall impact of dental insurance is to increase the regular consumption of dental care from, for example, 30% to 70% of the population, then the general effect, even taking into account caries reduction, may be a dramatic increase in dental care demand.

Unfortunately, most past available actuarial analysis performed for dental insurers in both the public and private sector concludes that the percentage of eligible persons actually seeking care is consistent with overall national statistics. Dental insurance help seems to expand the purchasing power of those individuals who are already predisposed to seek dental care. It has not yet significantly altered the behavior of a large segment of the population that, for reasons often having to do with aversive consequences, decides not to seek regular care. Some such consequences may be treatments to reduce pain or infection or injection of local anesthetic to allow cutting of hard and soft tissues. There are some recent indications that individuals with dental insurance are beginning to exhibit a higher utilization of dental services.

An economic review by Cohen and Roesler tends to substantiate the view that price does not in itself regulate the demand for dental services. They found a highly variable price elasticity of demand for dental services. Price elasticity is an economic measure calculated by dividing percent change in demand for a product or service by the percent change in its price. Price elasticity measures the sensitivity of demand for a product or service against fluctuations in price. The review states that the demand for dental services by children was price elastic, but for adults the price was inelastic. Income was found to be a more consistent predictor of use of dental services. The factor the authors did not consider in this review is price elasticity given the impact of caries reduction.

Perhaps in the future a synergism will develop between caries reduction and increase in dental care insurance coverage. If a positive feeling of well-being can replace the association of aversive experiences, a larger portion of the population will seek dental care on a regular basis. The net impact of reduction of aversive treatments and the increase in purchasing power may lead to increased dental care demand, resulting in higher patient volume.

Dental insurance may also provide the impetus in extending the service line in dental care use. In traditional or preinsurance private practice, fees could more accurately be described as true market prices or an equilibrium price between market supply and demand functions. Not long ago dentists would provide a free examination as a loss leader so that monetary issues would not interfere in establishing good communication with the patient. Once patient rapport was established and a total treatment plan accepted, certain service lines such as dentures would be a "net gain," which would compensate the dentist for the loss leader examination. Most dentists realized that the most important aspect of initial patient contact was to establish rapport and confidence that would eventually lead to patient acceptance of treatment options. The unfortunate consequence of this pricing and consumption pattern was the traditional fee schedule's emphasis on the dentist's role as provider of tangible services such as fillings, dentures, and crowns, rather than as diagnostician.

Dental insurance should influence this traditional use pattern and revenue and service mix. With the advent of partial or full coverage for

diagnostic service, there should be an observable yet gradual increase in the percent of dental practice revenue derived from these services. In addition, most dental plans largely, if not fully, cover preventive services; therefore, with the decline of dental caries, a larger percentage of practice revenue should also be derived from preventive services.

Is there any evidence for such revenue shifts? Analysis of the claims and patient copayment experience for six separate union management benefit trust funds involving approximately 100,000 eligible enrollees throughout the Commonwealth of Massachusetts indicates sufficient evidence. Table 5-2 compares the 1977 percent expenditures derived from Table 5-1 with the 1995 percent expenditures as derived from the union claims data for general practitioners.* Although such comparisons are open to charges that the populations are not comparable, the union data reflect the consumption pattern of a professional, skilled, and unskilled labor pool of an industrial northeastern state. The enrollment base of 100,000 individuals ensures that the consumption pattern observed is unlikely to be grossly atypical or subject to adverse selection.

As Table 5-2 indicates, according to the 1995 data, diagnostic and preventive services represent an 14.8% increase compared with the 1977 percent of revenue. By contrast, operative and fixed prosthodontic services indicate a decline of 18.7% for the general practitioner. The other interesting and not unexpected observation is that in 1977 periodontics was almost a negligible 0.8% of total revenue. The 1994 combined union trust fund data indicate that periodontic services now represent a more respectable 12.9% of total private practitioner revenue. A reasonable conclusion from Table 5-2 is that the countervailing forces of caries reduction and increased dental insurance do appear to have an impact on the service mix of consumer demand.

*Claims analysis provided by the author, October 1996.

Table 5-2. Percent expenditure by dental service type comparing 1977 U.S. data with 1995 Massachusetts union data

Service type	% 1977	% 1995	Net change (%)
Diagnostic	8.2	15.9	+7.7
Preventive	7.7	14.8	+7.1
Restorative	27.9	21.8	− 6.1
Fixed prosthetics	34.5	21.9	− 12.6
Removable prosthetics	9.6	2.0	− 7.6
Endodontics	6.4	7.3	+0.9
Periodontics	0.8	12.9	+12.1
Surgery	3.9	1.4	− 2.5
Orthodontics	1.1	2.0	+0.9

Modified from Douglass CW, Day JM: Cost and payment of dental services in the U.S., *J Dent Educ* 43:7, 1979.

Market forces: the supply side
BACKGROUND

As previously discussed, the economics of health care delivery have evolved from a system of private transactions between physician and patient to one involving various third parties. This development certainly will have its impact on the demand side, or consumption of dental services, but what was unforeseen was its impact on the supply of dental services, more specifically, the organization and structure of the financing and delivery of dental services.

The growth of insurance is not the only major force to shape and foster changes in dental care delivery. The other factor is the 1976 Supreme Court decision maintaining that state-organized restrictions on advertising by professions is a violation of the First Amendment.

Dentistry, along with other similar professions, maintains that the doctor-patient relationship is sacrosanct and therefore is separate from other types of economic activity. What is evolving is not a repudiation of this concept but a clearer definition of the doctor-patient relationship that is consistent with economic reality and constitutional law.

When the payment of services was primarily a private transaction between doctor and patient, all aspects of the therapy environment were private in nature. In today's economy, dental care payments are becoming benefits derived from an employer. In reality they have become another factor in computing labor costs for the production of goods and services in the U.S. economy. It is unrealistic to believe that industry—both labor and management—will not attempt to use its scarce resources to maximize benefits for its workers. If doing so requires a more active role in the payment and delivery of dental services, it will be pursued. The U.S. economy is now facing aggressive worldwide competition, and it is inevitable that all costs of the factors of production will be periodically reviewed. If, for example, a particular industry finds that by maintaining its own health clinics it can reduce labor costs by a certain amount, the economic choice is clear. Maximize production efficiency so prices are competitive.

Of course, what is evolving is not as simple as industry starting clinics and hiring doctors but payment reimbursement by various types of third parties representing a range of financial arrangements between industry and the health care sector. It should be added that the union or company clinic is an option that some industries have pursued, but the main thrust is not to get involved in the delivery of services but to negotiate an acceptable financing structure. Some of the new third parties in health care are health maintenance organizations (HMOs) and their dental counterpart, the prepaid group dental practice. In this particular arrangement the provider of services and insurer of care are the same organization.

This and other types of arrangements will increase competition in the third-party marketplace. It is in essence this competition between traditional insurance companies and other third-party arrangements that will encourage efficiency in the health care delivery system.

To flourish, these newer organizations must be free to develop marketing strategies that both penetrate the existing dental prepayment market and attract persons now without coverage. However, there has been a good deal of professional resistance to the idea of marketing health services. Until 1976 most state court decisions upheld states' rights to inhibit advertising for professional services. For example, in two court decisions, *People v Duben* (10 NE 2d 809 Ill 229) and *Cherry v Board of Regents of the State of New York* (44 NE 2d 405 NY 148), the Supreme Court stated and reaffirmed the states' right to limit advertising by physicians and dentists. With this legal precedent, most professional organizations, including dentistry, traditionally restricted professionals from using various forms of advertising.

With the evolution of new third parties who may advertise for plan members, the question that would naturally have arisen concerns the ethics of physicians and dentists who are employed by or contract with organizations that in turn advertise on their behalf. This would have been an area of new litigation, but the

Supreme Court in 1976 made it a moot issue. The U.S. Supreme Court decided a case on appeal from the Supreme Court of Arizona, *John R. Bates and Van O'Steen Appellants v The State Bar of Arizona* (76-316 4873, 4896) and upheld the right of attorneys to advertise their fees for certain services. The state's rule prohibiting this was found to be in violation of the First Amendment. The court considered six arguments for restricting price advertising: (1) the adverse effect on professionalism, (2) the inherently misleading nature of attorney advertising, (3) the adverse effect on the administration of justice, (4) the undesirable economic effects of advertising, (5) the adverse effect of advertising on the quality of service, and (6) the difficulties of enforcement. The court was not persuaded that any of them was an acceptable reason to inhibit attorneys' First Amendment right to announce to the public their prices for basic services. However, the court did not hold that advertising by attorneys may not be regulated in any way.

Given these economic and legal trends, the practitioner-patient relationship should and must be properly defined so that professionalism and quality of care are fostered. How a particular patient seeks and pays for service from a particular health care provider does not affect the ethical responsibility of that provider. Salaried dentists should maintain the same level of professionalism as those who work in the more traditional private practice setting. It is the role of the dental schools and professional organizations to define clearly and promulgate the concept of professional responsibility.

SUPPLY SIDE RESTRUCTURING

Several options are available to industry relating to the administrative and provider reimbursement structure for various health care benefits, including dentistry. Organizational arrangements outlined in this chapter are defined in a broad generic sense. It is beyond the scope of this discussion to analyze the finer details of specific organizations.

There are choices industry can and will make concerning the financial management structure of health care benefits. At present the three possible basic organizational arrangements are as follows.

1. Indemnification of dental benefits through an insurance carrier
2. Self-indemnification and self-administration of the benefit
3. Self-indemnification but with use of a third party to administer the benefit

Insurance option

To establish the proper framework for analysis, a few basic concepts should be discussed. As the list indicates, insuring involves several choices, including the indemnification of annual benefit costs through an insurance carrier.

In the attempt to explore the underwriting of health care programs such as dental care through an insurance carrier, there should be a clear idea of the potential benefits to industry and how they can be achieved. The simplistic idea of "let the insurance company handle everything" may be more costly to industry in the long run.

The use of an insurance carrier to indemnify or protect against possible damage or losses is at best a short-term risk-ameliorating option. In the long term the insurance company passes all costs on to its customers, in this case, industry. However, there are certain advantages. This type of indemnification makes annual budgeting for benefits much more predictable and efficient, and the technical expertise of insurance underwriters and actuaries can be useful in analyzing a program's economic impacts. The insurance company also assumes the more burdensome operational tasks such as claims processing, thus freeing management to concentrate on long-term strategic planning.

Undeniably, the growth of dental prepayment has been marked by an increasing role of the traditional insurance company in the financing of dental services. The insurance company maintains the appropriate administrative talent and resources to maintain large-scale benefits administration. Certainly, for particular industries this option makes the most sense, and currently most dental benefits are administered under this arrangement.

Self-indemnification and self-administration

Another approach to benefits administration is to self-insure and self-administer the benefit. Usually a union-management trust fund is established, and the fund pays for care directly rather than paying premiums to an insurance company. In a true self-administered benefit, the trust fund handles all aspects of benefit program administration. There are two main advantages to this approach. The trust fund has complete control of the benefit program, from policy initiation to implementation, and can invest earmarked benefit dollars to expand the resource base or dollars available for future benefits.

If this type of administrative structure is totally maintained by a particular company or union, the cash flow from benefit dollars will remain in its bank accounts until needed to pay for services and will not automatically be sent to the insurance company in regular premium installments. However, as pointed out previously, there is a price for maintaining this level of control. Industry's management must be responsible not only for long-term policy planning and analysis but also for large-scale day-to-day operational activities. The latter responsibility inhibits policy reformulation and creativity. Once a large-scale initiative has been completed, for example, when a computer database management system is set up, it becomes very difficult to change direction quickly and consider new economic and benefit policy directions.

Role of the third-party administrator

In the private sector a new type of administrative structure has evolved. Known as third-party administrator (TPA), it attempts to bridge the gap between indemnifying and administering through an insurance carrier and self-indemnification and self-administration. This option has the advantage that ultimate budgetary control is in the hands of those who pay for the services. In the private sector this means that if a company self-indemnifies but contracts with a TPA for claims processing and other program management activities, the money budgeted for health care is still in the control of the company for its own cash flow until services are rendered and claims must be paid. The advantage to industry is that the tedious aspect of program management is contracted out, but the analytical and long-term policy tasks remain the responsibility of industry benefit administrators.

Provider reimbursement structure

MEDICAL ECONOMICS AND INSURANCE

Once again, we must look to the concept of insurance and what it means for ambulatory care programs such as dental care.

The development of benefit packages and premium calculations for prepaid dental care programs differs greatly from similar work for insurance-type programs. The standard definition of an *insurable risk* contains three essential elements: (1) the loss or incident occurs infrequently, such as a flood; (2) the potential loss is very great, for example, destruction of home by fire; and (3) any single individual cannot affect the risk or frequency of the event in the community. Hospitalization is an insurable risk and meets these three criteria. However, expenditure for dental care, and for that matter most ambulatory care, is not an insurable risk. Dental disease is common. Dental care is not expensive, at least not when compared with the cost of hospitalization, and individuals generally know what their level of need is. This last point is the reason that dental care plans

cannot be marketed on an individual basis in the private sector. Adverse selection would result from all those persons with heavy accumulated dental needs joining the plan at the same time that those who have maintained their oral health do not join. This type of adverse selection would eliminate any element of cost sharing, forcing premiums up to an unmarketable level and causing closure of the prepaid plan.

Prepaid dental care plans are essentially a budgeting type of arrangement in which predictable expenditures are planned where groups are large enough. The real economic dilemma occurs when providers, who have considerable leverage over use, have no economic incentive to initiate courses of treatment consistent with budgeted premium dollars. With traditional private sector insurance, the third party is to assume risk for dental claims and the role of the consumer and the provider is to maximize benefits derived from the plan.

CHANGES IN THE MARKETPLACE

The introduction of the concept of risk sharing in prepaid programs is a product of the past decade. In its purest form, the insurers of care and the providers of services fuse into one umbrella organization. This is the HMO concept in which the provider is also given an incentive to initiate courses of treatment consistent with premium dollars.

Are the same forces at work in the dental care marketplace as in the HMO movement for medical care? Around the country, indemnity dental insurance plans are beginning to lose ground to capitation and other provider-type arrangements as large insurers speculate that the market is on the brink of some major shifts. The nature of the more common arrangements follow:

1. Fee-for-service (FFS): open panel
2. Fee-for-service: participating provider (no provider restriction)
3. Fee-for-service: independent practice association (IPA)/preferred provider orga-

nization (PPO) model (selected provider participation)

4. Capitation: staff model groups
5. Capitation: independent practice association model

RANGE OF CHOICES
Fee-for-service options

Fee-for-service open panel. This choice is the structure of the typical indemnity commercial insurance plan. The basic contractual arrangement is between the insurance company and the insured, whereby the insurance company indemnifies for losses from dental claims as outlined in the policy's list of coverage. Policyholders are free to select the dentist of their choice and can either pay the dentist directly for services rendered and later collect from the insurance company or assign such payments directly to the dentist. The insurance company in turn reimburses for care based on a table of allowances or usual and customary fees up to the 90th percentile. Dentists are free to collect from the patient any differences between their fee and that allowed under the terms of the insurance policy.

Fee-for-service: participating provider (no provider restriction). This is the structure of the typical professionally sponsored insurance plan, such as the Blue Cross/Blue Shield and Delta plans. The basic contractual arrangement is between the insurance underwriter and the provider of services, in this case the dentist. This type of coverage is usually termed *service benefits,* in contrast to the *indemnity benefits* of the previous commercial insurance structure. With the Delta plan as a typical example, providers submit their fee schedule with the carrier and cannot charge the patient more than the agreed-on fees. Becoming a participating provider usually entails signing a provider agreement with the insurance carrier, locking the provider into an agreed-on fee schedule that the provider submits. This agreement has caused much controversy because

most providers (both dentists and physicians) want the ability to bill patients directly for the difference when their fees exceed the fee schedule of the service-benefit contract. "Balance billing" has been the topic of much litigation and legislation.

Currently a large percentage of providers have become participating providers, usually with the insurance carriers reducing the reimbursable fee by 5% because of guaranteed payment. This has given the Blue Cross/Blue Shield and Delta plans some leverage in the marketplace, but the commercial carriers have countered this economic advantage by offering a more varied product line and packaging it with other types of insurance.

Fee-for-service: IPA/PPO model. Recently IPA or PPO networks have been observed in the marketplace. These organizations are participating-provider service-benefit insurance arrangements, but with the clear intention of negotiating a reduced fee with the providers. To entice providers to reduce their fees as much as 15% to 20%, the concept of a closed panel is introduced. This means that only a few offices will be selected to participate in any given geographic area, thereby guaranteeing each office a greater volume of patients than would otherwise be obtainable.

Fee-for-service spectrum. In the spectrum of fee-for-service options, if cost containment becomes of greater importance, the most likely solution is to contain, if not reduce, reimbursable fees. There is simplicity and ease in using this approach. Essentially, the problem is tackled by modifying the structure established long ago with a considerable amount of accumulated experience and professional acceptance in the marketplace today.

However, modifying the structure in this way leaves the fee-for-service option intact, and the concept of risk sharing is not used. It has been found that providers in the closed-panel PPO arrangement will maintain their contractual fee arrangements, but they are not deterred from trying to expand their service options with the patient or increase fees for noncovered or partially covered services. Once again, the third party is at risk, and the provider and patient have an economic incentive to maximize benefits, in this case dollars from the program.

Risk-sharing options

Dental capitation programs have grown in popularity during the past two decades. Most of the major dental insurers, including companies such as Prudential and Connecticut General, have established capitation programs. These companies would not have ventured into this area of the marketplace if they did not believe that doing so was in their best interests.

The essential feature of capitation is that the provider receives a predetermined fixed revenue and must budget his or her time accordingly. The typical industry standard for rate setting is to budget according to the cost of delivering dental services in the typical office. Fees do not play a role in the pricing mechanism.

Given that a fixed cost-based payment will be received, the provision of preventive and maintenance services is preferable to the more complex rehabilitation services that are usually associated with higher fees in the marketplace. One of the main advantages is that each dentist can base the treatment assessment on his or her own diagnosis, and a prior authorization or review by an insurance carrier consultant becomes superfluous.

The main criticism of this approach is that the provider will not have an incentive to perform needed dental work and may in fact collect the capitation payments without delivering the services. However, with adequate monitoring and utilization review, most providers will follow accepted treatment standards. As with any system of reimbursement, there will be a small percentage who abuse the system for personal gain.

Capitation: staff model groups. Prepaid capitation group practice is the HMO concept as applied to the delivery of dental services. In one setting the patient can receive all required dental services. The economic incentive of this concept is to improve the oral health status of the enrolled population, and the patient has the advantage of one-stop shopping for dental care. Although this option is enticing, there is a problem in the widespread application of this approach. Approximately 88% of the delivery of dental services is by solo practitioners. Large multispecialty groups are not the mainstay of dental care delivery; however, with the growth of retail-based dental centers, this is rapidly changing. From the perspective of benefits administrators, there are dental care delivery units that do have the potential for this type of arrangement, such as the growing number of group practice outlets in various shopping malls.

Capitation IPA model. The IPA model has the advantage of fitting the benefits of risk sharing of capitation with the dental care delivery system as it presently exists. At first glance it seems a perfect match; however, it does introduce a few problems. How does one handle the issue of specialist services? Should capitation payments go to the general practitioners, who in turn pay the specialists? Should the specialists be capitated directly, or should they be kept on a closely monitored fee-for-service system? In the private sector there are several variations of this arrangement, and each seems to work as intended.

Dental plan standards

Various combinations of financial and provider reimbursement structures for dental plans currently exist in the marketplace, although traditional indemnity fee-for-service plans dominate. The growth and design of individual dental plan products has simply evolved with the purchasing employer group on its own in the selection of a specific plan design. Recently a movement has emerged to establish standards for dental plan coverage. Two national organizations have attempted to establish standards for dental plans. The ADA and Health Policy Agenda have developed dental plan designs for both a limited-cost or basic plan and an expanded plan. The Health Policy Agenda is a coalition of medical, labor, and employer organizations that devises basic benefit packages to serve as benchmarks that employers and subscribers could use to evaluate health insurance plans including dental insurance. The ADA has similarly established standards for dental care plans.

The two organizations have developed coverage standards for four major categories of dental services: (1) diagnostic-preventive, (2) routine, (3) complex, and (4) orthodontic. Both urge that there should be no deductibles or co-payments for diagnostic, preventive, and emergency services. According to the Health Policy Agenda, these out-of-pocket expenses tend to discourage the patient from entering the system.

The ADA suggests full coverage for two examinations and prophylaxes per year. Bitewing radiographs are to be provided annually and complete radiographs are to be provided every 5 years. Topical fluoride treatments twice per year are suggested for patients under age 18; sealants and emergency care should be provided as needed.

The basic and expanded model plans developed by the Health Policy Agenda differ somewhat from the recommendations of the ADA. Under its basic plan, examinations, prophylaxes, and fluoride treatments are allowed annually rather than every 6 months. However, both organizations suggest that as the treatment becomes more complex, patient cost-sharing features should be included. The Health Policy Agenda maintains that cost sharing for complex care should be high enough to motivate employees and their dependents to maintain their oral health.

The model dental plans of the ADA and the Health Policy Agenda may differ in specific coverage details, but their development and promulgation are a natural consequence of changes in the financing of dental care. As third-party participation in dental care increases, two national organizations that have established standards have come to the forefront. These standards are to help guide constituents, whether they are employees, dentists, or consumers, to select from the myriad dental plan products now available.

Conclusion

This chapter discussed the factors that have led to changes in dental care delivery and the economics of dental care. We are currently in a period of transition, during which alternative modes of delivery of services and financing of these services will evolve. This chapter also discussed the potential impact of caries reduction in dental care delivery.

The reduction of dental caries and the role of fluorides have been well documented by the dental profession. The first step in its understanding occurred in 1902, when Frederic S. McKay gave systematic attention to the mottling he found in his patients. The unfolding of the fluoride story is a classic case study in chronic disease epidemiology. The dental profession can point with pride to its role in significantly preventing a disease that a few years ago was considered ubiquitous and its treatment an almost insurmountable task.

In this decade dental care delivery is also influenced by the unfolding of historical events that at first appear to have no bearing on current dental practice. The growth of fringe benefits is one such factor. Fringe benefits developed during World War II, when the federal government prohibited nearly all wage increases. War industries attracted workers by offering benefits in addition to wages. For example, many employers paid part of the cost of food served in their cafeterias. Later, companies offered medical insurance, life insurance, and accident and disability insurance. Since then, fringe benefits have grown in importance. Labor and management have introduced new benefits, including dental care and stock purchase plans. Unions often accept fringe benefits instead of higher wages because most benefits are not subject to income tax.

Dental professionals must and will adapt to this changing environment. Our responsibilities will not diminish; instead, we must remain involved to ensure the public of the highest standards of care and professionalism.

OUTCOME MEASURES TO EVALUATE DENTAL PLAN OPTIONS

The Massachusetts Public Employees Health and Welfare Fund (hereafter, the Fund) was established on January 3, 1984, as a result of collective bargaining between the Commonwealth of Massachusetts and a coalition of trade unions representing 36,000 state employees. The union coalition consisted of the American Federation of State, County, and Municipal Employees (AFSCME) Council 93 and the Service Employees International Union (SEIU) Locals 254, 285, and 509. The union coalition had seen similar jointly managed Health and Welfare Funds deliver cost-effective employee benefits in both Pennsylvania and New York and made the creation of the Fund a major issue during contract negotiations with the state. The Commonwealth of Massachusetts, mindful of escalating health care costs, wanted to share responsibility for managing future employee benefit costs with the unions and they endorsed the creation of the Fund to self-insure dental benefits.

The Fund's trustees consciously designed a dental program that would encourage lower-income plan beneficiaries, without a history of regular clinical dental care, to visit the dentist. After reviewing a variety of dental care plan options available to the Fund, the trustees concluded that creating their own preferred provider network would allow them both to provide more dental services to eligible members at a lower price and to monitor the quality of care. Some trustees, particularly those who represented higher paid state employees, thought that some type of indemnity program would be necessary, if only to serve workers in remote locations. Consequently, the trustees created a self-insured, dual-choice dental program featuring a fixed reimbursement schedule indemnity plan (hereafter, the Open Plan) and a preferred provider plan (hereafter, the Closed Plan).

By creating a preferred provider network, the trustees had to become involved with both patient care and fiscal planning. In early 1985, when the trustees first issued a request for proposal (RFP) to administer their dual-choice plan, only one bidder was prepared to take on the assignment. In all of New England there were no plans with comparable structure and size from which the trustees could learn. The Fund's first plan administrator started the plan on July 1, 1985, with a network of only 30 preferred providers.

During the last 10 years the trustees have successfully managed the plan. Member utilization of the dental plan is high, cost savings from preferred provider contracts have stretched scarce public resources as far as possible, and the preferred provider network has grown to include more than 400 general dentists and specialists. In 1993, when the Fund issued another RFP for administrative services, the trustees could receive 10 responsive bids and could choose from an array of excellent potential administrators.

UTILIZATION TRENDS

Since the inception of the dental plan, the trustees have received periodic reports of service utilization on a per patient basis. All dental claims from the start of the plan have been stored on computer tape at Boston University. In 1993, to facilitate claim analysis by the Fund administrator and the Fund's dental consultant, the claim files were transferred to personal computer diskettes. The claims data source, a service specific data file, was converted into a patient-specific compilation of claims information. Over the years the trustees had received summary reports of patient-specific dental service utilization that chronicled plan modifications including increased coverage for the Open and Closed Plan, reimbursable fees, and the number of offices that participated in the Closed Plan.

Since 1985 the Fund's dental plan administrators had been contractually required to perform periodic office audits of preferred providers and to perform an annual dental claims analysis. These quality assurance programs were needed to provide the trustees with feedback about both the quality and the cost-effectiveness of the dental plan. The trustees have always tried to maximize the benefits available under the Closed Plan as a way to both monitor quality and to encourage members to seek care from dental offices with contractual fee limits. For this reason it was especially important to ensure the trustees that the care delivered and paid for by the fund in the Closed Plan met basic quality standards and was sufficient to meet the needs of the enrolled population.

The periodic claims analyses and office audits have provided valuable feedback to the trustees and, as standards, can be termed *process measures*. Aggregate dental claim assessments are not direct measurements of oral health but are, at best, indicators of needs being met. Office and patient record audits review the process of patient care and determine whether professional standards are being met. The implication is that if offices meet accepted professional standards, then one can assume that the quality of care they deliver also meets accepted professional standards.

The ultimate goal of the dental plan was to improve the oral health status of the membership and these process measures, carefully reviewed, can be indirect indicators of oral health. In 1994 the trustees decided to allocate the resources necessary to directly measure directly the oral health status of a group of Fund members. There was one main concern the trustees wanted addressed.

The trustees wanted to know if members who had received treatment from the Closed Plan, with its lower fee structure, actually achieved a level of oral health similar to the level of oral health exhibited by Open Plan participants. As an adjunct to this question, the trustees wanted to know if Closed Plan preferred providers were basing their treatment choices on the maximization of their claim reimbursement rather than on the oral health and treatment needs of plan participants.

OVERVIEW OF RESEARCH PROJECT

Given the major concern listed above, it was decided that the best way to proceed was with a pilot project that asked the most fundamental question concerning a difference in oral health status between members of the Open and Closed Plans. Once completed and results analyzed, the pilot could then serve as a basis to obtain federal or foundation support to continue to pursue the other issues raised by the trustees.

In the pilot project the primary emphasis was to determine the performance of the delivery system as it relates to the oral health of Open and Closed Plan members. This assessment was accomplished by comparing the oral health status of a sample of patients in each of the two plans and who were comparable in demographics and dental treatment history. The pilot sought to determine whether Closed Plan members different systematically in oral health status compared with Open Plan members. This has important policy implications for the trustees. Over the years managed care has been the standard that guided the trustees' offerings of dental plan options. All past analyses have essentially supported this emphasis, but always in the background was the question that claims and process measures only *infer* the outcome of oral health but do not directly *measure* it. With this pilot project came the opportunity to select a sample of patients and directly measure health outcome.

In the process of accomplishing this phase there was also the occasion to start the learning curve in establishing the methods and procedures to conduct this evaluation. To this end, examination sites were established, examiners calibrated, examination instruments developed, clerical and organizational tasks outlined, and analytical methods tested and implemented. With the pilot project completed, the trustees also now have an assessment of the oral health of two groups of enrollees who have participated in both the Closed Plan and the Open Plan. The methods and procedures derived to date have provided the trustees the ability to tackle larger and more complex questions to insure top-quality care and improved oral health. The completion of this pilot represents the implementation of a statewide evaluation of the largest managed dental care program in New England.

EXAMINATION SITES

Given the size of the dental plan membership, the team decided to recruit examination sites throughout Massachusetts. Given extensive knowledge of membership utilization patterns throughout the commonwealth, the team targeted selected areas of the state as locations convenient for most members to undergo their oral examinations. During the summer of 1994, the team contacted preferred provider dental offices to determine their willingness to participate. The dentists were asked to donate an operatory for several days and were informed that an examiner hired and trained by the Boston University research team would perform the oral health assessments.

POPULATION AND SAMPLE

The eligible base for the Fund is a very diverse population in terms of demographics, culture, job category, and income. The Boston University research team proposed focusing their hypothesis on the dental health status of two homogeneous sample groups. One group included members enrolled in the Open Plan for at least 3 years, and the other group included those in the Closed Plan with the same length of enrollment criterion. The pilot study involved the direct examination and survey of a sample of 233 plan members.

The team acknowledged that the Fund's Closed Plan participants differed demographically from participants in the Open Plan. With the introduction of the Closed Plan, many members, because their economic barriers had been greatly reduced, for the first time obtained a full range of dental services. Open Plan members on the other hand tend to be those at the higher pay scale and who have a history of regular maintenance care. Members of this group are more likely to remain with their own dentist and not transfer to the Closed Plan.

To avoid selection bias and maintain this study as a pilot that concentrated on the issue of the delivery system, the team limited the sample of subjects to those of equivalent demographic and economic background. The SEIU Local 509 members were more homogeneous than the Fund's full membership and was also a group easier to contact and more willing to appear for an oral examination. Each member selected for participation was contacted by letter to explain the goals and purpose of the study. That letter was followed by telephone contact to determine willingness to participate and to provide a location and a phone number to call to schedule an oral examination. Arrangements were made to conduct the dental examinations at 20 dentist's offices located throughout Massachusetts.

MEASURES

A single dental examiner conducted all 233 of the examinations (direct dental examination). The examiner did not know in which of the two dental plans the members were enrolled. Two oral health status measures were used: (1) The Oral Health Status Index (OSHI) and (2) The number of decayed, missing, and filled teeth (DMF). The team used direct clinical measures of oral health to avoid the need for bite-wing and full series x-ray examinations. The OHSI, developed by Marcus, Koch, and Gershen, was the principal instrument to compare Open and Closed Plan participants. Use of this measure yields a score between 1 and 100 for each subject, 100 being perfect oral health.

Before the examinations, the principal investigator trained the study examiner in the use of the OHSI developed by Marcus and associates. There was a total of three full-day training sessions spent on examining nonstudy patients in a private dental office, a setting similar to the examination sites recruited for the project.

The developers of the OSHI have indicated many applications for the use of this index. In the words of the authors: "The most important applications of the index, however, will be for cost-effectiveness analysis. The index formulation provides a point system for outcome assessment by allowing the computation of dollar costs per points in index improvement."

The BU team believed that this tool could enable the Trustees to determine the return of improvement of oral health status as a function of dollar investment.

In addition to the OHSI, the number of DMF permanent teeth was computed for each subject. DMF has been a standard measure of dental morbidity for many years. The DMF includes filled teeth as a measure of past disease morbidity, whereas the OSHI treats filled teeth as a positive gain of treatment. In the adult application the OSHI measures variables that relate systematically to disease and missing teeth along with a positive factor of replaced teeth. It again takes into account the positive impact of treatment.

RESULTS

A total of 502 postcards were returned, indicating respondents' willingness to participate in the study; 211 responses were from the Open Plan and 291 from the Closed Plan members and their spouses. Examinations were successfully completed on 233 individuals (108 Open Plan and 125 Closed Plan members and their spouses). To explore differences between those examined and not examined, data available from past dental claims experience was used, namely age, number of procedures in the past year, and annual cost of the procedures performed. Table 5-3 shows, for each of the Open and Closed Plan groups, this comparison of those examined with those who returned postcards but were not examined. There seems to be a general trend that the means for each of these three characteristics are slightly higher in those not examined than in those examined. The differences, however, are indeed small, and there appears little indication of bias among those who completed the examination compared with those who had returned the postcard.

A more important consideration is whether the claims experience of the examined subjects are comparable with the overall claims experience of the plan during the prior plan year. It is clear that in terms of plan experience and age there appears to be a difference. Total plan averages for age, number of procedures and total claims cost are consistently less than for study subjects. This is to be expected because Local 509 S.E.I.U. members are atypical of total membership. This was clearly understood at the outset of the study but the purpose was to compare similar subjects who differ primarily in plan membership.

Table 5-4 shows the demographic characteristics of each of the Open and Closed Plan examinees. The overall distributions show that

Table 5-3. Mean and standard deviation (SD) of age, number of procedures, and cost for those examined, those not examined, and total plan adult members by plan type

Characteristic	Open			Closed		
	Examined	Not examined	Total plan	Examined	Not examined	Total plan
No.	108	103	14,908	125	166	26,295
Age						
Mean	47.5	47.5	45.1	43.9	43.8	40.2
SD	9.0	10.4	8.8	8.1	8.3	9.9
No. of procedures	5.2	5.3	4.9	6.5	6.6	6.1
SD	3.8	3.1	2.9	3.6	4.2	3.4
Cost						
Mean	$156	$161	$146	$268	$287	$240
SD	$205	$131	$219	$268	$287	$309

Data from Boffa J, Brouder J, Colton T, Kassler H: *Evaluation of managed dental care—final report,* Boston, Nov 1995, Massachusetts Public Employee Fund.

Table 5-4. Sociodemographic characteristics of those examined by type of plan

Characteristic	Open (n = 108)	Closed (n = 125)
Gender: female	58%	61%
Age (years)*		
Under 40 years	20%	29%
40-49 years	45%	50%
50 & Older	34%	22%
Mean ± SD*	47.5 ± 9.0 yr	43.9 ± 8.1 yr
Race: White	93%	88%
Marital status		
Married	70%	61%
Other	30%	39%
Education		
Less than bachelor's degree	12%	17%
Bachelor's degree	43%	48%
Postgraduate	45%	35%

Data from Boffa J, Brouder J, Colton T, Kassler H: *Evaluation of managed dental care—final report,* Boston, Nov 1995, Massachusetts Public Employee Fund.
*P <0.01.

the examinees were mostly female, predominantly white, the great majority married, and most with at least a bachelor's degree. The only demographic characteristic that differed statistically between the two examined groups was age, with the Closed Plan examinees on average 3.6 years younger than Open Plan examinees. Although somewhat more of Open compared with Closed Plan examinees were married (70% versus 61%) and had a postgraduate education (45% versus 35%), neither of these differences was statistically significant.

A single, trained examiner, unaware of the plan choice of each subject, conducted all the examinations. The findings of the examinations appear in Table 5-5 with regard to OHSI, number of teeth with 4 to 6 mm bone loss, and the percentage for whom the most recent visit was for periodontal therapy. Because of the difference in age between the two examined groups, Table 5-5 presents age-specific findings—within each of the three decades of age that characterized the subjects.

In terms of overall OHSI score, there was no statistical difference between the Open and Closed Plan; this held true for all three age strata listed. When OHSI components were examined, none showed a statistical difference except for the average number of teeth that exhibited moderate bone loss (between 4 and 6 mm). When stratified by age, in the 40- to 49-year stratum, the difference was statistically significant. This stratum represent 50% of the subjects examined. Also in terms of those who reported their most recent dental visit for periodontal services, a significant difference was found in that stratum. As age increases, the number of teeth that exhibit moderate bone

loss also increases. The exception is subjects aged 41 to 49. Closed Plan members in this age group exhibited a significantly lower mean number of teeth with moderate bone loss compared with their Open Plan counterparts. At the same time, note that this same group reported a significant higher number of recent dental visits for periodontal services.

Seventy-five percent of the subjects reported that they visit the dentist every 6 months. Table 5-6 examines the reported utilization of dental services by age. Table 5-6 indicates that for pa-

Table 5-6. Reported recent visit for periodontal services for subjects who seek dental care every 6 months

Age (yr)	Open (n = 82)	Closed (n = 93)
<40	0	5.6%
40-49	2.4%	12.9%*
50+	3.1%	14.8%

Data from Boffa J, Brouder J, Colton T, Kassler H: *Evaluation of managed dental care—final report*, Boston, Nov 1995, Massachusetts Public Employee Fund.
*P < 0.01.

Table 5-5. Outcome measures by age group and type of plan

Outcome measure	Open (n = 108)	Closed (n = 125)
Mean OHS score		
<40 years	95.7	95.5
40-49 years	92.3	91.2
50+ years	83.3	83.2
Mean no. teeth with 4-6 mm bone loss		
<40 years	3.5	3.0
40-49 years	4.9	3.6*
50+ years	5.4	5.2
Most recent visit for periodontal service		
<40 years	2.1%	2.2%
40-49 years	1%	15%*
50+ years	<1%	5%

Data from Boffa J, Brouder J, Colton T, Kassler H: *Evaluation of managed dental care—final report*, Boston, Nov 1995, Massachusetts Public Employee Fund.
*P < 0.01.

tients who seek care every 6 months, a statistically higher percent of Closed Plan members reported recent visits for periodontal services. This is consistent at all three age strata.

A multiple regression analysis was also conducted with OHSI as the dependent variable and the following as independent variables: plan type, age, gender, marital status, and education. The only variate found statistically significant was age, with a negative regression coefficient ($P <0.0001$). This indicates the strong relationship that exists for OHSI to decrease as age increases. This is to be expected because the effects of dental disease are cumulative and certain components of the OHSI reflect this fact. For example, decayed teeth can be restored to a healthy condition but if an individual experiences periodontal disease with alveolar bone loss, even if gingival and bone conditions can be stabilized, the bone loss still exists. This is the same for missing teeth. Prosthetic replacement of missing teeth only partially offsets the negative impact of missing teeth.

Commentary

With regard to overall oral health status, the Boston University team found no difference between the participants who were enrolled in the Open Plan and the participants who were enrolled in the Closed Plan. The one significant difference that emerged in subgroup analysis, by age, was that Closed Plan participants between age 41 and age 50 exhibited, on average, fewer teeth with moderate bone loss. In addition, based on the questionnaire responses, Closed Plan members reported more frequent periodontal treatment. When members are stratified by age, the greater use of periodontal services is restricted to Closed Plan participants between age 41 and 50. This observation coincides with this age group's better average periodontal health component score of the overall OHSI. It is concluded that among those

dental plan participants age 41 to 50, a greater proportion of Closed Plan members than Open Plan members avail themselves of periodontal services and consequently exhibit better average periodontal health status scores. However, for those plan members who visit the dentist every 6 months, a consistently higher proportion of Closed Plan members reported their most recent visit to be for periodontal services. Regular dental visits for anyone over age 40 is primarily for the prevention and of treatment periodontal disease. Closed Plan members who reported regular 6 month visits were the ones seeking routine periodontal visits.

Discussion

The Fund's underlying dual-choice dental plan design encourages members to participate in the Closed Plan by capping member copayments for dental services. In the Open Plan the Fund reimburses members a fixed dollar amount per procedure performed, regardless of the actual price charged by the dental practitioner. As a result of this policy, a Closed Plan member almost always pays considerably less out-of-pocket for needed periodontal services than does an Open Plan participant. It is possible that Open Plan participants would receive more periodontal treatment and that the periodontal health of Open Plan participants would show improvement if additional (but scarce) resources were committed in that area.

The trustees are also interested in knowing whether the results from this pilot project can be extrapolated to the Fund's full membership. The specific local union chosen for the pilot project contained an older, better-educated, higher-paid and more female workforce than the Fund as a whole. The trustees hope to draw their next sample from the full membership. This will provide a representative mix of the total membership. It is hoped that the next project will contain a longitudinal component, starting with new members whose progress can be followed over time. Such an examination of newly eligible members would allow the trustees to better understand the motivations and oral health level of newly eligible persons joining the perspective dental plans.

Finally, this study has potentially important implications for the dental insurance industry and for dental public health professionals. It is relatively easy and relatively inexpensive to measure the oral health status of populations, at least compared with the difficulty and expense involved in measuring medical health status of those same populations. Accurate ongoing measurement of oral health status could be a way for insurance companies, employee benefit managers, and dental public health programs to directly measure the affect of dental treatment spending on the oral health of populations. For this reason it is hoped that similar studies will continue to be done.

BIBLIOGRAPHY

American Dental Association, Council on Dental Care Programs: Council report, Chicago, March 1984.

American Dental Association: Study shows Americans' oral health improving, *ADA News,* June 10, 1996.

American Dental Association, Council on Dental Care Programs: What is the cost of compliance? *J Am Dent Assoc* 125:682, 1994.

Bell N: Managed care and dentistry: a perfect fit, *Business and Health,* Special report, 1991.

Boffa J, Brouder J, Colton T, Kassler H: *Evaluation of managed dental care—final report,* Boston, Nov 1995, Massachusetts Public Employee Fund.

Burnelle J, Carlos J: Changes in the prevalence of dental caries in U.S. school children, 1961-1980, *J Dent Res* 61:1347, 1982.

Cohen DM, Roesler TW: The effect of dental insurance and patient income level on the utilization of dental services and implications for future growth in dentistry, *J Dent Pract Admin* 3:4, 1986.

Delta Dental Plans: *Survey of dental insurance,* Fall 1994.

Douglass CW, Day JM: Cost and payment of dental services in the U.S., *J Dent Educ* 43:7, 1979.

Eilers RD: *Actuarial services for a dental service corporation,* Washington, DC, 1967, US Department of Health, Education and Welfare, Public Health Service.

Glass R: Secular changes in caries prevalence in two Massachusetts towns, *Caries Res* 15:448, 1981.

Leverett P: Fluorides and the changing prevalence of dental caries, *Science* 217:23, 1982.

Manninen DL, Dugan MK, Pearce S: *Dental outcomes study: comparison of capitation and fee-for-service dental plans,* Seattle, June 1994 (final report), Battelle Centers for Public Health Research and Evaluation.

Marcus M, Atchison KA: Oral health status: comparison of provider and patient perspectives, *J Dent Res* 72:521, 1992 (IADR abstract).

Marcus M, Koch A, Gershen J: Construction of a population index of adult oral health status derived for dentists' preferences, *J Am Dent Assoc* 43:284, 1983.

Marcus M, Koch A, Gershen J: Introduction of a practical oral health status index for adult population, *J Am Dent Assoc* 110:729, 1985.

Moen B, Poetsch V: Survey of dental services rendered 1969: more preventive less tooth repair, Bureau of Economic Research and Statistics, *J Am Dent Assoc* 81:25, 1970.

Praiss IL and others: Changing patterns and implication for cost and quality of dental care, *Inquiry* 16:131, 1979.

Spencer's Research Reports: *Basic elements of dental plan design as recommended by ADA and health policy agenda,* Chicago, 1991, Spencer's Research Reports.

Weisfeld R: *National preventive dentistry demonstration program, the Robert Wood Johnson demonstration program,* Special Report No 2, 1983.

SECTION II

Demographic shifts and dental health

CHAPTER 6

Recognizing cultural differences

Diana L. Mercado Galvis

Because of the increasing ethnic diversity of the population, dental health practitioners will need to become aware of cultural differences that relate to the oral health of the community. These differences will inevitably have an impact on how dental care is delivered. Currently, access to dental health care varies by socioeconomic status, and dental care to the underserved and to minority populations is limited.[1,2] Individuals from different cultural backgrounds bring to the clinical setting varying sets of values, beliefs, and practices that must be managed in an effective manner.[3] This chapter focuses on information related to the delivery of dental health services for an increasingly diverse U.S. population. The topics include U.S. demographic trends, definition of terms and concepts related to multiculturalism, oral health issues related to diversity, health beliefs and culture, and intercultural competence.

United States demographic trends

The U.S. population census of 1990 reveals a trend toward a more diverse population.[4] Dr. Harold Hodgkinson, a demographer, believes that the U.S. population will become more diversified, and he predicts that the current U.S. majority population will become the minority population by the year 2050.[5] The Asian/Pacific Islander, Hispanic/Latino, American Indian, and African-American populations demonstrated significant growth for the period 1980 through 1990; these population groups demonstrated a growth rate of 107.8%, 53%, 37.9% and 13.2%, respectively. As shown in Fig. 6-1, the Asian/Pacific Islander population is currently the fastest growing minority population in the United States. Asian/Pacific Islanders are characterized by a large group of recent immigrants and those whose families have been in the United States for many years. The Chinese, primarily located in California and New York, are the largest subgroup and comprise 23% of the total U.S. Asian/Pacific Islander population. The second and third largest subgroups are the Filipino at 19% and the Japanese at 12%, and both groups are located primarily in Hawaii and California. Asian Indian, Korean, and Vietnamese are the next largest populations. They are primarily located in California, New York, and Texas.[5] By the year 2000, a 400% growth rate is anticipated for the Asian/Pacific Islander population.

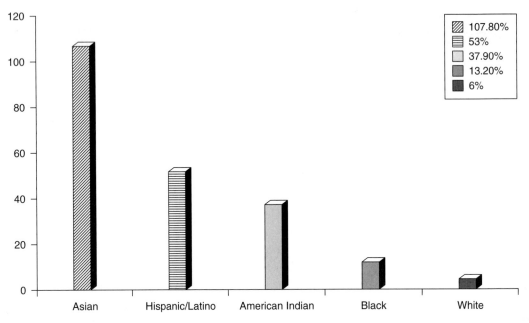

Fig. 6-1. U.S. population growth trends, 1980-1990.

With current growth rates, it is expected that the Hispanic/Latino population will become the largest minority population of the United States between the years 2000 and 2010. Today, 90% of Hispanic/Latinos live in 10 states, namely, California, Texas, New York, Florida, Illinois, New Jersey, Arizona, New Mexico, Colorado, and Massachusetts. The largest Hispanic/Latino populations are located in California (25.8%), Texas (25.5%), New York (12.3%), and Florida (12.2%). An important characteristic of U.S. minority population groups is that they are comprised of numerous subgroups. For example, the U.S. Hispanic/Latino population has more than 30 subgroups, whose common origin is the Spanish language. The Mexican population represents 61.2% of the total Hispanic/Latino population. The other subgroups include Puerto Ricans, 12.1%; Central Americans, 6%; South Americans, 4.7%; Spaniards, 4.4%; Cubans, 4.8%; Dominicans, 2.4%; and other Hispanic/Latinos 3.9%.

Patterns during the last two decades have demonstrated an increase in the numbers of immigrants from Pacific Rim countries, Panama, El Salvador, Guatemala, Colombia, Honduras, the People's Republic of China, Vietnam, Laos, and Cambodia.[6] There is no doubt that the shifts in cultural orientation will have an impact on the delivery of dental health care in the United States.

Definition of terms and concepts

The dental health care provider brings a set of beliefs and assumptions to each patient encounter. These beliefs and assumptions belong to a particular cultural group of which the dental health care provider is a member. What occurs when the beliefs and assumptions of the dental health care provider and the patient are different? For the purpose of exploring cultural differences, the following definitions and concepts will be used.

Race and *ethnicity* are similar in that they relate to the basic divisions of humanity. *Race* refers to varieties of humanity with different physical characteristics. These groups are known as the Caucasoid, Mongoloid, and Negroid groups. The Caucasoid is the group with very light to brown skin color. The Mongoloid group has white to yellowish-brown skin color, and the Negroid group has brown to black skin color. In the United States and around the world interracial/ethnic marriages have made it increasingly more difficult to categorize individuals according to these terms. *Ethnicity* refers to the divisions of a heterogeneous population as distinguished by customs, language, and so on.[7]

Diversity is the condition of being different or having differences.[8] *Diversity* is an inclusive term used to describe not only existing cultural differences but also differences regarding sexual orientation, gender, physical and mental disabilities, and age differences. In this chapter the term *diversity* is used in the context of describing cultural differences. *Culture* is a term that describes the characteristics of a group of people over a given time. This definition does not project the depth of the term adequately. According to Gary Althen, culture can be viewed as a collection of values and assumptions that blend together to shape the way a group of people perceive and relate to the world around them. Culture guides an individual throughout his or her life, provides the framework for decision making, and serves as a lens through which to visualize and interpret the world. Culture is dynamic in nature; it evolves, adapts, and recreates itself from generation to generation. *Subculture* refers to a group of persons who have developed different interests or goals from the primary culture, on the basis of factors such as occupation, sex, age, social class, or religion. *Acculturation* refers to learning the rules of another nonnative culture. It differs from *assimilation* in that it is an additive, rather than a subtractive, process.[9] To assimilate is to replace traditional cultural values with those of another culture.

It is important to recognize that all persons are influenced by culture; however, dental health care providers should not assume that individuals possess certain characteristics or traits because they are members of a particular group. *Stereotyping* is a common problem that fails to recognize an individual's uniqueness. Although general cultural characteristics are described for different cultural groups, not all members of a cultural group follow the norms of their group entirely. *Ethnocentrism* is a term that describes one group's belief that their culture is superior to that of others. A reasonable goal of a diverse society (or world) is to create an environment that accepts *multiculturalism* or promotes the mutual respect of different cultures.

Developing an awareness of differences increases the level of cultural *sensitivity* of the dental health care provider. Persons of the same culture generally demonstrate an ability to react appropriately within the context of a specific interaction. This is known as *cultural competence*. Dental health care providers need to develop the skill of *intercultural competence*, which is the ability of two or more individuals to reinforce culturally different identities that interplay during the health care encounter. The expectation is that individuals of different cultures can maintain their identity throughout an intercultural communication.

Effective communication requires an understanding of those values, beliefs, and assumptions held by the different parties and especially the values, beliefs, and assumptions of the dental care provider. Values, beliefs, and assumptions are ideas about what is right and wrong, proper and improper, and normal and abnormal. These ideas are specific for different cultural groups. For the most part U.S. health care providers are influenced by Western cultural values and beliefs and scientific principles regarding current and acceptable standards of care. The oral health practices of patients may be rooted in their own culture rather than in scientific fact. Dental health care providers must be able to recognize and deal with the beliefs of others if they are to be successful practitioners.[8]

Issues related to diversity

Patient care issues related to diversity are directly influenced by culture. Culture has an impact on the client's view of the world, communication, trust, health practices and behaviors, concepts of wellness and illness, pursuit of mainstream health care, and mainstream health care compliance. Cultural beliefs play a major role in the health assumptions and practices of an individual. What are the expected dental health behaviors of the patient that are held by the dental health care provider? What are the expected professional behaviors of the dental health care provider held by the patient?

Verbal and nonverbal communication patterns represent important differences among different groups. Language differences present a barrier for many new immigrants, as well as those who have chosen to maintain their native tongue. Verbal communication is not always dependable because differences in conceptual frameworks may interfere with the meaning of words. Translators are sometimes reluctant to translate what they perceive as ignorance or superstition on the part of the patient.[10]

What constitutes trust and compliance for individuals of diverse backgrounds? Dental patients of diverse backgrounds may exhibit behaviors that are interpreted as noncompliant by a U.S. dental health care provider. A lack of trust is experienced by many individuals if the health care provider is not a member of their own culture. The gender of the health care provider also may be an issue for some patients. It has been stated that most health care practitioners possess ethnocentric biases that are in conflict with patient health practices and beliefs. If the beliefs and assumptions held by

the dental health care provider and the patient are in conflict, how does this conflict affect the manner in which dental care is delivered? In 1984 Ahia observed that individuals behave according to the "limitations bias," the "generalizations bias," or both. The limitations bias means that people generally do not consider as important concepts those with which they are not familiar. Generalization bias occurs when a health care provider perceives that a certain approach to care for one individual is applicable to the entire population of which the patient is a single member.[11] Generalization bias in this context becomes stereotyping and should be avoided. Exhibiting biases and stereotyping are common problems among all groups, but they are especially serious when exhibited by the dental health care provider. A number of studies have concluded that if health professionals are interculturally competent then the patient's response is enhanced.[12-27]

Health beliefs and culture

How do individuals from diverse backgrounds view health, illness, and the world around them? Does their view of health, illness, and the world have an impact on their oral health status? A review of the sociologic literature reveals major differences in health beliefs by various cultures. Some general cultural characteristics of the white middle class in the United States will be contrasted with the beliefs of other cultural groups. This information is essential to intercultural competence.

The cultural and health beliefs of the American white middle class can generally be described with the following terms: *individuality, belief in progress, ideals of freedom, the use of time, and things that are factual.* Emphasis is placed on the ability of the individual to control and to be responsible for his or her destiny. Issues regarding privacy are highly valued and an individual's privacy is protected through laws of confidentiality. The family is referred to as the immediate or nuclear family and consists of a mother, father, and children. The nuclear family prepares the children for adulthood, and at this time (between the ages of 18 and 21) the young adult is encouraged to become independent. Other members of the family, such as grandparents, aunts, uncles, and cousins, are considered to be relatives and are not connected to the nuclear family. The nuclear family is extended in other cultures. Youth is valued over age.[28]

An important characteristic of American white middle-class belief is its focus on the future, especially as it relates to progress. References to the future are expressed in everyday communication; for example,"I am looking forward to," is a common phrase that is used frequently in verbal and written forms of communication. There is less of an emphasis on history. This can be explained in part by the relatively brief history of the United States. Punctuality and keeping appointments are expected because time is regarded as a valuable resource. Americans expect to be advised 24 hours in advance if an appointment will not be kept or if someone will be 10 to 15 minutes late. Time is often equated with a monetary value, as demonstrated by the statement, "My time is worth money." In business-like interactions Americans are known for getting to the point and exhibiting behavior that is action oriented. In contrast, open and frank approaches to resolving issues and accomplishing objectives is sometimes perceived as cold and unfriendly by other cultures.[29]

Gender roles in the United States have changed considerably over the years, with women assuming positions traditionally held by men. Although there may be exceptions to the rule, laws are in place to protect the equality of the genders. The white middle class generally believes that people have the right of access to education, freedom of speech, religion, political convictions, and friendship with any sex. Other cultures are not as accepting of the

woman's role in society and are generally guided by a hierarchical view of society that establishes difference among people on the basis of gender or other attributes. In the United States individuals are addressed by the titles of Miss, Missus, or Mister or another earned title, such as doctor or professor, and not by titles that are inherited. This custom demonstrates the value that is placed on the acknowledgment of an individual's hard work. Other cultures may maintain titles related to social class.

Belief in things that are factual versus emotional appeals is another cultural difference. The American white middle class typically uses hyperbole to describe its accomplishments, such as the *largest* building in the world, the *best* armed forces, the *most* developed nation, the *best* medical attention, and so on. Consequently, Americans find comfort in the use of numbers and percentages for substantiating claims and supporting the facts. Scientific research is the basis for finding the facts, which in turn make things credible and valid. These facts are necessary to make logical decisions and are not to be clouded by feelings or sentiments. Since the U.S. white middle class believes that health equals freedom from disease, they take a proactive approach to seeking information, facts, options, and second opinions. It is commonly believed that professional people can help individuals solve their health problems.[30] Health care providers trained in the United States practice within the context of Western scientific and cultural values and beliefs. Common health problems that are encountered are cardiovascular disease, gastrointestinal disease, cancer, suicide, and chemical abuse. Remedies that may be used have been influenced by several European cultures.

As mentioned earlier in this chapter, the Hispanic/Latino population comprises many cultures that are linked by the common origin of their language. It should be noted that culture is comprised of many elements, some of which are apparent and others that are not. Elements that are apparent include dress, diet, dance, drama, art, and language. Those that are not apparent include notions of modesty, conceptions of beauty, patterns for handling emotions, conceptions of justice, decision making patterns, and the conception of self. Therefore it is erroneous to assume that all persons whose language origin is the same belong to one culture. Language is merely one element of which culture is composed, and avoidance of the generalization bias is necessary to avoid misunderstandings.

History and religion have played an important role in the evolution of the various cultures of the Hispanic/Latino group, and for this reason there is an underlying respect for tradition. Health beliefs are characterized by the notion that health is a result of good luck or God's gift. Family members provide support for the nurturing of the young and care for the sick and elderly. Illness is thought to result from bad luck or God's punishment and may be viewed as a sacrifice that is helpful to salvation. Some Hispanic/Latino cultures explain illness through influences of an "evil eye," and they believe that spirits can protect and harm people or prevent and cause illness.[6] The three most common causes of disease are (1) natural and supernatural forces, (2) imbalances of heat and cold, and (3) emotions. Illnesses can be prevented by proper diet, wearing amulets, use of candles and incense, avoiding harmful people, and magical powers. The common health problems affecting this population in the United States include diabetes, poor nutrition, and lactose enzyme deficiency.[31,32]

A wide range of cultural beliefs and practices is representative of the many subcultures that stem from African origin. It is noteworthy to understand the cultural diversity that exists among blacks and the importance of avoiding stereotyping of individuals because of skin color. Black cultural beliefs and practices vary among black subcultures. For instance, those individuals whose African cultural heritage was influenced by the Spanish or Caribbean Island Indian tribes are different from those that were not.

In the United States Asian/Pacific Islanders represent at least 30 subcultures and specific cultural characteristics are extremely difficult to describe. The Filipinos are probably the most diverse of all the Asian cultures. The Phillippines is comprised of subcultures speaking 87 languages and dialects and inhabiting some 500 islands. In 1990 Raul S. Manglapus, Secretary of Foreign Affairs for the Republic of the Philippines said, "There is no other country in Asia as ethnically diverse as the Philippines." In his text *Considering Filipinos*, Theodore Gochenour notes that Filipinos have a Western orientation to the extent that *Asianness* is not a common identifying description among them.[33] A major problem of Native Americans is that they are seen by the U.S. majority as "one people" despite the fact that there are 500 federally recognized tribal and native groups in the United States.[34] It is important to note that they comprise distinct groups with observable differences in governance, language, and culture. Most Native Americans do not reside in reservations; approximately 48% live on or adjacent to Indian reservations.[35] Those who remain on the reservation may not want all the "advantages" of the mainstream culture and may prefer not to assimilate.[36]

Cultural characteristics of a Native American who demonstrates less contact with the mainstream culture might include a general preference to use the native language, maintain social relations with an extended family, practice the native religion, retain a sacred view of land and rituals, and retain traditional health beliefs regarding etiology and healing. Suspicion and distrust are not unique to them as a minority U.S. culture. On the other hand, a fully accultured Native American may show a preference for English as the primary language, maintenance of a nuclear household arrangement, conversion to a nonnative religion, and acceptance of mainstream explanations for illness and the use of American institutional health services.[9]

Native American attitudes and beliefs regarding health are based on the notion that all creation has a spiritual basis. All things in nature are viewed as possessing spirits, and the spirit world communicates with the physical world. Health is defined as harmony in body, mind, and spirit and therefore depends on a healthy physical and spiritual state. If one of the three parts is out of harmony, all parts will be affected.

Intercultural competence
UNDERSTANDING DIVERSITY

Intercultural competence among dental health care providers progresses through the following: a personal level of multicultural knowledge, an ability to provide health messages in a manner that is compatible with patients' cultural values and beliefs, appropriate dental health education for diverse populations, and appropriate dental health care.

Kluckholn and Strodtbeck[37] proposed five problems or questions that all cultures must deal with; these questions represent a framework for understanding differences among diverse groups. First, how do humans relate to one another? This question includes consideration of an individualistic orientation versus a collectivist approach. Second, what is the character of innate human nature? In other words, are humans innately good, evil, or more complex (i.e., a combination of good and evil). Third, what is the temporal focus of human life? This question includes consideration of orientation. Are individuals concerned with the past, present, or future? Paying attention to

the past carries a strong sense of tradition. Emphasis on tradition may hamper the willingness to change. Fourth, what is the focus of human activity? This question considers the goals of human activity. For example, some Hispanic/Latino cultures believe that human beings are born with innate worth and importance (a "being" orientation) and are not to be held accountable for their life situation. The Native American culture is more likely to reflect the " be-in-becoming" orientation. This approach is concerned with who we are, not what we can or have accomplished. The American white middle class culture epitomizes the "doing" orientation, which highlights the kind of activity that results in measurable accomplishments. Fifth, what is the relation of man to nature? This question considers human's relationship to the environment. Different cultural approaches would emphasize mastery over nature, harmony with nature, or subjugation to nature.

Sociologists also approach diversity through a cultural framework known as "high" or "low." One example of "high"-context culture is one in which everyone knows who takes credit for a successful outcome; another is that, when meeting for the first time, everyone knows who is the first to speak. On the other hand, in a " low"-context culture, there are many ways to accomplish a goal and group members feel constrained if there are too many rules. The exact guidelines for behavior are not clear in a low-context culture.[38]

COMMON CULTURAL COURTESIES

Table 6-1 depicts some of the common cultural courtesies that have been documented for specific cultures. These may be especially important in developing dental practice routines, whether it be welcoming the patient or establishing an appointment. For further information, the following resources are suggested: Terri Morrison's *Kiss, Bow, or Shake Hands*[39] and

Table 6-1. Common cultural courtesies

Country	Forms of address	Negotiation strategies	Courtesies
China	Sensitive to status and titles	One's feelings are primary source of truth	Nod or bow slightly when greeting
	Order of names is generational, then given name	Facts are accepted if not in conflict with one's feelings and faith	If handshake is to occur, allow Chinese person to extend hand first
	Married women retain their maiden name		Do not use hand gestures to speak
			Punctuality is valued
			Do not like to be touched by people they do not know
			Use open hand instead of finger to point
			Do not dislodge food with fingers from mouth or bite nails
Japan	Use last names plus *san*, meaning Mr. or Mrs.	Rely on feelings more than facts	Avoid gum chewing or yawning
		Insist on consensus within their group	Deny compliments graciously
		"I'll consider it" may mean "no"	Bow is traditional greeting
		U.S. "O.K." means $	May greet Westerners with a handshake
			Avoid nonverbal gestures when speaking
			Beckoning done with palm down
			Nose blowing not acceptable in public
			Male/female touching unacceptable in public
			Keep a smile even if upset
			Silence is valued
Philippines	Addressed by title and surname	Rely on feelings for truth	Handshake greetings
	Wives of husbands with important tiles are addressed as Mrs. (husband's title)	Some faith rests on ideologies	Middle finger used to point is an insult
			Things are not pointed at; use a glance or pursed lips
	May use two surnames (Hispanic influence)		The number 2 is indicated by the ring and little fingers
			Staring is negative

Modified from Morrison T, Canaway WA, Borden GA: *Kiss, bow, or shake hands: how to do business in sixty countries*, Holbrook, Mass, 1994, Adams Media Corporation; and Henderson G: *A practitioner's guide to understanding indigenous and foreign cultures*, Springfield, Ill, 1989, Charles C Thomas.

Table 6-1. Common cultural courtesies

Country	Forms of address	Negotiation strategies	Courtesies
			Hands on hips is an aggressive posture
			No male/female touching in public
			Attract attention by brushing person's elbow
Spain	Two surnames are used. Formal word for "you" as an adult is *usted*, and *tu* is for the child	Truth through subjective feelings. Faith in ideologies	Handshake greetings
			Men can hug and pat on back
			Women embrace and share a cheek touch and light kiss in air
			Many gestures are used
			Snapping hands down emphasizes a point
			OK gesture is rude
			Shorts not accepted in public
			Bullfighting is considered an art
			Give free advice—do not be offended
			Relationships are more important than expertise
Mexico	Two surnames are used: Sr., Sra., Srta. Formal word for "you" as an adult is *usted*, and *tu* is for the child	Truth is subjective. Objective facts used by those with higher education. Must know person before doing business with him/her	Handshake for greetings and departure with all members present in the room
			Slower pace valued
			Personal friendship important
			"Maybe, we will see" can mean "no"
Kenya	Personal contacts rather than phone calls or letters	Appointments are made in advance	Firm handshake greetings
			Punctuality is appreciated
			Women should not wear shorts in cities
Nigeria	Titles are used before surnames	All business is discussed face to face	Respect for older adults
			Value hard work and responsibility
			Avoid using greetings such as "Hi" or "What's happening?"
Ghana	Refer to ethnic group, not "tribe"	Superior attitudes are offensive	Handshake greetings
			Children are taught to be quiet and to avoid eye contact
			Can be late

G. Henderson's *A Practitioner's Guide to Understanding Indigenous and Foreign Cultures.*[31]

STRATEGIES FOR THE FUTURE

Intercultural competence education for all community health care practitioners is an important step in raising the intercultural sensitivity of the practitioner. Some strategies to consider are the following:

1. Reflect on your own cultural values and beliefs. Self-awareness is the first step in developing intercultural competence.
2. Take courses in intercultural communication.
3. Learn commonly used terms for the language of your patients. A chairside translator has been developed for dental health professionals who need a quick reference guide to frequently used dental terms in Spanish.[40]
4. Acknowledge the patients' experiences and interpretations of their condition and be prepared to negotiate culturally relevant care.
5. Present direct advice that places the patient's problem in a familiar framework.[41]

In *Experiencing and Counseling Multicultural and Diverse Populations,* Marilyn Jemison Anderson and Robert Ellis[36] make the following recommendations:

1. Recognize that diverse cultures approach life with a different set of expectations, values, and interpretations, and that their approach can be as satisfying and as rich to them as any other culture is to any other person.
2. Become familiar with those specific cultural values of your patients so that you can begin to understand and appreciate the pressures being faced by them.
3. Resist the temptation to interpret a particular behavior or problem as if it emerged in a manner typical of that problem in the majority culture.

4. Appreciate that culturally diverse patients want minimal stress and aggravation in their lives.
5. Consider culturally diverse patients with an attitude of respect rather than paternalism.

Summary

This chapter has focused on the importance of intercultural competence among dental health care practitioners. Demographic changes and the consequences of those changes have been described in terms of a major shift in the ethnic/cultural composition of the U.S. population in the twenty-first century. Definitions of terms and concepts have been provided. Issues related to diversity have been identified, and cultural and health beliefs were described in a general way. Strategies for the future were recommended. As the field of community dental health prepares for the twenty-first century, it is faced with the needs of an increasingly diverse population. U.S. dental health care providers will be challenged to provide culturally relevant oral health care programs in multicultural health environments. The effectiveness of these future programs will depend on the multicultural knowledge and intercultural competence of the dental health care team. Success of health care delivery depends on the ability of practitioners to know more about the world as a result of their experiences with a variety of cultures. In the words of Samuel Betances: "You cannot tell a person to forget what they know, you cannot argue that it is better to know less rather than more."

REFERENCES

1. Caplan DJ, Weintraub JA: The oral health burden in the United States: a summary of recent epidemiological studies, *J Dent Educ* 57(12):853-862, 1993.

2. Bolden AJ, Henry JL, Allukian M: Implications of access, utilization and need for oral health care by low income groups and minorities on the dental delivery system, *J Dent Educ* 57(12):888-898, 1993.

3. Clark LW: *Faculty and student challenges in facing cultural and linguistic diversity*, Springfield, Ill, Charles C Thomas, 1993.

4. United States Bureau of Census: *1990 Census of the population*, Washington, DC, 1991.

5. Hodgkinson H: Keynote speaker, Kappa Delta Pi, International Convocation 1994 (videotape).

6. Gordon L: Southeast Asian refugees migration to United States. In Faucet J, Carino B, editors: *Pacific bridges: the new immigration from Asia and the Pacific Islands*, New York,1987, Center for Migration Studies, pp 243-273.

7. *The American Heritage Dictionary*, New York, 1983, Dell Publishing.

8. Samovar LA, Porter RE: *Intercultural communication: a reader*, ed 7, Belmont, Calif, 1994, Wadsworth.

9. Pipes AP, Westby CE, Inglebret E: Profile of Native American students. In Clark LW, editor: *Faculty and student challenges in facing cultural and linguistic diversity*, Springfield, Ill, 1993, Charles C Thomas.

10. Fitzgerald FT: How they view you, themselves, and disease, *Consultant* 28:65-77, 1988.

11. Ahia C: Cross-cultural counseling concerns, *Personnel Guidance J 62:339-41, 1984.*

12. Leininger MM: Transcultural nursing: an essential knowledge and practice field for today, *Can Nurs* 80(11):41-45, 1984.

13. Adams LM, Knox ME: *Traditional health practices: significance for modern health care.* In Van Horne WA, Tonnesen TV, editors: *Ethnicity and health*, Milwaukee, 1988, University of Wisconsin.

14. Farley E Jr: *Cultural diversity in health care: the education of future practitioners.* In Van Horne WA, Tonnesen TV, editors: *Ethnicity and health*, Milwaukee, 1988, University of Wisconsin.

15. Boyle JS, Andrew MM: *Transcultural concepts in nursing care*, Glenview, Ill, 1986, Scott, Foresman.

16. Leininger MM: Leininger's theory of nursing: cultural care diversity and universality, *Nurs Sci Q* 1:152-160, 1988.

17. Lyons S: Learning the language of public health, *Access* 3(12):7-12, 1989.

18. Giger JN, Davidhizar RE: *Transcultural nursing: assessment and intervention*, St Louis, 1991, Mosby.

19. Huttlinger K, Wiebe P: Transcultural nursing care: acheiving understanding in a practice setting, *J Transcultural Nurs* 1:27-32, 1989.

20. Leininger MM: Transcultural nursing: an overview, *Nurs Outlook* 32:72-73, 1984.

21. Leininger MM: A new generation of nurses discover transcultural nursing, *Nurs Health Care* 8:263, 1987.

22. Muecke M: Caring for Southeast Asian refugee patients in the USA, *Am J Public Health* 73:431-438, 1987.

23. Niederhauser VP: Health care of immigrant children: incorporating culture into practice, *Pediatr Nurs* 15:569-574, 1989.

24. Reinert B: The health care beliefs and values of Mexican-Americans, *Home Healthcare Nurs* 4(5):23-31, 1986.

25. Sands RF, Hale SL: Enhancing cultural sensitivity in clinical practice, *J Natl Black Nurs Assoc* 2:54-63, 1987.

26. Spector RE: *Cultural diversity in health and illness*, ed 2, Norwalk, Conn, 1985, Appleton-Century-Crofts.

27. Westberg J: Patient education for Hispanic Americans, *Patient Educ Couns* 13:143-160, 1989.

28. Althen G: *American ways: a guide for foreigners in the United States*, Yarmouth, Me, 1988, Intercultural Press.

29. Condon JC: *Good neighbors: communicating with the Mexicans*, Yarmouth, Me, 1985, Intercultural Press.

30. Vacc N, DeVaney S, Wittmer J: *Experiencing and counseling multicultural and diverse populations*, ed 3, Muncie, Ind, 1995, Accelerated Development.

31. Henderson G: *A practitioner's guide to understanding indigenous and foreign cultures*, Springfield, Ill, 1989, Charles C Thomas.

32. Spector R: *Cultural diversity in health and illness*, ed 2, Norwalk, Conn, 1985, Appleton & Crofts.

33. Gochenour T: *Considering Filipinos*, Yarmouth, Me, 1990, Intercultural Press.

34. Reeves MS: The high cost of endurance, *Education Week*, Aug 2, 1989, pp 2-4.

35. Bureau of Indian Affairs: *American Indians today: answers to your questions*, Washington, DC, 1991, Department of the Interior.

36. Anderson MJ, Ellis R: On the reservation. In Vacc N, DeVaney S, Wittmer J, editors: *Experiencing and counseling multicultural and diverse populations*, ed 3, Accelerated Development–A Francis Taylor Group.

37. Kluckholn FR, Strodtbeck FL: *Variations in value orientation*, New York, 1961, Row, Peterson.

38. Brislin R: *Understanding culture's influence on behavior*, Orlando, Fla, 1993, Harcourt Brace.

39. Morrison T, Canaway WA, Borden GA: *Kiss, bow, or shake hands: how to do business in sixty countries*, Holbrook, Mass, 1994, Bob Adams, Inc.

40. Hispanic Dental Association: *Spanish chairside translator: quick reference sheet*, Chicago, 1992, Hispanic Dental Association.

41. Mercado Galvis DL: Clinical contexts for diversity and intercultural competence, *J Dent Educ* 59:1103-1106, 1995.

CHAPTER 7

Geriatric oral health

Rima Bachiman

The aging phenomenon emerges as the most significant health issue of the twenty-first century. In the coming years the nation's social and health institutions will continue to be challenged by changing demands for social and health services as a result of the anticipated growth in the number of elderly Americans. This demographic imperative is expected to have a major impact on the dental profession and the delivery of oral health services. The oral and general health status and needs of the older adult reflect a complex interaction of the age-related physiologic changes, their psychosocial concomitants, and the various pathologic processes that occur with increasing frequency in aging. This chapter reviews some of the social and economic issues, as well as the biologic and psychologic considerations that affect the oral health of the elderly. It considers what is currently known about the oral health of older adults and what the profession might expect in the future. Emphasizing the concept of the interdisciplinary team approach to care, the chapter also provides a framework for managing the oral health needs of older adults in various settings.

Demographic and socioeconomic trends

Significant changes in the demographic characteristics of the older population have occurred in recent years.[1,2] The size of the geriatric population, persons 65 years of age and older, has increased dramatically during the twentieth century and is expected to continue to increase well into the next century. Since the turn of the century, the percentage of Americans 65 years of age and older has more than tripled, from 4.1% in 1900 to 12.7% in 1994, and the number has increased nearly 11 times, from 3.1 million to 33.2 million individuals. As Fig. 7-1 demonstrates, the older population will continue to grow in the future. The growth is expected to slow somewhat during the 1990s because of the relative decline in the birth rate during the Great Depression of the 1930s. The most rapid increase is expected between the years 2010 and 2030, when the "baby boom" generation, persons born between 1946 and 1964, reaches age 65. By the year 2030 there will be about 70 million older persons, representing 20% of the population.

Another important trend is the change in the ethnic composition of the elderly population.

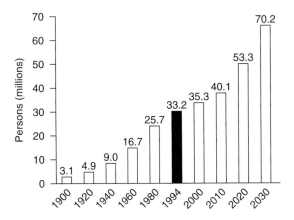

Fig. 7-1. Number of persons aged 65+ years (in millions): United States 1900-2030. *(Data from US Bureau of the Census.)*

In 1994 about 14% of persons 65+ were minorities. Eight percent were African-American, 2% were Asian or Pacific Islander, and less than 1% were Native American or Native Alaskan. Persons of Hispanic origin represented 4% of the older population. Minority populations are projected to represent 25% of the elderly population in the year 2030. Between 1990 and 2030 the white non-Hispanic population 65+ is projected to increase by 93% compared with 328% for older minorities, with the Asian and Pacific Islander group experiencing the largest increase. The burgeoning elderly minority population will have major implications for the dental profession. It will necessitate an increased sensitivity to, and a heightened awareness of, the unique cultural issues affecting the planning and provision of oral health care in the various ethnic subgroups (see Chapter 6).

Of particular interest and concern with respect to the provision of health care and other social services is the increase in the number of very old people. The older population itself is getting older. In 1994 the 65- to 74-year-old age group (18.7 million) was 8 times larger than in 1900; but the 75- to 84-year-old group (10.9 million) was

14 times larger and the 85+ group (3.5 million) was 28 times larger, making it the fastest growing segment of the elderly population.

Longevity varies considerably with the gender of the person and is greater for American women than men. As the population ages, the distribution by sex also changes. The elderly population is composed of many more women than men. At age 65 there are 122 women for every 100 men. The sex ratio increases with age; at 85 there are 259 women for every 100 men. Of the women over age 65, 47% are widows and 43% are married. Of the older men, only 10% are widowers and 77% are married.

The majority (68%) of older noninstitutionalized persons live in a family setting, and about 30% live alone. Although a small segment (5%) of the over-65 population lives in nursing homes, the percentage increases dramatically with age, ranging from 1% for persons 65 to 74 years to 6% for persons 75 to 84 years and 24% for persons 85+.

Social Security is the major source of income for older individuals (40%), followed by income from assets (21%), public and private pensions (19%), earnings (17%), and all other sources (3%). The poverty rate for persons 65+ is 11.7%, about the same as the rate for the younger adult population. However, it is higher for older women and minorities. Although most older adults are retired, approximately 12% are still in the labor force either working or actively seeking work.

As a group older adults have significantly less formal education and a higher illiteracy rate than younger adults. Still, the educational level of older Americans has increased in recent years. Among noninstitutionalized elderly who are 65 years and older, the median level of education rose from 8.7 years in 1970 to 12.2 years in 1991. The percentage of older Americans who had completed high school rose from 28% in 1970 to 62% in 1994. The percentages are substantially lower for African-Americans and Hispanics. These numbers are expected to continue rising as the difference between educational levels of the young and old decreases.[3]

If the demographic trends visible in successive cohorts of the elderly persist, the elderly people whom the dental profession of today will need to care for in the future will be significantly different. They will certainly be older, and more will be women. There will be more minorities, and most patients will be better educated.

The increase in the number and proportion of the elderly in the population has been attributed to three basic phenomena: (1) the decline in birth rate, (2) the aging of the "baby boomers," and (3) the substantial increase in life expectancy during the twentieth century. As Table 7-1 demonstrates, the overall decline in age-specific death rates has led to increases in life expectancy at birth and also at 65, 75, and 85 years of age. The decline in mortality among the very old has been greater than that for any other age groups. An important issue for health care professionals is the relationship between changes in the mortality experience of the elderly population, and coincident changes in the underlying morbidity and disability experiences. Will future increases in longevity be associated with prolongation of dependency? Or will active life expectancy increase as health promotion and disease prevention strategies for the elderly become increasingly more effective?[4] Currently an argument can be presented for either view.

Aging, function, and dependency

Aging can be viewed best as a biopsychosocial process, in which changes occur at various levels in all three components of the biopsychosocial system.[5] From the biologic perspective, gradual declines in the physiologic reserves of most major organ systems begin during the third or fourth decade.[6] In addition, there is an increasing probability of specific age-related diseases that also contribute to the loss of physiologic reserves. Within the psychologic component, age-associated alterations in perceptual[7] and cognitive[8] capabilities also occur. From the social perspective, the aged are faced with different societal attitudes and are confronted with a higher likelihood of losses within their support network as a result of retirement or the deaths of family and friends.[9] From a clinical standpoint these changes become most significant when they break through the clinical threshold and begin to impair the functional status of the individual.[5] Because of the great variability in functional status among people aged 65 and older, it is more appropriate to address the health needs of older adults according to their level of function.

Table 7-1. Life expectancy at birth and at 65, 75, and 85 years of age, by gender: United States, 1900 and 1991

	1900			1991		
Age	*Both sexes (yr)*	*Male (yr)*	*Female (yr)*	*Both sexes (yr)*	*Male (yr)*	*Female (yr)*
At birth	47.3	46.3	48.3	75.5	72.0	78.9
At age 65	11.9	11.5	12.2	17.4	15.3	19.1
At age 75	7.1	6.8	7.3	11.1	9.5	12.1
At age 85	4.0	3.8	4.1	6.2	5.3	6.5

Data from National Center for Health Statistics: *Trends in the health of older Americans: United States, 1994,* Vital and Health Statistics, US Department of Health and Human Services, series 3, no 30, Washington, DC, 1995.

Functioning is a critical indicator of health and well-being in the older person. It is more important than the presence of specific diseases. Impairments in physical and cognitive functioning predict mortality and institutionalization among the elderly and the amount of services they receive.

The most common way of assessing functional capacity is evaluating limitation in activities of daily living (ADLs) and instrumental activities of daily living (IADLs), which generally indicate an inability to live independently.[10] ADLs include bathing, dressing, eating, transferring from bed or chair, walking, getting outside, and toileting. IADLs include preparing meals, shopping, managing money, using telephone, and doing housework. It is apparent that ADL and IADL levels would affect the older adult's ability to access and maintain oral health care.

Several scales are used to determine the level of orientation, memory, and cognitive ability.[11] The most commonly used scales are the Short Portable Mental Status Questionnaire (SPMSQ) by Pfeiffer,[12] the Mini-Mental State by Folstein et al.,[13] and the Mental Status Questionnaire by Kahn et al.[14] These brief mental status screening tests can be administered in a dental setting as part of the mental assessment of potentially impaired patients. Poor scores usually indicate an increased probability that a cognitive or dementing disorder is present. Although screening test scores alone do not measure presence of a disorder, they alert the dental practitioner to request a comprehensive medical evaluation.

Two types of conditions most frequently cause disability among the elderly: those that are also the leading causes of death (heart disease, cancer, and cerebrovascular disease) and chronic conditions that are generally nonfatal (dementia, arthritis, orthopedic, visual, and hearing impairment).[15] Although more than 4 of 5 people age 65 or older have at least one chronic health condition, their disability ranges from minimal problems to total dependence.[10] Fig. 7-2 lists the top 10 chronic conditions that

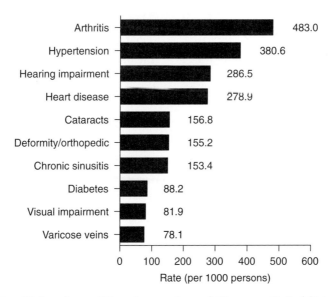

Fig. 7-2. The top 10 chronic conditions for people aged 65+ years: United States, 1989. *(Data from National Center for Health Statistics:* Current estimates from the National Health Interview Survey, 1989, *Vital and Health Statistics series 10, no 176 [October 1990].)*

affect people 65 years of age and older. Based on their functional status and level of dependence, older adults have been described as being either independent, frail, or functionally dependent.[16] Independent older adults are those who reside in the community and require no assistance in their necessary ADLs. These individuals comprise 80% of the elderly population and are able to access dental care as would younger individuals. The frail elderly have chronic debilitating physical, medical, and emotional problems and are able to maintain some independence in the community only with assistance. Approximately 10% to 15% of the elderly are frail and depend on various support services. Most of these individuals reside in the community; a small percentage are institutionalized. The functionally dependent are those who are seriously impaired and unable to maintain themselves. About 5% to 10% of the elderly are unable to function independently and are either homebound or institutionalized. Based on the functional status and level of dependence, the oral health status, dental needs, utilization of services, and mode of delivery vary from group to group. The present dental care delivery system is least effective in caring for the homebound and institutionalized segment of the elderly population, and they remain the least served.

The elderly can also be characterized according to the historical, cultural, and social events in their lives, as well as their past experiences with the dental care system.[17] Accordingly, the "young old," individuals between 65 and 79 years of age, are better educated, more politically aware, and more demanding of health services. Having benefited from the availability of fluoride and prevention, they have retained more of their teeth and have been using dental care services at a higher rate than their older cohorts. Characteristically, the "old old," individuals age 80 and older, have experienced dentistry in an era of mass extractions. Consequently the majority of this cohort is edentulous and still believe that losing one's teeth is an inevitable consequence of aging. They are more likely to have medical conditions and take medications that affect their oral health. They have grown up with the notion that dentistry is a luxury, and therefore they tend to be low utilizers of dental services.

Use of dental services

Table 7-2 demonstrates the steady increase in the use of dental services by the general popu-

Table 7-2. Percent of population with dental visit in the past year in the United States by age and year of survey

Year	All ages* (%)	25-44 years (%)	45-64 years (%)	65+ years (%)
1957-58	36.6	44.1	32.3	16.2
1970	46.8	52.3	44.2	25.8
1975	50.3	54.5	48.2	30.3
1981	50.1	54.2	49.6	34.6
1986	57.1	60.4	54.6	41.7
1989	55.4	60.1	56.8	43.2

From Jones JA and others: Gains in dental care use not shared by minority elders, *J Public Health Dent* 54:39-46, 1994. (Copyright American Association of Public Health Dentistry. Reprinted with permission.)
*All ages except under age 2.

lation during the past three decades. The percentage of persons of all ages reporting use of dental care during the previous year has increased from about 37% in 1957-1958 to 55% in 1989.[18,19] Similarly, in 1989, 43% of persons 65 years of age and older reported using dental care compared with 16% in 1957. The mean numbers of visits per person per year for all individuals aged 65 years and older have also increased from 0.8 to 2.1 visits over the same period.[18,19] Data from the 1990 survey of dental care utilization by adults 18 years of age and older are even more encouraging. Approximately 49% of the elderly reported using dental services at least once during the past year, compared with 63% of the overall population.[20] This increase has not been attributed to changes in the dental delivery system: it is more indicative of changes in the socioeconomic status and dental profile of the younger cohort of older adults. However, with the possible exception of children under the age of 6 years,[21] the elderly as a group still have the lowest utilization rate of dental services. Studies also indicate that reported dental care use among minority elders has not increased parallel with elders of all races and ethnic origins.[22] In 1957-1959 17% of white elders versus 9% of nonwhite elders had seen a dentist within the past year. By 1989 the percentage for whites had improved to 45%, but only to 22% for African-Americans and 40% for Hispanics. Given the expected future growth in minority elders, attempts should be made by the profession to identify and alleviate barriers to care and to improve access to necessary dental services.

The low utilization of dental services cannot be explained solely by conventional sociodemographic variables such as age, gender, ethnicity, residence, education, and income. The variables tend to interact in a complex pattern with other factors, particularly attitudinal factors. Schou divided the factors reported to directly and indirectly influence older persons'

utilization of dental services into four main categories: (1) ill-health related factors, (2) sociodemographic factors, (3) service-related factors, and (4) attitudinal or subjective factors. The variables most frequently found within these four categories are listed in Box 7-1.[23]

Studies comparing users and nonusers of dental services often report the dentate status of the elderly as one of the most significant factors related to utilization of dental care.[24-28] The 1985-1986 National Institute for Dental Research (NIDR) survey discovered that among 5000 well elderly, approximately 55% of the dentate elderly had visited a dentist within the past 12 months. Only 13% of the edentate elderly had seen a dentist during the same period. The well dentate elderly used the services of a dentist at about the same rate as working adults and the population as a whole.[29] Use of dental services seems to be highly related to presence of teeth. When dentate status is controlled, visit rates are similar between older and younger persons.

Poor general health and functional limitation have been reported as barriers to seeking oral health care by institutionalized[30] and frail, homebound elderly.[31] However, other studies have shown that variables such as functional impairment[32] and the presence of health problems[33] are not as conclusive in predicting or explaining utilization behavior in the elderly; presence or absence of teeth remains the key factor in utilization of dental care.

The traditional barrier, cost for services, was found by Kiyak to have only a slight influence on the utilization of care in the elderly.[34] The same investigator suggested that lack of perceived need is the primary reason for not seeking dental care.[35] This was confirmed in a study by Tennstedt et al.,[28] who reported that one quarter of nonrecent dentate utilizers and only 5% of all dentate subjects cited treatment cost or lack of dental insurance as a problem. Although these elders, consistent with other findings, cited a lack of need as the most fre-

---

BOX 7-1

FACTORS INFLUENCING OLDER PERSONS' DEMAND FOR AND UTILIZATION OF DENTAL SERVICE

Ill-Health Factors
Dental health status
   Edentulousness
   Number of teeth
Experiencing discomfort
General ill health
Mobility, functional limitations

Sociodemographic Factors
Place of residence
Education
Income
Age
Gender
Cultural
Ethnicity

Service-Related Factors
Accessibility
   Financial
   Spatiotemporal
   Psychosocial
Dentist behavior
Dentist attitude
Price of service (cost)
Insurance coverage
Satisfaction with service
Transport
Lack of regulations, policies

Attitudinal Factors
Personal beliefs
Feeling no need, perceived need
Perceived importance
Fear and anxiety
Resistance to change
Perceived economic strain
Satisfaction with dental visits

From Schou L: Oral health, oral health care, and oral health promotion among older adults: social and behavioral dimensions. In Cohen LK, Gift HC, editors: *Disease prevention-sociodental sciences in action,* Copenhagen, 1995, Munksgaard. (Copyright Munksgaard. Reprinted with permission.)

quent reason for nonuse of dental care, clinical examinations provided objective evidence of the need for treatment in the dentate subjects. These investigators concluded that lack of importance attributed to oral health and perceived need for oral health care are significant barriers to utilization. This finding underscores the importance of oral health promotion and education in the older adult population.

Because perception of treatment needs affects utilization of services, the discrepancy between actual and perceived need for treatment is a major concern. Treatment needs are generally described in terms of professionally established clinical criteria. The elderly, however, have different standards in evaluating their oral health status and tend to have different expectations for the outcomes of therapy. Because oral health status is influenced by clinical, socioeconomic, and behavioral factors, need assessment, therefore, cannot be based solely on clinical measures. To improve assessment of needs in older persons, a better understanding of the role of social and behavioral factors is definitely needed.[23]

The use of dental services by the elderly is also partly determined by the education and attitudes of the dental professionals. Surveys of dental professionals indicate that many have little or no training in geriatrics and most accept popularly held aging myths.[36,37] Surveys on dental education reveal continuing efforts at both the predoctoral and postdoctoral levels to remedy this situation. The lack of geriatric sophistication by dental professionals often results in dental offices that are poorly located or poorly designed for the purpose of accommodating the needs of the elderly. Adequate nearby parking is often missing. Ramps to assist those who are physically disabled or hallways of sufficient width for the passage of wheelchairs may not be provided.[38,39] Many professionals believe that the elderly or the chronically ill cause discomfort for other patients. Treatment of the elderly is perceived as being more difficult and more time-consuming than treatment of other groups. The enactment of the Americans with Disabilities Act is expected to lessen some of these barriers to care encountered by the functionally disabled elderly.[40] The law requires that private dental offices serve persons with disabilities and that dentists make reasonable modifications to facilitate access to dental offices.

The utilization of dental services by older adults is closely related to oral health status. The decision to access the dentist appears to be based on a variety of sociodemographic and perception-of-need variables. The most regularly cited factors associated with dental utilization include age, income, education, ethnicity, the presence of one or more teeth, and a perceived need for dental care.

Dental disease and oral health status

The pattern of dental disease in the older population has changed during the past 40 years. However, the epidemiologic literature describing the oral health status of older Americans is limited, especially regarding the oldest old (85+). Although older adults were sampled in national surveys such as The National Health Examination Survey (NHES)[41] of 1960-

1962 and the National Health and Nutrition Examination Survey (NHANES)[42] of 1971-1974, individuals over the age of 79 were not included in NHES, and those over the age of 74 were not included in NHANES. The NIDR Survey of 1985-1986[29] included a sample of adults between 65 and 99 years of age who attended senior centers, but the sample was not representative of the entire older adult population. Regional studies among rural elderly Iowans,[43,44] elderly in North Carolina,[45] and the New England Elders Dental Study (NEEDS)[46] have contributed to the knowledge of the epidemiology of dental disease in the elderly and have further documented the change in oral disease pattern.

TOOTH LOSS

Despite the general decline in edentulism over the last four decades, the prevalence of edentulism is still high in the older population. Table 7-3 demonstrates the consistent decline in edentulism in each age group including those older than age 65. Approximately 41.1% of adults aged 65 and older were found edentulous in the 1985-1986 NIDR survey.[29] Edentulism tends to increase with age and is associated with low income, less education, and belonging to a minority group. A substantial decline in edentulism is projected in the year

Table 7-3. Percent of edentulous adults in the United States by age, sex, and year of survey

Age (yr)	NHES[41] 1960-1962		NHANES[42] 1971-1974		NIDR[29] 1985-1986	
	Male	Female	Male	Female	Male	Female
45-54	20	20	15	17	7	11
55-64	35	38	32	35	16	15
65-74	45	53	45	47	35	38
65-79	56	66	—	—	53	41
80+	—	—	—	—	51	43

—, Data not available.

2024 for the 65- to 74-year-old cohort, which is the 15- to 24-year-old cohort in the 1986 survey, a group that has benefited from preventive activities and advances in dental treatment.[47]

Although the elderly continue to share a disproportionate burden of the problems associated with tooth loss, there is substantial evidence that older adults are maintaining a greater number of teeth into later years. Among dentate older adults, the NHES survey[41] of 1960-1962 reported a mean number of teeth present of 10.6 for the age group 65 to 74; the NIDR number was almost 18 for the same age group. For the age group 75 to 79, the mean number of teeth retained was 7.1 in 1960-1962[41] and 16.8 in the 1985-1986 survey.[29]

DENTAL CARIES

The prevalence of coronal caries is decreasing in children and young adults. However, it is difficult to draw conclusions about the prevalence of coronal caries in older adults. Although the mean number of decayed and filled teeth among the age group 65 to 74 increased from 1960-1962[41] to 1985-1986,[29] as shown in Table 7-4, the increase is probably the result of greater retention of teeth within this cohort and may not represent a true increase in disease prevalence. Because of the increase in the retention of natural teeth and the greater utilization of dental services, dentate elderly remain at risk for coronal caries, especially in its recurrent form. Coronal caries, once thought to decrease after young adulthood, have been found to continue to threaten the dentition as long as the teeth are present.[48,49] The same studies showed that the likelihood of developing coronal caries was significantly linked to the development of root caries, which indicated common causative risk factors.

In addition to continued coronal caries activity in adults, root surface caries, in their primary and secondary forms, account for a significant amount of dental decay experienced by the aged. The 1985-1986 survey found the average percentage of adults aged 18 to 64 with at least one decayed or filled root surface was 21.2. Among seniors aged 65+, the average percentage of individuals with at least one decayed or filled root surface was 62.6. The age association of the disease is evident in Fig. 7-3, which shows the prevalence of root caries by age and gender among dentate employed persons and seniors in the United States from the 1985-1986 NIDR national survey.[29]

Large studies of the incidence of new coronal and root caries have not been performed. Among a sample of 451 dentate Iowans older

Table 7-4. Mean number of decayed and filled teeth among dentate adults in the United States by age, sex, and year of survey

Age (yr)	NHES[41] 1960-1962		NHANES[42] 1971-1974		NIDR[29] 1985-1986	
	Male	Female	Male	Female	Male	Female
45-54	7.1	8.1	9.3	9.4	11.0	11.4
55-64	5.7	7.1	8.3	8.9	9.7	10.6
65-74	4.3	6.0	6.2	7.7	7.4	8.4
75-79	2.7	5.0	—	—	6.4	7.6
80+	—	—	—	—	6.0	6.5

—, Data not available.

than age 65, a mean of 0.87 new surfaces of coronal decay per person per year and a mean 0.57 new surfaces of root decay per person per year were noted.[43] Therefore coronal and root caries were still active in this group. Beck estimated that the annual incidence of root caries among older Americans is in the order of 1.6 surfaces per 100 surfaces at risk.[50] Tooth survival results in continued exposure to environmental factors and therefore continued risk of disease. Root caries is found only where loss of periodontal attachment has led to exposure of the roots to the oral environment.

PERIODONTAL DISEASE

Contrary to previously held views, periodontitis is not considered a disease of aging. The greater prevalence and severity of the disease seen in older people in cross-sectional surveys do not reflect greater susceptibility but rather the cumulative progression of lesions over time.[51,52] In the NIDR survey[29] 7.6% of employed adults had at least one site with 6 mm or more loss of periodontal attachment (LPA),

compared with 34% of the population aged 65 or older. The NIDR data show that with increasing age there is a gradual decrease in the proportion of sites with 2 to 3 mm LPA and a gradual increase in the proportion of moderately affected sites (4 to 6 mm LPA). The extent of severe disease ($\geq$6 mm LPA), however, remains relatively low even in the oldest groups.[53]

Longitudinal data to describe the progression of periodontal disease with age are few. Data from a study of a group of tea workers in Sri Lanka who received virtually no dental treatment for 15 years showed that the condition worsened with age for the most susceptible individuals but that among the nonsusceptible age did not seem to be a factor.[54]

Analysis of the data from the NEED Study indicated that of the examined variables, gender, number of dentate arches, and socioeconomic status emerged as the important predictors of periodontal destruction in older adults. Age was not significantly associated with periodontal destruction in this elder population. The investigators further stated that what previously was considered an age effect may be related to cohort differences. The great increase in number of teeth in the elderly is the primary difference among cohorts of older person. With greater tooth retention comes a higher risk of moderate periodontal disease. Longitudinal studies are needed to document these relationships in the best way.[55]

ORAL CANCER

Cancers of the oral cavity and pharynx are diagnosed in approximately 30,000 persons in the United States and cause nearly 8,000 deaths per year.[56] Oral cancer, like most cancers, is a disease related to older age. About 95% of all oral cancers occur in persons over 40 years of age, and the average age at the time of diagnosis is approximately 60. Oral cancer occurs more frequently in men, but the male/female ratio, which in 1950 was approximately 6:1, is

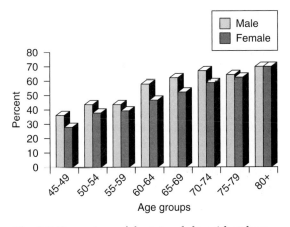

Fig. 7-3. Percentage of dentate adults with at least one decayed or filled root surface by age group and gender. *(Data from NIDR: Oral health of United States adults, the national survey of oral health in US employed adults and seniors: 1985-1986, NIH Pub No 87-2868, Washington, DC, 1987.)*

now approximately 2:1 and declining. The increase in smoking among women and the greater number of women in the over-65 age group are offered as explanations for the reduced ratio.[57] The highest incidence rate is reported for African-American men.[56]

The tongue is the most common site for oral cancer in both men and women. Eighty-five percent of all oral cancers occur in the tongue, oropharynx, floor of the mouth, and lips; 8%, in the gingiva; 3%, in the buccal mucosa; and less than 2% in the hard palate. The remainder occur in unspecified areas in the mouth.[58] Oral cancer incidence has remained stable relative to the occurrence of all newly diagnosed cancers, with absolute numbers increasing each year. The only exception is cancer of the lip, which has shown a 5% reduction. This trend may reflect public education regarding the dangers of exposure to ultraviolet light and the use of sunscreens.[57] In spite of advances in treatment of cancerous lesions, 5-year survival rates remain poor. Therefore improvement in prevention and control of oral cancer is critical. Both public and professional awareness of the disease is fundamental for minimizing the time from onset to appearance of signs or symptoms to diagnosis.

In a discussion of oral health status, treatment needs, and treatment strategies in the older adult population, it is very important to recognize the great diversity of this population. Variations in health, functional status, and lifestyle influence the oral condition and treatment options and contribute to the challenge of treating this population.

Management of the older adult patient

The elderly differ from other age groups in important respects, and these differences demand a multidisciplinary approach by the dental practitioner that is geared to the special needs of the individual patient. The proper management of the older adult patient depends on an understanding of the aging process, the diseases that affect the elderly, their treatment and sequelae, and the elderly themselves.

THE AGING PROCESS

The process of aging is a multifactorial one in which tissues, organs, and cells age at different rates, with much individual variation. The major results of the aging process are (1) a reduced physiologic reserve of many bodily functions (e.g., cardiac, respiratory, and renal), (2) an impaired homeostatic mechanism by which bodily activities are kept adjusted (e.g., fluid balance, temperature control, and blood pressure control), and (3) an impaired immunologic system, as well as a related, increased incidence of neoplastic and age-related autoimmune conditions.[59] The reduction in physiologic reserve and the impairment of the homeostatic and immunologic systems contribute to the increased vulnerability of the elderly to disease during acute illness, trauma as a result of burns, major surgery, and administration of medications. Visits to the dentist or dental hygienist, of course, are potential sessions of increased stress, and the practitioner must modify the management of the patient accordingly.

Many common geriatric diseases, disorders, impairments, and their management necessitate alterations in the provision of dental treatment. It is beyond the scope of this chapter to review all geriatric medical conditions, their treatment and sequelae, and influence on the dental treatment. Instead an attempt will be made to provide the dental care provider with key principles and a general framework for the management of the older patient.

PATIENT ASSESSMENT

Assessment is the key to developing a comprehensive, appropriate treatment plan. The assessment is a comprehensive multidisciplinary evaluation in which several domains of the elderly patient—physical, mental, social, economic, and functional—are reviewed and integrated into a coordinated plan of care.

The general goals of the assessment are to (1) determine the patient's current general and oral health status and diagnosis, (2) establish a database against which future developments and changes can be compared, (3) establish a good relationship with the patient and the patient's family and caregivers, and (4) determine the priorities for management and intervention to prevent or alleviate disease and improve the quality of the patient's life.

The practitioner performing the assessment needs to adopt the following two principles:

1. *Oral health is an integral part of total health.* Therefore oral health care is an integral part of comprehensive care. Oral health is linked to the overall health of the older patient because oral diseases and conditions have consequences that extend beyond the confines of the oral cavity.

2. *The interdisciplinary team approach to care is the safest and most effective way of providing appropriate dental care to older adult patients.* Communication among the patient's multidisciplinary care providers is key to the development of an appropriate treatment plan and the proper coordination of care. In addition, regular communication among providers tends to educate and sensitize nondental providers to the dental aspects of the patient's overall health care and treatment needs, thus optimizing treatment outcomes.

The following elements are incorporated into the assessment process: (1) review of the patient's biopsychosocial systems, (2) determination of the patient's functional status or capacity (both physical and mental), and (3) assessment of the patient's oral health status.

COGNITIVE FUNCTIONING

Because of the multiplicity of factors that relate to the treatment of the elderly, it is important to evaluate the ability of the patient to communicate and to understand, consent to,

and participate in the treatment. The practitioner must determine, either through a psychologic evaluation or through an interview, the capacity of the individual to respond to treatment. Although instances of senile dementia are not common, they do increase in frequency as the individual ages. Prevalence starts at about 1% at age 60 and then doubles approximately every 5 years, reaching 32% at age 85.[60] Data from the National Nursing Home Survey suggest that among inhabitants of nursing homes about 47% have some sort of dementing disorder.[61]

The most common type of dementia in the elderly is senile dementia of the Alzheimer type. It has a prevalence rate of 50% to 75% of all dementias.[62] This disease is characterized by a gradual deterioration of almost every function of the brain. The patient progresses through a series of behavioral changes and losses. Cognitive skills and competency in the life skills decline. There is loss of intellectual prowess, and the patient experiences language difficulties, memory loss, concentration difficulties, aberrant emotionality, and altered spatial-motor performance. Verbal and nonverbal communication are affected.

The second most common cause of dementia in the elderly is multiinfarct dementia or vascular dementia, accounting for 15% to 25% of cases.[62,63]

TREATMENT PLANNING

Treatment planning decisions for the older patient are more complex. The dental practitioner must consider the normal and pathologic aging changes and their great individual variability; the impact of the presence and interaction of multiple disorders, medications, and psychosocial issues; and the effects of years of accumulated oral changes. The appropriate level and type of dental care for the older patient is based on the individual's capacity to understand, withstand, and maintain the care planned. In order for the dentist to provide the most appropriate and effective care with successful outcomes, the treatment plan must be based on the patient's functional capacity, with the primary goal of maintenance or enhancement of function and quality of life. Given future functional decline and uncertainties in some outcomes of the older person's life, the treatment plan should also have great flexibility and strong emphasis on prevention.

PREVENTION AND ORAL HEALTH PROMOTION

Prevention of oral disease—through frequent recalls, regular updating of vital information, and ongoing assessment of the patient's functional status—is the cornerstone of geriatric care. In addition to promoting and monitoring the basic oral hygiene practices (brushing with a fluoride dentifrice, flossing, and maintaining a nutritious well-balanced diet, low in refined carbohydrates), the clinician should be vigilant of the changing physical, psychologic, socioeconomic, and medication status of the older patient and should be ready to intervene and make necessary modifications in the prevention protocol. The most effective strategy for prevention of caries has been increasing tooth resistance through the use of systemic and topical fluorides. Systemic and topical fluoride application has been deemed by many researchers the single most important preventive and treatment modality older adults can use to prevent dental caries.[64] The concentration, method, and frequency of application depend on the level of risk and the ability of the individual to manage the regimen.

Older adults and their caregivers need to be educated to enhance their knowledge and modify their attitudes regarding prevention, regular professional care, use of appropriate oral hygiene devices and chemotherapeutic agents, and the important relationship of oral health to general health. In addition, dental health professionals, as part of the health care team, have a responsibility to evaluate the health status and health risks of their older patients and make the proper referrals.

Oral health in long-term care settings

Long-term care refers to health, social, and residential services provided to chronically disabled persons over an extended time.[65] These services may be provided in a variety of settings including nursing homes, chronic disease hospitals, mental health facilities, rehabilitation centers, residential facilities, and the individual's own home. With the projected growth of the older population, particularly the 85+ cohort, the demand for long-term care is expected to increase in the future. In 1990 approximately 7 million older people needed long-term care. By the year 2005, the number will increase to almost 9 million. By the year 2020, 12 million older people will need long-term care at home, in the community, or in a nursing home.[66]

The provision of dental care to the nursing home and the homebound elderly presents a special challenge to the oral health care delivery system because the mode of care usually requires that the patient travel to the dentist's private office. The nursing home and homebound elderly are characterized as being frail or functionally dependent as the result of at least one chronic, long-standing physical, mental, or emotional disability. Therefore their dental treatment needs differ somewhat from those of the functionally independent cohort. As a group, nursing home and homebound elderly experience many barriers to dental care and are currently underserved.

Cognitive decline, lack of motivation, physical impairment, and other chronic medical problems all contribute to a decrease in self-care ability and subsequent increased risk of oral diseases. In addition, difficulties with transportation to the dentist, accessing the dental office, lack of perceived need, preexisting attitudes and expectations, and financing the care are some of the barriers for accessing dental services in this population.

The homebound and nursing home elderly have been characterized as having high rates of edentulism, coronal and root caries, poor oral hygiene, gingivitis and periodontal disease, and soft tissue lesions.[67,68] Table 7-5 depicts the type and prevalence of oral conditions in a sample of dentate nursing home residents.

Poor oral hygiene has been identified as the most significant problem among nursing home residents.[69-72] This is not surprising given the functional impairment affecting most nursing home residents. It does, however, underscore the importance of the regular involvement of caregivers in the residents' oral hygiene maintenance, and the need for in-service training of the nursing staff.

Homebound and nursing home elderly also have other characteristics in common that affect the delivery of dental services. As a group, they are older (mean age 80), predominantly female (approximately two thirds), and physically disabled with respect to basic ADL (more

than 90%). In addition, 63% have some disorientation or memory impairment, and in 47% dementia has been diagnosed.[73] Although it is important to recognize the general characteristics shared by nursing home residents, the dentist, as a member of the professional team, needs to be cognizant of the individual needs of each resident. Decisions regarding treatment planning, level of care, and modality of care are usually based on the condition of the resident, other treatment goals and the anticipated length of stay in the facility.[73]

Delivering dental care to the homebound population presents a different practice environment, and a different set of challenges, than the nursing home setting. The type and range of dental services provided are limited by the type of equipment and delivery system used. It is important to remember that a dentist in a homebound setting has no backup support available. Complicated and invasive procedures are therefore not appropriate in a homebound setting.[73] This mode of dental service delivery is still in its infancy as far as regulations and funding mechanisms.

Table 7-5. Number of percentage of nursing home residents with natural teeth who have oral problems

Rank order of problems	n = 445	%
1. Poor oral hygiene	321	72.1
2. Sore or bleeding gums	191	42.9
3. Root caries	160	36.0
4. Coronal caries	117	26.3
5. Retained root tips	105	23.6
6. Significant tooth mobility	80	18.0
7. Dry mouth	44	9.0
8. Toothache	34	7.6
9. Intraoral swelling or suppuration	27	6.1
10. Soft tissue lesions	20	4.5

From Kiyak AH, Grayston MN, Crinean CL: Oral health problems and needs of nursing home residents, *Community Dent Oral Epidemiol* 21:49-52, 1993. Copyright Munksgaard. Reprinted with permission.

FEDERAL NURSING HOME REGULATIONS

As a result of the nursing home reform law of the Omnibus Budget and Reconciliation Act (OBRA) of 1987, all nursing homes that accept Medicaid and Medicare payments were held to providing a new, higher standard of care focusing on the residents' "highest practicable physical, mental and psychosocial well-being."[74] The new law imposed some additional dental care requirements on nursing facilities. In addition to the annual comprehensive assessment, which must include the resident's present dental condition, the final regulation requires that facilities: (1) assist residents in obtaining routine and 24-hour emergency dental care, (2) provide or obtain from an outside resource routine and emergency dental services to meet the needs of each resident, (3) may charge a Medicare resident (but not a Medicaid resident) an additional amount for routine and emergency dental services, (4) provide to Medicaid residents emergency dental services and routine dental services (to the extent covered under the state plan), (5) assist the resident in making appointments and by arranging for transportation to and from the dentist's office, and (6) promptly refer residents with lost or damaged dentures to a dentist. A nursing home also must ensure that a resident who is unable to carry out ADLs receive the necessary services to maintain good nutrition, grooming, and personal and oral hygiene.[74]

DENTAL DELIVERY SYSTEMS

There are four basic types of dental care delivery systems available for the homebound and institutionalized elderly: (1) the private dental office, (2) on-site dental programs, (3) portable dental programs, and (4) mobile van dental programs.

Private dental office

The private dental office that has been appropriately designed to receive frail and functionally dependent older adults is the ideal delivery system for those elderly individuals who can be easily transported. This modality is the most ideal and cost-effective for the dentist because no travel or setup and breakdown time is involved. It also allows the dentist to treat the patient in the comfort of an equipped office, with the help of auxiliary personnel. However, this type of delivery system is expensive and time-consuming for the nursing home, which often must have a staff member accompany the resident. Therefore nursing facilities do not favor such an arrangement.

On-site dental programs

On-site dental facilities are appropriate options in very large nursing homes, where the economy of scale renders them cost-effective. They are less disruptive to the functioning of the facility. The disadvantage of on-site facilities is that they cannot be moved to treat bedridden residents; they need to be supplemented with a portable dental unit.

Portable dental programs

These are self-contained dental units and instrument kits that can be transported by the provider into the facility or the person's home. This type of delivery system is ideal for homebound and bedridden individuals.

Mobile van dental programs

Mobile dental care vans are modified to accommodate built-in dental equipment, supplies, a dental team, and patients. A mobile dental office has all the advantages of the private office in addition to the ability to visit nursing facilities and private homes. Transporting patients to the vehicle may still be a problem, however, especially those patients who are bedridden.

The appropriate use of portable dental equipment and mobile setups is encouraged by the American Dental Association,[76] and dentists have been providing dental services to homebound or institutionalized patients for several years. However, the majority of dentists, like other health professionals, are not attracted to working in institutions such as nursing homes. The apparent reluctance of dentists to treat elderly patients outside the conventional practice has been attributed primarily to low reimbursement levels, inadequate treatment facilities in the nursing home, and inadequate training in gerontology and geriatric dentistry.[77]

Financing geriatric oral health

Financing of oral health services for the older population differs from financing in younger groups and from financing for general health services.[31] Dental care, unlike medical care, is heavily financed through the private sector. In 1990 out-of-pocket spending and insurance plans' share combined accounted for approximately 97% of the total dental care expenditure for the elderly and the general population alike. Government programs paid less than 3%.[77,78] In contrast, government programs covered 63% of the health expenditures for older persons, compared with only 26% for the population younger than 65.[1]

Out-of-pocket payment remains the dominant method of paying for dental services. However, the proportion of persons insured for dental services has increased dramatically since the mid-1960s. Currently about 45% of Americans have some form of dental insurance.[79] Unfortunately, few of these programs offer prepaid coverage after the insured reaches retirement age. It had been reported that by age there was a descending rate of dental insurance coverage among the elderly; that is, 36% in the 60 to 64-year age group, and only 7% in the 80 and older age group.[80] The 1985-1986 NIDR survey[29] found that approximately 52% of all employed adults age 60 or older had dental care coverage and only 34.5% of nonemployed seniors had similar coverage. The

differential in coverage between employed adults and the elderly has occurred as the elderly retired and left the workforce.

As a group, older adults account for only 10% of the national dental expenditures.[81] However, when they used dental services, the average amount expended was found to be higher than that expended for all age groups. In 1987 an average of $311 was expended by those older adults making one or more visits, compared with $295 of mean annual dental expenditure for all ages. However, the elderly had the lowest proportion of dental expenses reimbursed by private dental insurance—10% compared with 35% for all ages—and the highest percentage of out-of-pocket dental expenses—79% compared with 56% for all ages.[81]

Another survey in 1990 showed that 44% of persons 66 years and older used dental services and, among users, 88% of the average total expenditure of $378 was paid out-of-pocket.[82]

Public programs are not a major source of payment for dental services. Medicaid, or Title 19 of the Social Security Act, enacted in 1965, provided federal funds to be distributed among the state public assistance programs. The intent of the program was to provide health benefits to the indigent. Some services were required under this program. However, dentistry was not a required service. When dentistry was included, it was usually underfunded and limited in benefits, especially for adults.

Medicare, or Title 18 of the Social Security Act, also enacted in 1965, was a program intended to provide health insurance for those over age 65. The program was to pay for hospital and physician services. Dental services, unless provided under special circumstances, were not to be included.

Medicare does not pay for dental services, except for limited medically necessary oral health care. Medically necessary oral health care is oral and maxillofacial care that is a direct result of, or has a direct impact on, an underlying medical condition or its resulting therapy. In 1987 only 3% of elderly dental expenditures were paid by Medicaid and Medicare.[81]

There have been a few unsuccessful initiatives to expand dental coverage for the elderly through Medicare and private insurance. Private plans, however, are unlikely to assume programs for the elderly for the following reasons: (1) the uncertainty of cost as a result of inflation increases the insurer's risk, and there is fear of dollar losses; (2) administrative costs are high, especially if only a fraction of the population is involved; (3) current programs, such as Medicaid and Medicare, would undercut the market for these programs; and (4) adverse selection, that is, the purchase of the insurance by high-risk groups, would drive premiums up and low-income individuals out of the plan. The only effective oral health care benefit plan for the older adult population is one that is part of a comprehensive benefits package developed with the understanding that oral health is an integral part of general health and that the two cannot be separated. An infection in the mouth needs to be considered the same way as an infection in any other part of the body.

The unlikely expansion of dental coverage under current health care reform initiatives, coupled with the potential loss of insurance benefits by retirees, may lead to a decrease in the number of elderly persons in the future that will have dental insurance. Thus expenditures for dental services are likely to remain a large source of out-of-pocket expenditures for elderly persons.

Geriatric training and personnel needs

Currently the majority of dental care for the older adult population is provided in the community by general practitioners. According to the American Dental Association, approximately 20% of dentists also provide some care in long-term care settings. With the projected increases in tooth retention and utilization rate, demand for a wider range of dental services by older individuals is also anticipated.

Although the majority of older individuals are relatively healthy and have oral needs similar to those of the adult population, a sizable group experience complex conditions and problems requiring intensive and sophisticated care. These individuals may live at home or in long-term care facilities. The two cohorts of elderly require different types of dental services, delivered by appropriately trained practitioners.

The 1987 Department of Health and Human Services (DHHS) report to Congress entitled, *Personnel for Health Needs of the Elderly Through the Year 2020,* recognized the need for three levels of professional training in geriatric dentistry.[83] Because the dental profession will be serving an increasing number and proportion of older patients, all dentists, dental hygienists, and dental assistants should receive basic training in gerontology and geriatric dentistry. To prepare dentists capable of serving functionally dependent older individuals, advanced postdoctoral training (e.g., residency programs with a dental geriatric emphasis) will be required. A small cadre of dental professionals, responsible for educational and research activities as well as specialized consultation, will also be needed. To develop competencies for this leadership group, formal programs of at least 2 years' duration in the form of fellowships or doctorate degrees are necessary.[83]

Projections by the American Association of Dental Schools and the American Society for Geriatric Dentistry indicate a need for about 7500 dental practitioners with advanced training in geriatric dentistry in the year 2000 and 10,000 practitioners in the year 2020. It is estimated that the leadership cadre may be about 20% of the group with advanced education in geriatric dentistry. These practitioners may number about 1500 in the year 2000 and 2000 in the year 2020. The leadership cadre usually will be located at dental schools and teaching hospitals. On the basis of the above projections, it appears that dentists with such advanced preparation will make up about 5% of all practicing dentists.[83]

Recognizing the deficiency in the supply of health care personnel adequately prepared to serve the elderly, in 1988 the federal government awarded funding to 23 medical schools to support 2-year fellowship training and 1-year faculty retraining programs for dentists and physicians who are interested in career preparations and professional advancement in geriatrics.[84] The programs offer interdisciplinary training in clinical care, research, teaching skills, and program administration.

Other learning opportunities in geriatric dentistry have evolved during the last 15 years.[85] Short-term intensive experiences offered by regional geriatric education centers have also emerged. They are federally initiated, university-based programs that offer and coordinate geriatric training for several different professions. Forty-one centers were in existence in 1993, and the majority had dental components. In addition, there are other continuing education experiences of shorter duration, offering mixed clinical and didactic training opportunities. There are currently four such programs in Illinois, Kentucky, Minnesota, and Washington.

Important progress has also been made in recent years in expanding geriatric educational efforts as part of the predoctoral and postdoctoral dental programs. Changes in the curricula were initiated by the Geriatric Dentistry Academic Awards Program between 1980 and 1984. This program was funded by the National Institute on Aging. The purpose of the awards was to assist the preparation of researchers and leaders in academic dentistry and to help develop and strengthen curricula in geriatrics. With a grant from the Bureau of Health Professions of the Health Resources and Services Administration in 1979, the American Hygienists' Association developed the Geriatric Curriculum for Dental Hygiene Education to expand geriatric training in the dental hygiene programs.

Summary and future trends

The aging of the nation's population and the apparent decrease in the prevalence of dental caries in children have shifted attention to the oral health needs of older adults. The oral health care professional of today and tomorrow will undoubtedly be called on to treat an ever-increasing number of older adult patients who differ from older cohorts in the past. The majority of the new cohorts of elderly will have more of their own teeth, visit the dentist more often, and demand more sophisticated care. It is important, however, to recognize that the elderly are not a monolithic group. They are a heterogeneous mix of individuals with various levels of functional, socioeconomic, and oral health status. The challenge for the dental profession will be to develop oral health promotion and disease prevention programs and treatment and financing strategies that will meet the unique needs of each subgroup.

With the shift of population toward an older composition with more chronic diseases and medications, there will be a need for expanded courses in internal medicine, pharmacology, gerontology, and geriatrics in the dental curriculum. In addition, the complex nature of the aging process will demand an increase in the interdisciplinary communication among health and allied health personnel to optimize treatment outcomes.

Finally, oral health care should be recognized as a primary health care service that is essential to the general health and well-being of older adults. It will therefore be imperative for oral health care professionals to act as agents to facilitate this change.

REFERENCES

1. American Association of Retired Persons: *A profile of older Americans,* Washington, DC, 1995, The Association.
2. National Center for Health Statistics: *Trends in the health of older Americans: United States, 1994,* Vital and Health Statistics, US Department of Health and Human Services, series 3, no 30, Washington, DC, 1995, US Government Printing Office.
3. Aiken LR: *Aging—an introduction to gerontology,* Thousand Oaks, Calif, 1995, Sage.
4. National Research Council: *The aging population in the twenty-first century—statistics for health policy,* Washington, DC, 1988, National Academy Press.
5. Becker PM, Cohen HJ: The functional approach to the care of the elderly: a conceptual framework, *J Am Geriatr Society* 32(12):923-929, 1984.
6. Rossman I: Bodily changes with aging. In Busse EW, Blazer DG , editors: *Handbook of geriatric psychology,* New York, 1980, Van Nostrand-Reinhold, p 125.
7. Marsh GR: Perceptual changes with aging. In Busse EW, Blazer DG , editors: *Handbook of geriatric psychology,* New York, 1980, Van Nostrand-Reinhold, p 47.
8. Seigler IC: The psychology of adult development and aging. In Busse EW, Blazer DG , editors: *Handbook of geriatric psychology,* New York, 1980, Van Nostrand-Reinhold, p 169.
9. Palmore E: The social factors of aging. In Busse EW, Blazer DG, editors: *Handbook of geriatric psychology,* New York, 1980, Van Nostrand-Reinhold, p 222.
10. US Senate Special Committee on Aging: *Aging america: trends and projections,* US Department of Health and Human Services, DHHS Pub No (FCoA) 91-28001, Washington, DC, 1991, US Government Printing Office.
11. Medalie JH, Pasem HR, Calkins E: Confusion (delirium). In Calkins E, Davis PJ, Ford AB, editors: *The practice of geriatrics,* Philadelphia, 1986, WB Saunders.
12. Pfeiffer E: A short portable mental status questionnaire for assessment of organic brain deficit in elderly patients, *J Am Geriatric* Soc 23:433, 1975.
13. Folstein MF, Folstein EE, McHugh PR: Mini-mental state: a practical method for grading the cognitive state of patients for the clinician, *J Psychiatric Res* 12:189, 1975.
14. Kahn RL and others: Brief objective measures for the determination of mental status in the aged, *Am J Psychiatry* 117:326, 1960.
15. Katz P, Dube D, Calkins E: Aging and disease. In Calkins E, Davis PJ, Ford AB, editors: *The practice of geriatrics,* Philadelphia, 1986, WB Saunders.
16. Ettinger RL, Beck JD: Geriatric dental curriculum and the needs of the elderly, *Special Care Dent,* 4(5):207-213, 1984.

17. Ettinger RL, Beck JD: The new elderly: what can the dental profession expect? *Special Care Dent,* 2(2):62-69, 1982.
18. National Center for Health Statistics: *Dental care: interval and frequency of visits, United States, July 1957-June 1959,* Public Health Service Pub No 584-B14 (Health statistics from the National Health Survey, series B, no 14, p 12), Washington, DC, March 1960.
19. Bloom B, Gift HC, Jack SS: *Dental services and oral health, United States, 1989,* DHHS Pub No (PHS) 93-1151. (Vital and health statistics, series 10, no 183) Hyattsville, Md, 1992, Centers for Disease Control and Prevention/National Center for Health Statistics.
20. National Center for Health Statistics: *Health promotion and disease prevention, United States, 1990* (Vital and health statistics, Series 10, No 185). Hyattsville, Md, 1993.
21. Jack SS: *National Center for Health Statistics: use of dental services: United States, 1983,* Advance data from Vital and Health Statistics, No 122, DHHS Pub No (PHS) 86-1250, Washington, DC, 1986, Government Printing Office.
22. Jones JA and others: Gains in dental care use not shared by minority elders, *J Public Health Dent* 54(1):39-46, 1994.
23. Schou L: Oral health, oral health care, and oral health promotion among older adults: social and behavioral dimensions. In Cohen LK, Gift HC, editors: *Disease prevention and oral health promotion,* Copenhagen, 1995, Munksgaard.
24. Holtzman JM, Berkey AB, Mann J: Predicting utilization of dental services by the aged, *J Public Health Dent* 50(3):164-171, 1990.
25. Grytten J: How age influences expenditure for dental services in Norway, *Commun Dent Oral Epidemiol* 18:225-229, 1990.
26. Ter Horst G, de Wit CA: Review of behavioral research in dentistry 1987-1992: dental anxiety, dentist-patient relationship, compliance and dental attendance, *Int Dent J* 43(3) Suppl:265-278, 1993.
27. MacEntee MI, Stolar E, Glick N: Influence of age and gender on oral health and related behaviour in an independent elderly population, *Commun Dent Oral Epidemiol* 21:234-239, 1993.
28. Tennstedt SL and others: Understanding dental services use by older adults: sociobehavioral factors vs need, *J Public Health Dent* 54(4):211-219, 1994.
29. NIDR, US Department of Health and Human Services, Public Health Service, National Institutes of Health: *Oral health of United States adults, the national survey of oral health in US employed adults and seniors: 1985-86, national findings,* NIH Pub No 87, 2868, Washington, DC, 1987, US Government Printing Office.

30. Merelie DL, Heyman B: Dental needs of the elderly in residential care in Newcastle-upon-Tyne and the role of formal carers, *Community Dent Oral Epidemiol* 20:106-111, 1992.

31. Jones JA and others: Issues in financing dental care for the elderly, *J Public Health Dent* 50(4):268-275, 1990.

32. Branch LG, Antczak AA, Stason WB: Toward understanding the use of dental services by the elderly, *Spec Care Dent*, 6(1):38-41, 1986.

33. Commission on Dental Education and Practice, Working Group 10: *FDI Technical Report No. 43: Delivery of oral health care to the elderly patient*, London, 1992, Federation Dentaire Internationale.

34. Kiyak HA: Recent advances in behavioral research in geriatric dentistry, *Gerodontol* 7:27-36, 1988.

35. Kiyak HA, Miller RR: Age differences in oral health attitudes and dental service utilization, *J Public Health Dent* 42:29-41, 1982.

36. Ettinger RL, Beck JD, Glenn RE: Some considerations in teaching geriatric dentistry, *J Am Soc Geriatr Dent* 13:7, 1978.

37. Gluck GM, Lakin LB: Determination of common myths among dental students and dental school faculty, unpublished data, 1985.

38. Epstein CF: Enhancing the dental office environment for the elderly, *Dent Clin North Am* 33:43, 1989.

39. Ettinger RL, Beck JD, Glenn RE: Eliminating office architectural barriers to dental care of the elderly and handicapped, *J Am Dent Assoc* 98:398, 1979.

40. *Americans with Disabilities Act, PL 101-336*, Americans with Disabilities Act Title III regulations, 28 CFR part 36, Nondiscrimination on the Basis of Disability by Public Accommodations and in Commercial Facilities, Washington, DC, 1992, US Department of Justice, Office of the Attorney General.

41. Johnson ES, Kelly JE, Van Kirk LE: *Selected dental findings in adults by age, race, and sex: United States 1960-1962*, US Department of Health, Education, and Welfare, Public Health Service, PHS Pub No 1000, series 11 No 7, Washington, DC, 1965, US Government Printing Office.

42. Harvey C, Kelly JE: *Decayed, missing, and filled teeth among persons 1-74 years, United States*, National Center for Health Statistics, Vital health statistics series 11 No 223, DHHS Pub No (PHS) 81-1673, Washington, DC, 1981, US Government Printing Office.

43. Hand JS, Hunt RJ, Beck, JD: Coronal and root caries in older Iowans: 36-month incidence, *Gerodontics* 4(3):136-139, 1988.

44. Hunt RJ and others: Incidence of tooth loss among elderly Iowans, *Am J Public Health* 78:1330, 1988.

45. Drake CW and others: Eighteen-month coronal caries incidence in North Carolina older adults, *J Public Health Dent* 54(1):24-30, 1994.

46. Douglass CW and others: Oral health status of the elderly in New England, *J Gerontol Med Sci* 48(2):M39-M46, 1993.

47. Weintraub JA, Burt BA: Tooth loss in the United States, *J Dent Educ* 49:368, 1985.

48. Hand JS, Hunt RJ, Beck JD: Incidence of coronal and root caries in an older population, *J Public Health Dent* 48:14, 1988.

49. Papas A, Joshi A, Giunta J: Prevalence and intraoral distribution of coronal and root caries in middle-aged and older adults, *Caries Res* 26:459-465, 1992.

50. Beck JD: The epidemiology of root surface caries, *J Dent Res* 69:1216, 1990.

51. Page RC: Periodontal diseases in the elderly: a critical evaluation of current information, *Gerodontol* 3:63, 1984.

52. Abdellatif HM, Burt BA: An epidemiological investigation into the relative importance of age and oral hygiene status as determinants of periodontitis, *J Dent Res* 66:13, 1987.

53. Burt BA: Epidemiology of dental diseases in the elderly, *Clin Geriatr Med* 8(3):447-459, 1992.

54. Loe H and others: Natural history of periodontal disease in man: rapid, moderate, and no loss of attachment in Sri Lankan laborers 14 to 46 years of age, *J Clin Periodontol* 13:431, 1986.

55. Fox CH and others: Periodontal disease among New England elders, *J Periodontol* 65(7):676-684, 1994.

56. American Cancer Society: *Cancer facts & figures—1993*, Atlanta, 1993, The Society.

57. Silverman S: Precancerous lesions and oral cancer in the elderly, *Clinics Geriatr Med* 8(3):529-541, 1992.

58. Silverman S: *Oral cancer*, ed 3, Atlanta, 1990, American Cancer Society.

59. Medalie JH: An approach to common problems in the elderly. In Calkins E, Davis PJ, Ford AB, editors: *The practice of geriatrics*, Philadelphia, 1986, WB Saunders.

60. National Center for Health Statistics: *Use of nursing homes by the elderly: preliminary data from the 1985 National Nursing Home Survey*, advance data 135, Washington, DC, 1987, US Government Printing Office.

61. Katzman R: Alzheimer's disease, *N Engl J Med* 314:964, 1986.

62. White L and others: Geriatric epidemiology, *Ann Rev Gerontol Geriatr* 6:215, 1986.

63. Cohen D, Eisdorfer C: Risk factors in later life dementia. In *Senile dementia outlook for the future*, New York, 1984, Alan R Liss.

64. Stamm JW, Banting DW, Imrey PB: Adult root caries survey of two similar communities with contrasting natural fluoride levels, *J Am Dent Assoc* 120:143, 1990.

65. Doty P, Liu K, Weiner J: Special report: an overview of long-term care, *Health Care Financing Rev* 6(3):69-78, 1985.

66. Department of Health and Human Services: *Healthy people 2000*, Public Health Service DHHS Pub No (PHS) 91-50212, Washington, DC, 1990, US Government Printing Office.

67. Berkey D and others: Research review of oral health status and service use among institutionalized older adults in the United States and Canada, *Special Care Dent*, 11:131-136, 1991.

68. Strayer M, Ibrahim M: Dental treatment needs of homebound and nursing home patients, *Commun Dent Oral Epidemiol* 19:176-177, 1991.

69. Kiyak HA, Grayston MN, Crinean CL: Oral health problems and needs of nursing home residents, *Commun Dent Oral Epidemiol* 12:49-52, 1993.

70. Weyant RJ and others: Oral health status of a long-term care veteran population, *Commun Dent Oral Epidemiol* 21:227-233, 1993.

71. California Dental Association: *California skilled facilities' residents: a survey of dental needs*, Sacramento, 1986, California Dental Association.

72. Empy G, Kiyak HA, Milgrom P: Oral health in nursing homes, *Special Care Dent* 3(2):65-67, 1983.

73. Henry RG, Ceridan B: Delivering dental care to nursing home and homebound patients, *Dent Clin North Am* 38(3):537-551, 1994.

74. National Citizens' Coalition for Nursing Home Reform: *Nursing home reform law: the basics*, Washington, DC, 1991, The Coalition.

75. Ettinger RL: Oral care for the homebound and institutionalized, *Clin Geriatr Med* 8(3):659-672, 1992.

76. Council on Access, Prevention and Interprofessional Relations: *Portable and mobile dentistry information*, Chicago, 1995, American Dental Association.

77. Olsen ED: Dental insurance and senior Americans, *J Am Coll Dent* 58:22-25, 1991.

78. US Health Care Financing Administration: National health expenditure, 1991, *Health Care Financing Rev* 14(2):1-30, 1992.

79. Health Insurance Association of America: *Source book of health insurance data*, Washington, DC, 1985, Health Insurance Association of America.

80. Meskin LH and others: Economic impact of dental service utilization by older adults, *J Am Dent Assoc* 120:665-668, 1990.

81. Center for General Health Services Extramural Research: *Expenditures and sources of payment for medical care*, 1987, *National medical expenditure survey*, Washington, DC, Agency for Health Care Policy and Research.

82. Kington R, Rogowski J, Lillard l: Dental expenditures and insurance coverage among older adults, *Gerontologist* 35(4):436-443, 1995.

83. National Institute on Aging: *Personnel for health needs of the elderly through the year 2020*, Public Health Service, Department of Health and Human Services, Bethesda, Md, Sept 1987.

84. Shay K, Berkey DB, Saxe SR: New programs for advanced training in dental geriatrics, *J Am Dent Assoc* 120:661-663, 1990.

85. American Society for Geriatric Dentistry: *Resource directory of postgraduate educational opportunities in geriatric dentistry*, Chicago, 1993, American Society for Geriatric Dentistry.

CHAPTER 8

Dental health of children and strategies for prevention

Benjamin Peretz, Eliezer Eidelman

Along with modern medicine, dentistry is advancing at a swift pace, especially as it relates to our understanding of the mechanisms of dental diseases and treatment methods. This progress has tremendous implications for all the associated dental disciplines, including pediatric dentistry and public health dentistry. This chapter discusses some aspects of pediatric dentistry, particularly those that are relevant to problems in public health. Before new insights in this important field are introduced, some aspects of tooth development are reviewed briefly.

Enamel formation

Enamel formation of the primary teeth begins with the incisors at approximately 11 to 14 weeks of fetal life.[1,2] The initial phase consists of matrix formation followed by calcification. These two processes begin in utero and are completed by the third postnatal month. Because enamel is a relatively stable structure, defects of the enamel of the primary teeth involving its matrix secretion maturation, or both, can act as a permanent record of insults occurring prenatally, perinatally, or early postnatally.

Birth itself leaves its mark on the developing teeth. The change from intrauterine life to extrauterine life causes the formation of the neonatal line.[3] This is a narrow line of hypoplasia, seen in the crowns of the primary incisors near the gingiva and in the primary molars in the middle portion of the crown. In a child born through a normal delivery, the neonatal line is seen only microscopically; however, after complicated deliveries the neonatal line is likely to be macroscopic and visible to the naked eye. A wide range of conditions may contribute to these hypoplastic/hypocalcified defects. Systemic maternal disorders associated with enamel hypoplasia of the dentition of the fetus/neonate include diabetes, kidney disease, and viral or bacterial infections. Systemic disorders of the neonate may include premature birth, Rh incompatibility, allergies, tetany, gastroenteritis, malnutrition, infectious diseases, and chronic diarrhea.[4-8] Some researchers have suggested that a common factor in all these conditions—both maternal and fetal neonatal—is transient hypocalcemia which may be a predisposing factor for dental caries. Others maintain that linear enamel hypoplasia is a predisposing factor to dental caries.[9] A possible correlation between hypoplastic defects and dental caries was proposed as early as three decades ago.[10,11] However, hypoplastic dental defects may be difficult to distinguish from caries caused by excessive bottle nursing,[12] especially when the caries is subsequent to the defect.

Dental caries

Dental caries is the most prevalent childhood dental disease. In the 1980s, studies of children up to age 12 in Western countries showed a dramatic decline in the prevalence of dental caries and an increasing number of children with caries-free dentitions.[13,14] However, a more recent study warned that the 50% caries-free characterization of U.S. schoolchildren was mythical because it failed to consider decayed primary teeth and it inappropriately averaged in children who were too young to have experienced decay.[15] When decay in primary teeth is also considered, roughly half of children have already experienced decay before first grade. It has been observed that the prevalence of dental caries continues to increase steadily with age until five of every six high school graduates are affected. In light of such opposing opinions, a review of some basic aspects of dental caries is in order.

Dental caries is caused by the demineralization of the dental enamel by organic acids that are the outcome of the metabolism of carbohydrates by microorganisms in the mouth. It is a multifactorial disease, involving four main factors:

1. *Microorganisms. Streptococcus mutans* is the principal microorganism involved in the carious process.[16] *S. mutans* is present in the mouth only after tooth eruption. Infants whose teeth have not erupted yet do not have this microorganism in their oral cavities.[17,18] Some researchers suggest that there is a continuous transmission of *S. mutans* from the parent's oral cavity to the infant's oral cavity through kissing, sharing of food, and other contact.[19-21] In caries-free children the *S. mutans* count was found to be negligible.[22]

2. *Substrate.* Carbohydrates in the diet provide the microorganisms with the substrate for organic acid production, which leads to enamel demineralization.[16,23] Sucrose has long been considered the arch-criminal of dental caries.[24,25] *S. mutans* accumulation strongly depends on the amount of sucrose.[26]

3. *Host—tooth enamel.* For caries to occur, a susceptible host is required so that microorganisms can adhere, colonize, and metabolize available carbohydrates. The tooth's morphologic condition and enamel structure are important in this respect; both food debris and microorganisms readily impact in the pit and fissure areas of molar teeth, making them highly susceptible to caries. Although smooth enamel tooth surfaces are not prone to caries development, bacteria accumulate and adhere onto irregular enamel surfaces, thus, accelerating the carious process. In general, the surface of the tooth is more acid resistant than its subsurface. Furthermore, the increase in fluoride content and the decrease in permeability of the enamel of the mature teeth make them more acid-resistant than is the immature enamel surface of young teeth. Thus, as a host, the enamel of a young tooth is more prone to dental caries than is the enamel of the mature tooth. In addition, as the tooth enamel matures, the tooth surface may be considered a reservoir of fluoride, thus increasing tooth resistance to caries.[27,28]

4. *Time.* Elapsed time determines the three previous factors. The longer the teeth are exposed to fermentable carbohydrates, the more acid will be produced. This phenomenon increases the probability that caries will occur.

Saliva is a major factor influencing the development or inhibition of dental caries. Saliva is to the tooth enamel what blood is to body cells. Just as body cells depend on the bloodstream to supply nutrients, remove waste, and protect the cells, enamel depends on saliva to perform similar functions. The beneficial actions of the saliva include:

1. Speeding oral clearance of food particles and dissolving sugars
2. Facilitating the removal of insoluble carbohydrates from the mouth by salivary enzymes
3. Neutralizing organic acids produced by plaque bacteria by salivary buffers
4. Inhibiting demineralization and enhancing remineralization by the action of salivary minerals on tooth structure
5. Recycling ingested fluoride into the mouth
6. Discouraging the growth of bacteria
7. Inhibiting both mineral loss and the adhesion of bacteria by adsorption of salivary proteins to tooth suraces[29,30]

Children as young as 6 months to 3 years old are already at risk for a distinctive pattern of dental caries known as baby-bottle tooth decay or nursing bottle caries. Baby-bottle tooth decay, caused by prolonged nursing from a bottle containing milk or other sweet liquid, is seen in epidemic proportions in the Third World, and among disadvantaged children in western countries.[31] Because it is so prevalent, baby-bottle tooth decay requires special attention from both clinical and public health perspectives.

Baby-bottle tooth decay

Baby-bottle tooth decay (BBTD) and *nursing caries* are terms that describe a form of rampant caries of the primary dentition caused by prolonged use of a bottle of milk or other liquid including carbohydrates.[12,31] Clinically, the decay is first found in the maxillary primary incisors; later it spreads to the maxillary molars, mandibular molars, and, rarely, the mandibular incisors. It has been postulated that this pattern of caries is related to the following factors:

1. The chronology of primary tooth eruption. With the exception of the mandibular incisors, teeth that erupt early are most affected. Therefore the maxillary incisors are affected most.
2. The duration of the harmful habit. The longer sweet liquid remains around the teeth, the more likely it is that it will be metabolized by oral microorganisms into organic acids that demineralize the tooth enamel.
3. The pattern of the muscular activity of the sucking infant. Because the teeth cannot be protected by the tongue, weak muscular activity results in the teeth being bathed in an increasingly large pool of liquid that cannot be effectively washed out by the available saliva.

Thus the occurrence of dental caries in cases of BBTD depends on all four factors: microorganisms, substrate, host, and time.

The contents of the feeding bottles must be considered in cases of BBTD. Most studies have reported that these bottles all contain some form of sugar.[32-35] How, for example, does milk affect the occurrence of BBTD? Cow's milk and mother's milk contain lactose, composed of glucose and fructose, both of which enhance cariogenic bacteria colonization and acid production.[36-38] Some studies report on BBTD in children who were fed with cow's milk only[32,39] and some on BBTD in children who were only breast-fed.[40-42] It has also been found that the high concentrations of calcium and phosphate in milk are caries protective.[43-45] Apparently, under normal diet conditions milk is not cariogenic and may even provide some protection against caries. However, the diets of most children with BBTD are not normal; prolonged exposure to milk leads to its stagnation around the necks of the teeth, especially the maxillary incisors, leading to high acidogenicity and subsequent enamel demineralization.[46] In addition to having sweet liquids from bottles, affected children are often given pacifiers dipped in sweets; an association has been established between the use of these comforters and BBTD.[47-49]

PREVALENCE

It is difficult to determine the exact prevalence of BBTD because every survey is seriously limited. Preschool-aged children with BBTD are less available for dental examination than are older children. In addition, those children who are examined may not necessarily represent the general population of this age. Instead, the population of children seen at a given dental clinic may be biased because their parents believed that their children had a dental problem.[39] Selection of survey samples from mother-child centers or from child health centers could skew the sample into a particular socioeconomic class.[50] In addition, because the patterns of infant feeding habits are largely culturally and ethnically influenced, survey samples of children from such cultural or ethnic backgrounds will be similarly skewed.[51] For all these reasons it is difficult to make an analogy from the prevalence of BBTD in one country with its prevalence in another country.[52-54]

The reported prevalence of BBTD may also be influenced by the fact that infants are difficult to examine. Not every pediatric dentist knows that a thorough dental examination of an infant requires that the infant lie with his or her head on the dentist's lap with the legs on the mother. Furthermore, the infant's distress and crying may trouble an inexperienced examiner so much that the examination may be superficial at best.

The diagnosing criteria of BBTD are somewhat controversial; some researchers claim that a minimum of one infected incisor is a sufficient criterion for diagnosing the condition.[52] Others maintain that a minimum of two teeth is required,[47,55] whereas some believe that at least three infected maxillary incisors are required.[51]

It is generally accepted that the prevalence of BBTD in predominantly Western-type cultures is approximately 5%.[34,39,47,48,50-55] In certain populations a higher prevalence has been found. In the United States Hardwick et al.[56] reported a 21% prevalence of BBTD for urban Hispanic children younger than 5 years. Barnes et al.[57] reported a 16% prevalence for urban children and a 37% for rural Hispanic children. In a preliminary study of children of Mexican-American migrant farmworkers, Weinstein et al.[58] found a 29.2% prevalence of BBTD among infants aged 27.6 months on the average. In a subsequent study the same research group found that in a sample of children with an average age of 17.1 months, 7% had at least one maxillary incisor with decay and more than 30% had at least one incisor with a white spot lesion.[59]

DISEASE PROGRESSION

BBTD has a predictable progression. Initially the teeth are seen to have white spots that are usually decalcification lesions, which may become frank lesions or caries within 6 months to a year. Such decalcification lesions do not necessarily progress to cavities because the process may be reversed and the teeth may become remineralized.[60] Undetected, and thus unchecked, early BBTD causes severe problems for the child, who may be in considerable pain and may have difficulty eating and talking. The disease is also a serious threat to the health of other primary teeth and subsequently to the health of the permanent dentition. Recently an association between BBTD and failure to thrive (FTT) has been found.[61] However, the results of this study do not distinguish clearly whether BBTD had caused the FTT or whether the FTT, caused by various general systemic conditions, was itself a predisposing factor in the development of BBTD.

The results of a new pilot study indicate a strong correlation between BBTD and maternal diseases or complications during pregnancy and/or delivery.[62] This study compared the pregnancies of the mothers of two groups of age-matched children with similar eating and feeding habits—they all were fed from bottles containing sweet liquids. Compared with the pregnancies of mothers of children with healthy teeth, the pregnancies of the mothers of children with BBTD involved more cases of vaginal bleeding, premature uterine contractions, episodes of viral or bacterial infections, and other indications of high-risk pregnancies. There were also more instrumental deliveries (vacuum or forceps) and cesarean sections. Therefore it seems clear that children born of high-risk pregnancies are more likely to have BBTD than are children of normal pregnancies.

TREATMENT

Treating frank lesions in very young children is invasive and most frequently requires crown preparation for the affected teeth and often pulp treatments. These treatments are most often carried out with the child under general anaesthesia or some form of sedation and thus are risky for the child. All such treatments are expensive, both from the point of view of the parent and as a general public health expense. In any case, before any invasive treatment is undertaken, the first necessary step in treating BBTD, as recommended by most practitioners and educators, is to stop the deleterious habit of unrestrained bottle nursing. It is important to note that not only would stopping the habit cause a decrease in the exposure to the cariogenic liquid, but it would also arrest the carious process and allow the pulp to produce reparative dentin. The formation of this dentin prevents the pulp from being exposed after caries removal. Protecting the pulp reduces the likelihood that the child will require pulp treatments such as pulpotomy or pulpectomy; it also conditions the tooth material so that new adhesives will be more likely to bond to it.[63]

PREVENTION

Most researchers agree that the only rational approach to the treatment of BBTD is prevention, which begins with education about oral self-care. Teaching oral self-care is extremely frustrating for health educators; thus it is not surprising that Weinstein et al.[64] call one of the chapters in their book "Why most plaque control programs do not work." Most traditional stand-alone health educational approaches provide general information about BBTD, focus on the bottle as the risk factor, and recommend immediate substitution of the cup for the bottle at all feedings by 12 months. Unfortunately this approach has not been very successful. Considering the seriousness of this disease and how unsuccessful most preventive programs have been, it is surprising how few alternative programs have been suggested.

The child's risk for BBTD should be assessed. As described here, a risk for BBTD could be caused by complications or diseases during the pregnancy or by instrumental delivery. Teeth that develop while these complications occur, especially the incisors, are especially at risk for BBTD.[62] When risks are high or when the results of the dental examination indicate the presence of BBTD, culturally appropriate interventions should be undertaken.

Although weaning to a cup at 1 year is recommended, it may prove difficult for parents who have a sick or temperamentally difficult child and who have little social support. It may also be culturally unacceptable.[65] In many societies, until they are several years old, infants are carried everywhere by their mothers and nursed by them. In other societies in which there are many children per family, it is difficult to encourage weaning from the bottle at an early age. In an attempt to overcome the problem of parents' noncompliance, Weinstein et al.[65] tried an original approach: they applied fluoride-containing varnish to the teeth of BBTD high-risk populations, a simple and effective method that requires only minimal parental cooperation. The varnish is brushed on dried teeth, and the procedure takes less than 2 minutes. Although the only compliance required from the parents is to bring the children for semiannual treatment, parents in the study demonstrated only about 50% compliance after 6 months. The rationale for this approach was to allow the fluoride to arrest the carious process and to enhance the formation of reparative dentin, thus keeping the tooth condition stable even though not restored. This approach is very close to the idea that stopping the habit would allow new reparative dentin to be formed. Attempts to enhance follow-up are needed, especially in migrant families living on subsistence wages and in families with more than one child because bringing in one child for a follow-up would entail providing care for the other children and is thus logistically complicated.

THE FETUS IS ALSO A PATIENT!

With the aim of improving the health education of the general public, health professionals are constantly searching for target populations at high risk for preventable diseases.[59,60,64,66-68] Within this framework, and considering the association between BBTD and maternal diseases or complications during pregnancy or delivery,[62] we propose that the dental profession adopt the concept that *the fetus is also a patient.* Because the quality of intrauterine life affects the quality of the infant's teeth, dental health educators should educate women who may experience complications during pregnancy or delivery about the dangers of BBTD and how to avoid it. For example, they could teach appropriate methods for infant bottle-feeding.

The rapid progress in medicine and the increasing ability of modern medicine to maintain high-risk pregnancies, as well as to keep newborns alive after complicated or instrumental deliveries, have resulted in many more infants whose teeth may be affected and could be more vulnerable to dental caries. Thus it is only natural that the dental profession will encounter more young patients at risk for BBTD. It is important to warn parents and prospective parents that maternal diseases and complications during pregnancy and delivery may predispose their fetus's/infant's teeth to BBTD. These parents in particular should be taught to avoid prolonged bottle-feeding of sweetened liquids to their infants.

General recommendations: caries prevention in infants and children

In this chapter we have chosen not to deal with the issue of water fluoridation, which has been discussed at length in the literature. However, we believe that the following recommendations should always be mentioned. It is recommended that an infant be examined soon after eruption of the first primary tooth.[68] This examination should include the soft tissues of the oral cavity, and the teeth to detect defects in the enamel or early carious lesions. At this time the dentist can teach the parents proper maintenance of oral and dental health. Tremendous success has been reported in educating parents for preventive dental treatment for children younger than 4 years of age.[69] A protocol for preventive procedures beginning early in infancy should include the use of fluoride and instruction in proper home dental care.[70,71]

Preventive measures can be divided into two categories: home care and professional dental care.

HOME CARE

Home care includes the following elements:
1. *Consistent visits to the dentist.* Preferably the first visit should occur before the eruption of the first tooth. Dental visits provide the dentist with the opportunity to teach the parents to wipe their infant's teeth clean with a small piece of gauze

held between their fingers. Because it has been found that bacteria are transferred from the parents to the child,[20] parents should be encouraged to keep their own teeth very clean during the time that their infant's teeth are erupting.

2. *Effective oral hygiene.* The infant's teeth should be brushed twice daily, with the whole dentition being brushed both after breakfast and before bedtime.[72]

3. *Use of home-fluoride modalities.* These treatments include fluoridated dentifrices, fluoride supplements (tablets or drops), and fluoride rinse solutions. The most common topical application of fluoride is obtained during brushing with a fluoride dentifrice. Fluoride toothpastes have contributed considerably to the recent decline in the incidence of caries in industrialized countries. Their effect is related more to the frequency of use than to the fluoride concentration.[73] Brushing with a fluoride dentifrice after breakfast and just before bedtime is recommended to maintain an intraoral reservoir of salivary fluoride ions for as long as possible. Such brushing and the use of fluoride tablets or drops require the establishment of a regular daily routine, in which the main responsibility is taken by the parents. Because this demands a high degree of health consciousness and concern by at least one parent, compliance for this regimen has been low.[74] When the fluoride tablets have been given at school, the coverage has been better, but such cases require a time commitment from the teachers, who are not always cooperative. Fluoride supplements should be considered for all children drinking fluoride deficient water (<0.6 ppm).[68] Before supplements are prescribed, however, it is essential to know the fluoride concentration of the patient's drinking water to avoid dental fluorosis. (For a discussion on dental fluorosis, see Chapter 9). Once the fluoride level of the water supply has been evaluated, the daily dosage schedule can be prescribed as shown in Table 8-1; other sources of fluoride or its removal through the use of in-house filtration systems need to be taken into account.

Fluoride rinse solutions are used to provide the tooth enamel surface with a constant supply of fluoride ions, which help to remineralize initial carious lesions. This method is recommended only for children 6 years of age or older because younger children may swallow the solution. For this reason fluoride rinse solutions are not appropriate for the treatment of infants with BBTD.

All home care methods depend on patient compliance. The child's socialization process and developmental framework must be considered, especially in the design of home care programs for children.

Table 8-1. Quantities of fluoride to be ingested daily by age of child and fluoride concentration in drinking water

Age	<0.3 ppm	0.3-0.6 ppm	>0.6 ppm
0-6 mo	0	0	0
6 mo-3 yr	0.25 mg	0	0
3 yr-6 yr	0.50 mg	0.25 mg	0
6 yr-16 yr	1.00 mg	0.50 mg	0

From American Academy of Pediatric Dentistry Manual, *Pediatr Dent* 17(Special issue):2, 1995-1996.

PROFESSIONAL DENTAL CARE

Professional dental care includes the following:

1. *Oral hygiene instructions.* In accordance with the child's developmental framework and socialization process, oral hygiene education should be integrated with general health education dealing with body cleanliness, grooming, and self-esteem.[75] It is also beneficial to involve the parents in health promotion programs for children.[76] Oral health for children should be supportive and cannot be achieved without parallel efforts for a healthy environment, which would support healthy choices and healthy behavior of the individual.

2. *Fluoride gel or varnish applications.* The application of topical fluoride to the teeth increases tooth resistance to caries. Constant and repeated applications of fluoride varnish have been highly successful in preventing BBTD.[65] Nevertheless, now that fluoride action is better understood, dentists must ask themselves if they should give fluoride treatments to all their patients. For example, is it possible that applying topical fluoride to the teeth of patients who have been caries-free for 1 or 2 years may be considered as overtreatment?

3. *Pit and fissure sealants.* The issue of pit and fissure sealants has become one of the most important and controversial topics in pediatric dentistry. Some researchers have recommended that sealants be placed over initial caries.[77,78] However, other clinicians and researchers have raised serious objections to this recommendation.[79-81] In any case, because the issue of pit and fissure sealants has enormous implications for public and community dentistry as a means of preventing dental caries in children and young adolescents, elaboration on the

subject from some practical viewpoints is necessary.

Occlusal surface pits and fissures increase the risk of primary and permanent teeth to the ravages of caries attack. Because these areas are least benefited by fluoride, treating them with pit and fissure sealants can be particularly effective for newly erupted noncarious primary or permanent molar and premolar teeth with deep pits, or fissures, or both and for the cingulum area of maxillary incisors with deep lingual pits and/or fissures.[68]

The issue of sealant retention is of utmost importance. Among the various factors affecting sealant retention, the most important is the ability to keep the tooth surface dry. Contamination of the tooth surface by saliva or gingival fluid may prevent the adhesion of the sealant. Therefore as soon as possible after the tooth erupts, sealants should be placed under conditions permitting sufficient isolation so that contamination of the tooth surface by moisture is prevented. Because gingival fluid can be spread and may interfere even more with the adhesion process, it is necessary that the eruption status of the tooth be such that no operculum covers the distal portion of the occlusal surface. Sealant retention is further affected by the position of teeth in the mouth (the sealants on the more anterior teeth are better retained), the skill of the operator, and the age of the patient (the behavior of younger children may make it difficult to maintain a dry field).[82] Sealants may be applied to the teeth of individual children, with the use of criteria such as caries history, patient's age, length of time the tooth has been exposed in the oral cavity, and tooth surface anatomy. Alternately, sealants may be used as a public health preventive measure, with members of the dental team applying the sealant under the dentist's supervision. The results of recent research on sealant retention rates indicate much higher retention when sealants are placed after mechanical preparation, that is, the fissures are widened with a bur before sealant placement.[83] Because auxiliary workers are not permitted to cut tooth structure, it would be necessary to have the dentist perform the mechanical preparation.

4. *Diet counseling.* In addition to reducing the incidence of dental caries by adequate oral hygiene immediately after the ingestion of cariogenic foods, reducing the consumption of cariogenic food can also be helpful.[84,85] However, because controlling dental caries through diet modification is complex, it has been only moderately successful. Furthermore, the precise cariogenicity of any food is not easily predicted. It should be noted that when there is a general decline in the incidence of caries, there is a weaker association between sugar consumption and the incidence of caries, especially when there is an optimal concentration of fluoride in the drinking water.[86] It seems that although most children realize that eating sugar may cause tooth decay, this realization does not cause them to modify their behavior. Community- or school-based programs directed at dietary changes have met with only short-term success,[86] leading to attempts to replace sugar with sugar substitutes in snack foods, beverages, and chewing gums at the population level.[87] As clinicians and educators, we have found that teenagers worried about their body image are more motivated than younger children to use sugar substitutes. Of course, it is important to consider the general health of the child and to modulate accordingly our recommendations for decreasing sugar in the diet or using sugar substitutes. The complexity of these individual behavior modifications or social changes suggests that population-wide oral health promotion based on diet modification is less practical than other caries prevention strategies.[86,87] All foods containing even small quantities of sugars or cooked starches can potentially lead to organic acid production by plaque bacteria.[88] This is one of the reasons that it is difficult to judge the relative cariogenicity of various foods. In general, it is more important to control the frequency of sugar consumption and whether it is consumed during daytime activity or immediately before bedtime and the length of time that residual food material remains in the mouth after eating.

Summary

This chapter has shown that BBTD is a serious and all too common disease. It has emphasized the risks for BBTD that are involved in maternal diseases and complications during pregnancy and/or delivery. By identifying populations at risk and using existing treatment modalities and appropriate educational approaches, dental caries in general and BBTD in particular may be controllable and even preventable. Other treatment strategies that are useful in the prevention of dental disease in children were also discussed.

REFERENCES

1. Kraus BS, Jordan RW: *The human dentition before birth,* Philadelphia, 1965, Lea & Febiger, p 102.
2. Lunt RC, Law DB: A review of the chronology of calcification of deciduous teeth, *J Am Dent Assoc* 89:599-606, 1974.
3. Shour I, Massler, M: Development of the teeth. In Brauer JC and others, editors: *Dentistry for children,* ed 4, New York, 1958, McGraw-Hill, p 65.
4. Infante PF, Gillespie GM: An epidemiologic study of linear hypoplasia in anterior teeth in Guatemalan children, *Arch Oral Biol* 19:1055-1061, 1974.
5. Noren J, Grahnen H, Magnusson BO: Maternal diabetes and changes in hard tissue of primary teeth, *Acta Odontol Scand* 36:127-135, 1978.
6. Smith DM, Miller J: Gastro-enteritis, coeliac disease and enamel hypoplasia, *Br Dent* J 147:91, 1979.

7. Suckling GW, Pearce EI: Development defects of enamel in a group of New Zealand children: their prevalence and some associated aetiological factors, *Community Dent Oral Epidemiol* 12:177-184, 1984.

8. Needelman HL and others: Antecedents and correlates of hypoplastic enamel defects of primary incisors, *Pediatr Dent* 14:158-166, 1992.

9. Nikiforuk G, Fraser D: The etiology of enamel hypoplasia: a unifying concept, *J Pediatr* 98:888-893, 1981.

10. Grahnen H, Larsson PG: Enamel defects in the deciduous dentition of prematurely born children, *Odont Revy* 9:193-204, 1958.

11. Rosenzweig KA, Sahar M: Enamel hypoplasia and dental caries in the primary dentition of prematurity, *Br Dent J* 113:279-280, 1962.

12. Johnsen DC: Characteristics and background of children with "nursing caries," *Pediatr Dent* 4:218-224, 1982.

13. Brunelle JA, Carlos JP: Changes in the prevalence of dental caries in U.S. school children, 1961-1980, *J Dent Res* 61(Special issue):1346-1351, 1982.

14. Hargreaves JA, Thompson GW, Wagg BJ: Changes in caries prevalence of Isle of Lewis children between 1971 and 1981, *Caries Res* 17:554-559, 1983.

15. Eidelstein BL, Douglas CW: Dispelling the myth that 50 percent of U.S. schoolchildren have never had a cavity, *Public Health Rep* 110:522-530, 1995.

16. Loesche WJ: Role of *Streptococcus mutans* in human dental decay, *Microbiol Rev* 50:353-380, 1980.

17. Berkowitz RJ, Jordan HV, White G: The early establishment of *Streptococcus mutans* in the mouth of infants, *Arch Oral Biol* 20:171-174, 1975.

18. Catalanoto FA, Shklair IL, Keene HJ: Prevalence and localization of *Streptococcus mutans* in infants and children, *J Am Dent Assoc* 91:606-609, 1975.

19. Berkowitz RT, Turner J, Green P: Maternal salivary levels of *Streptococcus mutans* and primary oral infection of infants, *Arch Oral Biol* 26:147-149, 1981.

20. Kohler B, Andreen I, Jonsson B: The effect of caries preventive measures in mothers on dental caries and the oral presence of the bacteria *Streptococcus mutans* and lactobacilli in their children, *Arch Oral Biol* 29:879-883, 1984.

21. Dasanayake AP and others: Transmission of mutans streptococci to infants following short term application of an iodine-NaF solution to mothers' dentition, *Commun Dent Oral Epidemiol* 21:136-142, 1993.

22. van Houte J, Gibbs G, Butera C: Oral flora of children with "nursing bottle caries," *J Dent Res* 61:382-385, 1982.

23. Kleinberg I: The role of dental plaque in caries and inflammatory periodontal disease, *J Can Dent Assoc* 40:56-66, 1974.

24. Newbrun E: Sucrose, the archcriminal of dental caries, *J Dent Child* 36:239-248, 1969.

25. Makinen KK: The role of sucrose and other sugars in the development of dental caries: a review, *Int Dent J* 22:363-386, 1972.

26. Loesche WJ: Nutrition and dental decay in infants, *Am J Clin Nutr* 41:423-435, 1985.

27. Nyvad B, Fejerskov O: Formation, composition and ultrastructure of microbial deposits on the tooth surface. In Thylstrup A, Fejerskov O, editors: *Textbook of cariology*, Copenhagen, 1986, Munksgaard, pp 56-57.

28. Newbrun E: *Cariology*, ed 3, Chicago, 1989, Quintessence, pp 52-54.

29. Peretz B, Sarnat H, Moss SJ: Caries protective aspects of saliva and enamel, *N Y State Dent J* 56:25-27, 1990.

30. Moss SF, and others: Insights into saliva action: A program for the International Association of Dentistry for Children, New York, 1994, Colgate Palmolive Co.

31. Ripa LW: Nursing caries: a comprehensive review, *Pediatr Dent* 10:268-282, 1988.

32. Picton DCA, Wiltshear PJ: A comparison of the effects of early feeding habits on the caries prevalence of deciduous teeth, *Dent Pract* 20:170-172, 1970.

33. Dilley GJ, Dilley DH, Machen JB: Prolonged nursing habit: a profile of patients and their families, *J Dent Child* 47:102-108, 1980.

34. Goose DH, Gittus E: Infant feeding methods and dental caries, *Public Health* 82:72-76, 1968.

35. Curzon MEJ, Curzon JA: Dental caries in Eskimo children of the Keewatin District in the Northern Territories, *J Can Dent Assoc* 36:342-345, 1970.

36. Koulourides T, and others: Cariogenicity of nine sugars tested with an intraoral device in man, *Caries Res* 10:427-441, 1976.

37. Brown CR, and others: Effect of milk and fluoridated milk on bacterial enamel demineralization, *J Dent Res* 56:210, 1977 (abstract 632).

38. Birkhed D, and others: Milk and lactose-acid production in human dental plaque, *J Dent Res* 60:1245, 1981 (abstract 6).

39. Powell D: Milk . . . Is it related to rampant caries of the early primary dentition? *J Calif Dent Assoc* 4:58-63, 1976.

40. Gardiner DE, Norwood JR, Eisenson JE: At-will breast feeding and dental caries: four case reports, *J Dent Child* 44:187-191, 1977.

41. Kotlow LA: Breast feeding: a cause of dental caries in children, *J Dent Child* 44:192-193, 1977.

42. Curzon MEJ, Drommond BK: Case report—rampant caries in an infant related to prolonged on-demand breast feeding and a lactovegetarian diet, *Int J Paediatr Dent* 3:25-28, 1987.

43. Bibby BG, and others: Protective effect of milk against in vitro caries, *J Dent Res* 59:1565-1570, 1980.

44. McDugall WA: Effect of milk on demineralization and remineralization in vitro, *Caries Res* 11:166-172, 1977.
45. Mor BM, McDugall WA: Effects of milk on pH of plaque and salivary sediment and the oral clearance of milk, *Caries Res* 11:223-230, 1977.
46. Rugg-Gunn AJ, Roberts GT, Wright WG: Effect of human milk on plaque pH in situ and enamel dissolution in vitro compared with bovine milk, lactose, and sucrose, *Caries Res* 19:327-334, 1985.
47. Winter GB, Hamilton MC, James PMC: Role of the comforter as an etiological factor in rampant caries of the deciduous dentition, *Arch Dis Child* 41:207-212, 1966.
48. Holt RD, Joles D, Winter GB: Caries in preschool children: the Camden study, *Br Dent J* 153:107-109, 1982.
49. Shannon Il, Edmonds EJ, Madsen KO: Honey: sugar content and cariogenicity, *J Dent Child* 46:29-32, 1979.
50. Currier GF, Glinka MP: The prevalence of nursing bottle caries or baby bottle syndrome in an inner city fluoridated community, *VA Dent J* 54:9-19, 1977.
51. Kelly M, Bruerd B: The prevalence of baby bottle tooth decay among two Native American populations, *J Public Health Dent* 47:94-97, 1987.
52. Cleaton-Jones P, Richardson B, Rantsho JM: Dental caries in rural and urban black preschool children, *Commun Dent Oral Epidemiol* 6:135-138, 1978.
53. Aldy D, and others: A comparative study of caries formation in breast-fed and bottle-fed children, *Paediatrica Indonesiana* 19:308-312, 1979.
54. Richardson BD, and others: Infant feeding practices and nursing bottle caries, *J Dent Child* 48:423-429, 1981.
55. Winter GB, and others: The prevalence of dental caries in preschool children aged 1 to 4 years, *Br Dent J* 130:271-277, 1971.
56. Hardwick FK, McIlveen LM, Forrester DJ: A comparison of nursing caries prevalence in Black and Hispanic children, American Academy of Pediatric Dentistry, 1991 (abstract).
57. Barnes GP, and others: Ethnicity, location, age, and fluoridation factors in Baby Bottle Tooth Decay: pilot study at a migrant farmworkers clinic, *J Dent Child* 59:376-383, 1992.
58. Weinstein P, and others: Mexican-American parents with children at risk for baby-bottle tooth decay: pilot study at a migrant farmworkers clinic, *J Dent Child* 59:376-383, 1992.
59. Domoto P, and others: White spot caries in Mexican-American toddlers and parental preferences for various strategies, *J Dent Child* 61:342-346, 1994.
60. Lee C, and others: Teaching parents at WIC clinics to examine their high caries–risk babies, *J Dent Child* 61:347-349, 1994.
61. Acs G, and others: Effect of nursing caries on body weight in a pediatric population, *Pediatr Dent* 14:302-305, 1992.
62. Peretz B, Kafka I: Biologic factors influencing BBTD, *J Dent Res* 75:34, 1996 (abstract 130).
63. Eidelman E, Ulmansky M, Michaeli Y: Histopathology of the pulp in primary incisors with deep dentinal caries, *Pediatr Dent* 14:1372-1375, 1992.
64. Weinstein P, Getz T, Milgrom P: *Oral self care*, ed 3, Seattle, 1991, University of Washington.
65. Weinstein P, and others: Results of a promising open trial to prevent baby bottle tooth decay: a fluoride varnish study, *J Dent Child* 61:338-341, 1994.
66. Dunning JM: *Principles of dental public health practice*, Cambridge, Mass, 1970, Harvard University Press.
67. Mushlin AI, Appel FA: Diagnosing patient noncompliance, *Arch Intern Med* 137:318-321, 1977.
68. American Academy of Pediatric Dentistry Reference Manual, *Pediatr Dent* 17(Special issue):2, 1995-1996.
69. Schneider HS: Parental education leads to preventive dental treatment for patients under the age of four, *J Dent Child* 60:33-37, 1993.
70. Goepfred SJ: Infant oral health: a protocol, *J Dent Child* 53:261-266, 1986.
71. Goepfred SJ: Infant oral health program: the first 18 months, *Pediatr Dent* 9:8-12, 1987.
72. Frandsen A: Mechanical oral hygiene practices: state-of-the-science review. In Loe H, Kleinman DV, editors: *Dental plaque control measures and oral hygiene practices*, Oxford, 1986, IRL Press, pp 93-116.
73. Naylor MN, Murray JJ: Fluorides and dental caries. In Murray JJ, editor: *The prevention of dental disease*, Oxford, 1983, Oxford University Press, pp 83-158.
74. Honkala E, and others: Dental health habits in Austria, England, Finland and Norway, *Int Dent J* 38:131-138, 1988.
75. Blinkhorn AS, Hastings GB, Leather DS: Attitudes towards dental care among young people in Scotland: implications for dental health education, *Br Dent J* 155:311-313, 1983.
76. Blinkhorn AS, Taylor I, Willcox GF: Report of a dental health education program in Bedfordshire, *Br Dent J* 150:319-322, 1981.
77. Mertz-Fairhurst EJ, Schuster GS, Fairhust CW: Arresting caries by sealants: results of a clinical study, *J Am Dent Assoc* 112:194-197, 1986.
78. Frencken JE, and others: An atraumatic restorative treatment (ART) technique: evaluation after one year, *Int Dent J* 44:460-464, 1994.
79. Eidelman E: Intentional sealing of occlusal dentin caries: a controversial issue, *Pediatr Dent* 15:312, 1993.

80. Brannstrom M: Infection beneath composite resin restorations: can it be avoided? *Oper Dent* 12:158-163, 1987.
81. Liebenberg WH: The fissure sealant impasse, *Quint Int* 25:741-745, 1994.
82. Ripa LW: Occlusal sealants: rationale and review of clinical trials, *Int Dent J* 30:127-139, 1980.
83. Shapira J, Eidelman E: Six-year clinical evaluation of fissure sealants placed after mechanical preparation: a matched pair study, *Pediatr Dent* 8:204-205, 1986.
84. Newbrun E: Sugar and dental caries: a review of human studies, *Science* 217:418-423, 1982.
85. Schou L: Social factors and dental caries. In Johnson NW, editor: *Dental caries, markers of high and low risk groups and individuals,* Cambridge, 1991, Cambridge University Press, pp 172-197.
86. Schou L, Currie C, McQueen D: Using a "lifestyle" perspective to understand toothbrushing behavior in Scottish schoolchildren, *Commun Dent Oral Epidemiol* 18:230-234, 1990.
87. Corbin SB: Oral disease prevention technologies for community use, *Int J Technol Assess Health Care* 7:327-344, 1991.
88. Firestone AR, Schmid R, Muehlemann HR: Cariogenic effects of cooked wheat starch alone or with sucrose, and frequency-controlled feeding in rats, *Arch Oral Biol* 27:759-763, 1982.

SECTION III

Distribution of dental disease and prevention

CHAPTER 9

The epidemiology of oral diseases

David G. Pendrys

Importance of oral epidemiology

It is important for oral health practitioners to have a fundamental understanding of general epidemiologic principles and the epidemiology of oral diseases. This knowledge helps practitioners, their patients, and society in several ways. A key component of the ethical, rational management of dental patients is an assessment of risk for future oral diseases. This assessment is the rational foundation for the development and implementation of individualized preventive strategies for the patient. An understanding of the epidemiology of oral diseases is an essential step in this risk assessment process. A knowledge of how a patient's past and current disease status compares with that of others of the same age and gender is a valuable first step in the process of assessing the patient's future risk of disease. A knowledge of current understanding of the underlying determinants of oral diseases (both risk and preventive factors), when compared with the patient's individual history, provides a basis for an individualized preventive treatment plan.

A basic understanding of general epidemiologic principles provides the foundation for the important skill of critically interpreting new information as it becomes available in the literature and via presentations. An understanding of the strengths and limitations of epidemiologic research and the relative potential of a particular study design to contribute to a judgment of causation is fundamental to this process. When combined with a basic knowledge of oral disease epidemiology, a knowledge of epidemiologic principles allows the practitioner to assess how consistent the new information is with past information, how coherent it is with current knowledge, and what its impact might be.

An awareness of the epidemiology of oral diseases by the practitioner can be of broader benefit to society. The practitioner may be called on to be a source of expert guidance to the community on public health matters related to oral health. Only by having an understanding of the distribution and determinants of oral disease within populations and subgroups of the population, along with knowledge of risk and preventive factors, will the oral health practitioner be able to provide that expertise. In addition, the alert practitioner with an understanding of the epidemiology of oral diseases may be the first to identify the presence of an unusual pattern of disease in the population. The result can be profound. A classic example is Frederick McKay, who shortly after graduation from dental school called attention to the presence of an unusually high prevalence of enamel staining among his patients in Colorado Springs.[1] His further observation that these same patients had a lower caries prevalence ultimately led to the discovery that optimally fluoridated drinking water could dramatically reduce the incidence of caries, arguably the most important discovery made in the history of dental public health.

Introduction to epidemiology

Epidemiology is a discipline that strives to understand the occurrence of disease among groups of people. One of the more widely cited definitions describes epidemiology as "the study of the distribution and determinants of disease frequency in man."[2] Oral epidemiology is the application of the science of epidemiology to the realm of oral diseases.

Epidemiologic investigations usually measure and report findings in terms of either the prevalence or incidence of disease. The *prevalence* of disease is the proportion of *existing cases* of a disease in a population at one point in time or during a specified period of time.[3] For example, one might report a caries prevalence of 20% in a population of adults, meaning that 20% of the population had existing caries at a particular point or period in time (e.g., spring 1996). The *incidence* of disease (also known as the *cumulative incidence*) is the number of *new cases* of a disease that occur in a population *at risk of the disease* during a specific time period.[3] For example, one might report the incidence of caries in a population to be 20% per year, meaning that 20% of the population at risk for caries had new caries during a 1-year period. Edentulous individuals in the population would not be part of this incidence calculation because these individuals, lacking any teeth, would not be at risk for caries.

Much of previous oral epidemiologic research has been descriptive in nature. *Descriptive* epidemiologic research asks several basic questions. The first, and perhaps most fundamental question, is: "What is the disease or health outcome under study?" In other words, what exactly defines one person as having the disease and another person as not having it. The formal terminology for this is to state a *case definition*. This is a critical, but not always successful, first step in the understanding of a disease, as will be seen in the discussion of specific oral diseases later in this chapter. Descriptive epidemiology also attempts to determine *who* is getting the disease (i.e., the young, the old, males, females) and *where* the disease is occurring (i.e., across the United States, a particular geographic region, urban versus rural settings). Descriptive epidemiology also seeks to determine the specific timing of disease occurrence or *when* it occurs (i.e., all the time, during tooth formation, after gingival recession).

Descriptive epidemiologic studies help to define the extent of disease in a population. In addition, the findings of these studies often provide the basis for the generation of hypotheses concerning disease causation and prevention, which can be further investigated epidemiologically. Epidemiologic investigations that test hypotheses about disease causation and prevention can be broadly grouped into two categories: *observational studies* and *experimental studies*.

Observational studies attempt to assess the relationship between exposures and disease by observing exposure-disease associations as they naturally occur in the population under study. This exposure-disease relationship is usually reported in terms of an estimate of the *relative risk* of disease associated with a particular exposure. The relative risk can be defined as follows[3]:

$$\text{Relative risk} = \frac{\text{Incidence of disease in exposed group}}{\text{Incidence of disease in unexposed group}}$$

Because the relative risk is a ratio, a relative risk of 1.0 (i.e., a 1:1 ratio) represents *no difference* in risk of disease associated with an exposure. Relative risk estimates above 1.0 suggest *increased risk* of disease associated with the exposure, whereas relative risk estimates between 0 and 1.0 suggest a *protective effect* associated with the exposure. Because of the potential for bias and general "noise" in the data that inherently exists in epidemiologic studies, as contrasted with laboratory studies, relative risk estimates that lie in the range of 0.7 to 1.0 and 1.0 to 1.5 are generally considered to be weak evidence of an association.[4] Similarly, relative risk estimates of more than 3.0 or less than 0.3 are considered estimates of a strong association (in the direction of increased risk or protective effect, respectively).[4]

There are three main types of observational, hypothesis-testing epidemiologic studies: the cross-sectional study, the case-control study, and the cohort study. The *cross-sectional study* looks at both the exposure of interest and the disease outcome at the same point in time. A *case-control study* identifies subjects on the basis of whether the disease of interest is present and then, by means of a history, looks for associations between the disease and one or more past exposures. The *cohort study* identifies subjects according to whether they have a particular exposure of interest and then follows them over time to see if an association exists between the exposure and the development of one or more diseases. Consider the fictitious hypothesis that eating a particular fruit reduces the risk of caries. If researchers chose to conduct a cross-sectional study, they might examine a group of children for caries, with a choice from a selection of fruits as a reward for each child, noting which children take the fruit of interest as they left the examination. The researchers could then determine if there was an association between the presence or absence of caries and choosing the particular fruit. Although the cross-sectional study is relatively quick and inexpensive, its potential is very limited because it cannot determine whether the exposure of interest (in this case, eating or not eating a particular fruit) occurred before the disease of interest. For example, the argument could be made that the children with caries were less likely to have chosen the fruit of interest because having tooth decay made it uncomfortable to eat it.

If the researchers had chosen instead to conduct a case-control study, subjects would have been split into two groups, those with caries and those without, based on an examination. To search for an association with a particular fruit, a history of past exposure to that fruit in the diet would be taken. Thus the case-control study can establish a temporal relationship between the exposure and disease of interest—in this case eating or not eating a particular fruit—and subsequent caries. This type of study is only as good as the techniques it uses to gain a good history of exposure. Also, because a case-control design ordinarily does not allow direct measurement of incidence rates, it must estimate the relative risk with a measure called the *odds ratio,* a valid but indirect estimator of the relative risk.[5]

If the researchers had chosen to conduct a *prospective* (forward-looking) cohort study, children would have been divided into groups based on their dietary habits (i.e., eaters and noneaters of the fruit) and then followed over time to see which children develop caries and which do not. As with the case-control study, the prospective cohort study can establish a temporal relationship between the exposure and disease of interest. However, the cohort design does not rely on a history to determine past exposure. Importantly, because the cohort study allows direct measurement of incidence rates, the relative risk of disease can be directly estimated with the formula listed. However, this study design does require that subjects be followed for a potentially long period, during which they might move away, decide to quit the study, or, in the case of our example, change their dietary habits.

A variation of the prospective cohort study that eliminates the need for this prospective follow-up is the *retrospective* or *historical* cohort study. It is similar to the prospective cohort in design except that the exposure is determined by past exposure records, so that the follow-up period has already occurred as the study is begun. The feasibility of conducting a study of this design depends on the availability of suitable records of past exposure. In some situations records will be available (e.g., records of past medical or dental treatments). In our example, it is unlikely that records of fruit ingestion would exist.

The second broad category of hypothesis-testing epidemiologic study consists of experimental studies. Experimental epidemiologic studies can be divided into two main types, the *clinical trial* and the *community trial*. Clinical trials are conducted to test new preventive or therapeutic agents, with subjects assigned by the investigator to different treatment groups, usually according to some form of random assignment. A new treatment is generally compared with either the current conventional therapy, if one exists, or with a placebo (a nontherapeutic intervention). Well-designed clinical trials use a double-blind design, in which neither the subjects nor the investigator knows to which group a subject belongs. This design helps to prevent the potential for a biased interpretation of treatment effect (better or worse), which might occur if either the subject or the investigator knew to which treatment group (e.g., placebo or experimental agent) a subject belonged. Clinical trials compare the incidence of disease and the side effects between the groups in the study to draw inferences about the safety and efficacy of the treatment(s) under investigation.

In situations in which an intervention can be practically evaluated only at the community level, a community trial can be conducted. In these studies treatment is assigned on the basis of the community rather than the individual. The more similar that the comparison communities are in all aspects except the intervention under study, the more validity this type of study will have. The Newburgh-Kingston water fluoridation trial is a classic example of a community trial.[6]

Although an epidemiologic study might identify an association between an exposure and a disease, that is not the same as proving that the exposure *caused* the disease. Demonstration of an association only indicates that there is some relationship between the exposure and the disease, of which one *possibility* is a causal relationship. In fact, no epidemiologic study can ever "prove" causation. Causation is a judgment that can be arrived at only after a consideration of all available evidence.[3] Over the years criteria have been developed to aid in the process of arriving at a *judgment of causation*. The first criterion is the demonstration of a *temporal relationship* (i.e., to establish that the exposure of interest has preceded the disease in time). The second criterion is the *strength of association* (measured as relative risk)—the stronger the association, the less likely that it is the result of some other biasing factor. However, this criterion does not mean that a weak association cannot be causal. The third criterion is *consistency* of findings reported from different investigations of different populations. The greater the number of different studies showing a particular association, the less likely that the association is the result of some bias or deficiency in study design because it becomes increasingly unlikely that all the studies would share the same particular bias or deficiency. A judgment of causation is further supported if the finding is *coherent* with existing knowledge, although it should be realized that existing knowledge is continuously changing. Inherent in the concept of a judgment, there is no hard-and-fast rule as to when it is appropriate for a judgment of causation to be made. Consideration of the consequences of accepting a judgment of causation balanced against the consequences of delaying acceptance is part of the process.

Epidemiology of dental caries
MEASUREMENT OF CARIES

Caries is the pathologic process of localized destruction of tooth tissues by microorganisms.[7] Dental caries can be described epidemiologically in several useful ways, each of which helps to understand caries activity within groups of people. The conventional method of defining dental caries in a population is to measure the number of teeth or tooth surfaces that are either *decayed, missing,* or *filled* as a result of caries. When this measure is applied to the permanent dentition, either the expression *DMFT* or *DMFS* is used to indicate the number of decayed, missing, or filled teeth or surfaces, respectively.[8] In the same way, when this measure is applied to the primary dentition, either the expression *deft* or *defs* is used, with the *e* representing a primary tooth indicated for extraction.[9] Because of confusion over how this *e* term should be interpreted and applied, recent surveys often simply report *dft* or *dfs* findings. Measuring caries by surfaces affected (i.e., the DMFS of dfs) is more precise than measuring caries by affected teeth since, for example, a tooth with five surfaces affected by caries would make the same contribution to the DMFT score as a tooth with only one affected surface. At the same time, however, the DMFT can be a useful public health measure because it is an indicator of the number of teeth that have had or require treatment. The *M* component of the DMFT(S) assumes that missing teeth have been lost as a result of caries. Although this assumption is reasonable for children, among adults, the older the population, the more likely it becomes that teeth may have been lost as a result of other causes, for exam-

ple, periodontal disease. For this reason a DFS is often used to measure caries in adult populations. Although this measure may underestimate total caries experience (because teeth missing as a result of caries are not included), it avoids a biased overestimate that would result by including missing teeth that were not lost because of caries.

Although the DMFS is a useful measure, it is often important to be more specific in the measurement of the presentation of caries in a population. One important measure with public health implications is the proportion of the overall DMFS that is untreated caries, or the *D* component of the DMFS or DFS. This ratio of D/DMFS (D/DFS) is often presented as a percent. It is a measure of the level of treatment need in a population. The higher the value for this ratio, the higher is the unmet need in the population under study.

A second important way to specify caries activity is on the basis of the type of tooth surface affected by decay. Thus the presence of caries in a population can be described in terms of *coronal pit and fissure caries, coronal smooth surface caries,* and *root surface caries.* Describing caries in this surface-specific manner can provide greater insight into potential risk factors and allow for more effective planning of preventive strategies.

A third important way to specify caries is to draw the distinction between *primary caries,* caries that occurs on unrestored tooth surfaces, and *recurrent* or *secondary caries,* caries that occurs adjacent to an existing restoration. The presence of these distinct types of caries can have different implications for the public health management of caries in a population.

DESCRIPTIVE FINDINGS: CARIES IN CHILDREN

Several demographic factors have been consistently shown to be related to the occurrence of caries. These factors are associated with either the *person* or the *environment* in which that person has lived. As with many diseases, *age* is directly and strongly associated with the prevalence of dental caries. This relationship between age and caries is illustrated in Fig. 9-1, drawn from the two most recent National Institute of Dental Research (NIDR) national surveys of the oral health of U.S. children and adults.[10,11] With increasing age the number of surfaces affected by caries increases, plateauing at around 50 years of age. This figure also illustrates the relationship between caries and *gender.* The mean DMFS for males lags behind

that of females by about 1 year. For example, 14-year-old boys have about the same mean DMFS as 13-year-old girls (i.e., 4.2 mean DMF surfaces). One explanation for this finding is the parallel finding that the dentition appears to erupt earlier in girls.[12,13] Thus at any given age the dentition in male patients has been at risk for a shorter period of time as compared with female patients.

The relationship between *race* and caries is more equivocal. Although in the past some

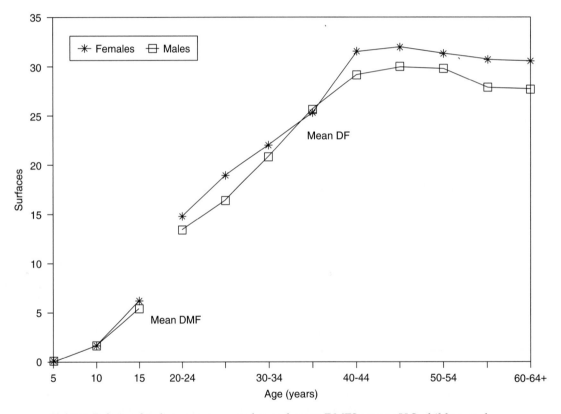

Fig. 9-1. Relationship between age, gender, and mean DMFS among U.S. children and mean DFS among U.S. adults. *(Modified from US Department of Health and Human Services: Oral health of United States children: the National Survey of Dental Caries in U.S. School Children: 1986-1987, National Institutes of Health Pub No 89-2247, Washington, DC, 1989, US Government Printing Office; US Department of Health and Human Services: Oral health of United States adults: the National Survey of Oral Health in U.S. Employed Adults and Seniors: 1985-1986, National Institutes of Health Pub No 87-2868, Washington, DC, 1987, US Government Printing Office.)*

studies reported a lower caries prevalence among African-American children compared with Caucasian children, others reported either a higher caries prevalence among African-Americans or no difference.[14] Two recent national surveys in the United States indicate little difference in caries prevalence between Caucasians and minority children.[10,13] However, consistent differences in the extent to which caries has been treated were found. For example, the National Health and Nutrition Examination Survey (NHANES) III survey reported that although the mean DMFS for Caucasian and African-American children was virtually identical, untreated decay was more than twice as high among African-American children.[13]

Historically, the prevalence of caries in the United States has varied by geographic region. This finding can be traced back to the time of the Civil War and continues today.[14] The advent of artificial water fluoridation has had a profound affect on the distribution of caries. Historically, the prevalence of caries would be as much as 60% lower in fluoridated areas compared with nonfluoridated areas.[15] Today this type of comparison is less meaningful because children living in areas not served by a fluoridated water supply may be indirectly benefiting from it, by drinking beverages manufactured in a fluoridated community and thus prepared with fluoridated water.[16] Recent national survey data show that the greater the number of fluoridated communities in a region, the less is the difference in caries prevalence between children living in fluoridated and nonfluoridated communities.[17]

There have been important long-term changes in the prevalence of dental caries in the United States and elsewhere. Fig. 9-2 shows findings drawn from four national surveys.[13,18] Two important trends can be seen in this figure. The first is that the prevalence of caries in the United States has been declining for at least the past 25 years. Although the mean DMFS for U.S. children aged 5 to 17 was 7.1 during

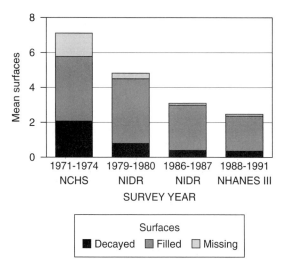

Fig. 9-2. Changes in DMFS prevalence among U.S. children: 1971-1991. (*Data from Brunelle JA, Carlos JP: Changes in the prevalence of dental caries in U.S. schoolchildren, 1961-1980,* J Dent Res *61:1346-1351, 1982; US Department of Health and Human Services:* Oral health of United States children: the National Survey of Dental Caries in U.S. School Children: 1986-1987, *National Institutes of Health Pub No 89-2247, Washington, DC, 1989, US Government Printing Office; Kaste LM and others: Coronal caries in the primary and permanent dentition of children and adolescents 1-17 years of age: United States, 1988-1991,* J Dent Res *75(Special issue):633-641, 1996.*)

the early 1970s, this value had dropped to 2.5 by the late 1980s, a 65% reduction. At the same time the proportion of DMFS that is either untreated caries or missing surfaces has also dramatically fallen during this period. As mean DMFS has fallen, the proportion of caries-free children has increased. For example, the percent of 12- to 17-year-old children in the United States who are caries-free has increased threefold—from 10.4% in the early 1970s to 32.7% in the late 1980s.[13,18] A similar decline in the prevalence of caries in the permanent dentition of children has occurred throughout other Western countries.[19,20] For example, in Australia the estimated mean DMFT among 12-

year-olds decreased from 4.8 teeth in 1977 to 1.2 teeth in 1992.[20]

These findings represent significant success on the part of national efforts to reduce the prevalence of caries, but it is important to remember that these values represent averages over a large age span (5 to 17 years). For example, although the mean DMFS for 10-year-old children in the 1986-1987 NIDR national survey was 1.7, the mean DMFS was four times as high (i.e., 8.0 DMF surfaces) among 17-year-olds.[10] Similarly, whereas 97% of 5-year-olds were caries-free, only 16% of 17-year-olds were caries-free.[10] There has also been a change in the contribution of specific surface types to the total DMFS. The proportion of DMF surfaces that were proximal smooth surfaces has decreased by half from 24% to 12% during the past 20 years, but the portion of the DMFS that involves occlusal and buccal lingual surfaces has proportionally increased.[10] Thus the greatest relative reductions in caries have occurred on the smooth surfaces, strongly suggesting the role of fluoride in the decline in caries prevalence.[21]

A decline in caries prevalence has also occurred in the primary dentition.[10,13,18] A comparison of the 1979-1980 and 1986-1987 NIDR national surveys shows mean dfs among 5- to 9-year-old children declining from 5.3 surfaces to 3.9 surfaces, a 26% decline.[10] The NHANES III 1988-1991 survey reported that 50% of 5- to 9-year-olds and 83% of 2- to 4-year-old children were caries-free in the primary dentition.[13] A similar decline in the prevalence of caries in the primary dentition has occurred in other Western countries.[19,20]

A distinct form of caries pattern in the primary dentition is *nursing caries*. Nursing caries is characterized by the rapid decay of many of the teeth of very young children, involving tooth surfaces generally considered to be at low risk for caries (e.g., the facial surfaces of the maxillary anterior teeth).[22] Nursing caries is the result of improper early feeding habits, specifically lengthy daily feeding, feeding during the night, and continuation of nursing (breast, bottle, or sweetened pacifier) beyond the usual period of weaning (age 1 year).[22] The majority of recent reports suggest that the prevalence of nursing caries in Western societies is 5% or less.[22] Nursing caries, referred to also as baby-bottle tooth decay, is discussed in greater detail in Chapter 8.

DESCRIPTIVE FINDINGS: CORONAL CARIES IN ADULTS

Nearly all dentate adults in the United States have at least one decayed or filled tooth.[11,23] Mean DFS continues to rise with age until around 50, after which it plateaus at approximately 30 DF surfaces,[11,23] as is illustrated in Fig. 9-1. Data from both recent U.S. national surveys of adults indicate that Caucasians have a significantly higher coronal DFS as compared with non-Caucasians. For example, the NHANES III survey reported that Caucasians had a mean coronal DFS twice as high as that of African-Americans (i.e., 24 surfaces and 12 surfaces, respectively).[23] However, although recent surveys have estimated that the proportion of untreated coronal caries for the entire U.S. population is less than 10%, this proportion is about three times higher in African-American adults than in Caucasians.[11,23]

The prevalence of coronal caries has declined during the past 25 years among U.S. adults younger than 45 years.[24] Actual prevalence estimates vary widely, but a decrease in the prevalence of coronal caries among adults has also been observed in other Western countries.[19,20,25]

DESCRIPTIVE FINDINGS: ROOT SURFACE CARIES

Wide variation in the methods used to diagnose and report root surface caries, in particular in the case definition used, has made the comparison of findings from different investigations challenging.[26-29] This had led to estimates of root caries prevalence that vary widely.[28] The two most recent U.S. national adult surveys suggest that between 20% and 25% of U.S. adults have at least one root surface that has been affected by caries.[11,23] This prevalence is virtually identical between Caucasians and African-Americans, as is the average root surface DFS, which is approximately equal to one surface.[11,23] The prevalence of root caries increases with age.[11,23,28,30] For example, the findings of the most recent national survey show the prevalence of root surface caries rising steadily from 7% among 18- to 24-year-olds to 56% among those 75 years and older.[23] In contrast to coronal caries, the proportion of untreated root surfaces caries can be quite high (e.g., 50% in the most recent U.S. national survey).[23] As is the case with coronal caries, minorities have a much higher proportion of untreated root surfaces compared with Caucasians.[23] It is important to note that, as with coronal caries, the prevalence and incidence of root caries are lower in areas served by fluoridated drinking water.[28]

In the absence of an underlying pathologic condition, root surfaces are not exposed to the oral environment and are therefore not at risk of carious attack. Thus although root surface DFS is a useful prevalence measure, root caries incidence is best measured in terms of root surfaces at risk.[29,31-33] The Root Caries Index (RCI), which counts only exposed root surfaces as being at risk for root surface caries, was developed to address this important issue.[31,32]

POLARIZATION OF CARIES AND RISK ASSESSMENT

Descriptive caries data indicate that in addition to a marked decrease in the prevalence of caries, there has been a change in the pattern of dental caries in the United States and other countries, with most of the caries occurring in 20% to 30% of the population.[13,34,35] For example, the recent NHANES III survey found that 80% of the total DMFT for children aged 5 to 17 years occurred within 25% of the children.[13] In recent years these findings have led to attempts to develop methods and models to identify those at high risk for future caries attack risk from a population generally at low risk.[36-45]

The concept that caries is a multifactoral disease has long been understood and accepted,[46] and individual factors affecting the risk for caries have been identified for many years. These factors include the presence of specific microorganisms, for example, *Streptococcus mutans*; dietary factors, such as the proportion and frequency of dietary carbohydrate; salivary factors, for example, salivary flow rate; and host factors, such as age and health behaviors.[36,47] In recent years a series of analytic epidemiologic investigations have been conducted in an effort to identify comprehensive models of future coronal caries risk[36-45]; however, the complex multifactoral nature of the caries process makes this a challenging task. To date, past caries experience (i.e., DFS), and salivary *S. mutans* and *Lactobacillus* levels have been found to be the best predictors of future coronal caries risk.[37-45] Studies have also identified sugar consumption as an indicator of future caries risk.[48,49] Studies indicate that factors such as fluoridation status, past root caries experience, age, number of teeth, gingival recession, number of decayed coronal surfaces, and use of sugared foods are predictors of root surface caries.[28,49,50]

Epidemiology of periodontal disease

Periodontal diseases have been defined by Loe as "a group of lesions affecting the tissues surrounding and supporting the teeth in their sockets."[51] The majority of periodontal disease cases can be classified as either *gingivitis* or *periodontitis*. Gingivitis is a disease characterized by inflammation restricted to the gingival soft tissues, with no loss of alveolar bone or apical migration of the periodontal ligament along the root surface.[52] Clinically, the signs of gingivitis are erythema, edema, and gingival bleeding.[52] Periodontitis is characterized by inflammation that extends beyond the gingiva to the periodontal structures, causing destruction of the periodontal ligament attachment and alveolar bony support and leading to migration of the junctional epithelium apical to the cementoenamel junction (CEJ).[53,54] The two main types of periodontitis are *adult-onset periodontitis* and *early-onset periodontitis*.[54] Clinically the signs of periodontitis can include loss of soft tissue attachment, gingival recession, tooth migration, mobility, and tooth loss.[52,55,56] Most cases of gingivitis and periodontitis occur as a result of the presence of bacterial plaque on the gingiva and subgingival tooth surfaces and calculus.[53] It is generally accepted that periodontal disease begins as gingivitis, which progresses, *only in some individuals,* to periodontitis.[52]

MEASUREMENT OF PERIODONTAL DISEASE

Historically, several indexes were developed in an attempt to provide a standardized method of measuring periodontal disease among groups of people in epidemiologic studies, most notably the Periodontal Index (PI),[57] the Periodontal Disease Index (PDI),[58] and the Gingival Index (GI).[59,60] The PI and the PDI both combine gingivitis and periodontitis into a single tooth score or average score for the individual or group. The PI identifies two levels of gingivitis, depending on its extent, and two severity levels of periodontal destruction, depending on the severity of periodontal destruction.[57] Criticisms of this index are that all assessments are made visually, with no periodontal probe being used, and that it combines the gingivitis and periodontitis scores.[61] The PDI, a modification of the PI, measures gingivitis and periodontitis separately, but, similarly to the PI, it combines these measures to generate an overall score

for the individual. The PDI differs from the PI in that it distinguishes three levels of gingivitis severity based both on the *extent* of the inflammation around the tooth and the *severity* of the inflammation.[58] The PDI also differs from the PI in its measurement of periodontitis by quantitatively measuring loss of attachment with a periodontal probe, defining degrees of periodontitis severity based on the amount of attachment lost. A total score for the individual is achieved by averaging the individual tooth scores.[58] The PDI suffers the same criticism as the PI in that it combines gingivitis and periodontitis measures into a common score.[61,62]

The GI was introduced to provide an index that solely measured inflammation of the gingiva and would allow a clear distinction to be made between the location or quantity of gingivitis and the severity or quality of the gingivitis.[59,60] The GI accomplishes this by applying a four-category qualitative assessment (normal, mild, moderate, or severe inflammation) to four sites on each examined tooth. These values can then be averaged to yield a score for the individual.[59,60] The GI has become a mainstay index of gingivitis over the past 30 years.[63] At the same time it has become generally accepted that periodontitis should be measured and reported separately from gingivitis, and quantitatively in terms of loss of periodontal attachment (LPA) measured in millimeters.[61] For example, recent U.S. national surveys have reported the prevalence and extent of periodontitis in terms of LPA measured in millimeters.[11,64]

Another index that has gained considerable international popularity in recent years is the Community Periodontal Index of Treatment Needs (CPITN), which was developed by the World Health Organization to provide a means to summarize treatment needs.[65,66] The CPITN combines an assessment of gingival health, pocket depth, and the presence of supragingival and subgingival calculus.[65,66] Proponents of the CPITN state that it allows for a rapid, simple, uniform method by which the average periodontal status and treatment needs of international populations can be determined with minimal equipment.[67] It has been further argued that the use of a widely understood index facilitates the formulation of international goals for periodontal health.[67] During the approximately 15 years since its introduction, the CPITN has been used in more than 100 countries to generate data for the WHO Global Oral Data Bank.[67] However, critics of the CPITN argue that the combination of gingival health, pocket depth, and the presence of calculus into a combined score is not consistent with current approaches to describing periodontal disease and that failure of the CPITN to measure gingival recession and pocket depth leads to an inaccurate estimate of attachment loss.[61]

The varied use of these different indexes in surveys of periodontal disease has made direct comparison of the findings from one survey to another difficult. In epidemiology this situation illustrates the importance of how a disease is measured and how a case of the disease is defined. Nevertheless, some broad conclusions can be drawn from these data. The two most recent U.S. national surveys (NIDR U.S. Employed Adult Survey[11] and the NHANES III survey[64]) used similar methodologies, allowing a comparison to be made. Although the NHANES III survey included a broader age range of individuals (younger as well as older) compared with the subjects in the U.S. Employed Adult Survey, the findings from the two surveys can be seen as fairly similar.

DESCRIPTIVE FINDINGS: GINGIVITIS

Both national surveys suggest that the prevalence of gingivitis declines from its highest during the second and third decades and remains relatively constant after the age of 30 years.[11,64] The surveys differ in their estimates of the prevalence of gingivitis; the U.S. Employed Adult survey reported an average gingivitis prevalence of 44%,[11] compared with the NHANES III estimated gingivitis prevalence of 63%.[64] These surveys also reported that from one half to two thirds of U.S. adults have subgingival calculus, affecting between 22% and 34% of available sites per person.[11,64]

DESCRIPTIVE FINDINGS: ADULT-ONSET PERIODONTITIS

Adult periodontitis (AP) is the most common form of that disease.[68] Significant disease associated with AP usually does not occur before the age of 35.[68] The two recent national surveys both suggest that the loss of some attachment is virtually ubiquitous among U.S. adults. The prevalence estimate for having at least one site with ≥1 mm of LPA was between 92.5% (NHANES III)[64] and 99.7% (U.S. Employed Adult Survey).[11] However, the two surveys are consistent in suggesting that both the prevalence and extent of more severe attachment loss are markedly lower.[11,64] Although the prevalence of LPA of ≥3 mm among U.S. adults is approximately 40% to 45%, the prevalence of LPA ≥5 mm is less than 15%.[11,64] Similarly, whereas between 7% and 10% of available sites had lost at least 3 mm of attachment, fewer than 3% had lost as much as 5 mm or more.[11,64]

Periodontal disease is recognized as an important cause of gingival recession.[56] The U.S. Employed Adult Survey reported 51% of individuals to have at least one site with ≥1 mm of recession, affecting on average 10% of available sites.[11] Similarly, the NHANES III survey reported this prevalence to be 42%, affecting 11% of available sites.[64]

In both surveys men were found to be more likely to have attachment loss and gingival recession.[11,64] The Employed Adult Survey reported African-Americans to have a higher prevalence of attachment loss and gingival recession compared with Caucasians.[11] The NHANES III data suggest that African-Americans were more likely to have more severe attachment loss (i.e., ≥3 mm) and more severe gingival recession (i.e., ≥3 mm) compared with Caucasians.[64] Socioeconomic factors appear to play an important role in these observed racial differences.[69]

Although most cases of adult periodontitis respond to therapies designed to remove bacterial plaque, some cases of AP are characterized by continued disease progression in the presence of low plaque scores.[70] The term *refractory periodontitis* was introduced to characterized this form of periodontitis that does not respond to plaque removal therapy.[70,71] However, the lack of a clear case definition, including an adequate description of its biologic and clinical features, has hindered the understanding of this form of periodontitis.[72]

DESCRIPTIVE FINDINGS: EARLY-ONSET PERIODONTITIS

Early-onset periodontitis (EOP) is a global category that refers to periodontitis that occurs before the age of 35 years, has a rapid rate of progression, and displays familial aggregation.[54,62] Several categories of EOP have been described, including periodontitis associated with systemic disease (prepubertal periodontitis), localized juvenile periodontitis, generalized juvenile periodontitis, and rapidly progressive periodontitis.[62,73] However, to date much of what is known about some of these diseases has been based on relatively limited case studies. Thus the case definitions and specific terminology associated with EOP have continued to evolve rapidly in recent years.

Prepubertal periodontitis (PP) is believed to have its onset shortly after the eruption of the primary teeth and affects both the primary and permanent dentition.[62] In the limited number of cases studied to date, PP demonstrates familial aggregation,[74] with most cases of PP associated with systemic disease, such as leukocyte adherence deficiency.[68] A recent position paper by the American Academy of Periodontology has placed PP under the heading of periodontitis associated with systemic disease, although the position paper acknowledges that

systemic disease has not been identified in all cases of PP.[73] The epidemiology of PP in the general population has not been determined.[62]

Juvenile periodontitis (JP) is characterized by gingival inflammation, severe angular bony defects, and marked loss of periodontal attachment during adolescence.[62] Two forms of JP have been identified, a localized form involving the incisors and first molars and a generalized form involving other teeth.[62] JP is a rare disease, with most reports indicating a prevalence of between 1 and 8 cases per 1000.[62,75-78] A recent U.S. national survey estimated that the prevalence of all forms of JP was 6.6 cases per 1000, 80% of which were cases of localized JP.[62] The incidence rate for all forms of JP among U.S. 14- to 15-year-olds was 1.3 cases per 1000 individuals at risk.[62] Familial aggregation of JP cases has been established.[79,80] Although some studies have suggested that the prevalence is higher in female than in male patients,[75,77] other studies have not found this relationship,[76,78] most notably the recent U.S. national survey.[62] Some studies have reported important racial differences in prevalence.[62,76] The recent 1986-1987 U.S. survey found African-Americans to be 15 to 22 times more likely than Caucasians to have JP, depending on whether it was localized or generalized.[62]

Rapidly progressive periodontitis (RPP) has been defined as occurring between puberty and age 35.[81] One challenge in the study of the epidemiology of RPP has been the difficulty in distinguishing it from the generalized form of JP.[68] The recent position paper of the AAP categorizes RPP as synonymous with generalized JP,[73] which would give it a prevalence in the United States of 1.3 cases per 1000.[62]

RISK ASSESSMENT INVESTIGATIONS

Although there has long been a consensus that bacteria are essential for gingivitis and periodontitis to occur,[51,82,83] there is also a consensus that most gingivitis does not become periodontitis.[52] Considerable attention has been given in recent years to attempting to develop models that will predict which *individuals* and which *sites within individuals* will progress to periodontitis. In this regard periodontitis is considered to have multiple risk factors. These factors can be divided into three groups: host factors, specific bacteria, and environmental factors.[83] Host factors include factors such as increasing age and the presence of systemic disease, for example, diabetes mellitus.[83,84] A number of specific bacteria have been found to be strongly associated with periodontitis, for example, *Porphyromonas gingivalis* and *Actinobacillus actinomycetemcomitans*.[81,82] Environmental risk factors for periodontitis include such factors as poor oral hygiene, the presence of subgingival calculus, and smoking, a habit that has been shown to be an important environmental risk factor for periodontitis.[85-88] Although specific factors associated with periodontitis have been identified, important questions remain. For example, it has been observed that specific bacteria often may be isolated from individuals with severe periodontitis, but these same bacteria can also be found in individuals free of disease.[82,83] Models that have been developed to date are not yet able to satisfactorily separate persons and individual sites within persons that are at high risk of future periodontitis from those that are at low risk,[89] although the extent of previous disease may be helpful in identifying persons who will experience further disease.[90] One complicating aspect of this search for a comprehensive model by which risk for periodontitis can be assessed has been the realization that there are likely multiple diseases currently existing under the name of adult periodontitis.[90] Thus an important step in the process of risk assessment for periodontitis may be a refinement of case definitions for periodontitis.

Epidemiology of tooth mortality

Tooth loss among children and adults in the United States has been declining for many years.[91,92] Edentulism has become uncommon, affecting 11% of all adults or less, depending on the survey.[11,92] More than 30% of U.S. adults retain all of their teeth (excluding third molars).[11,93] Tooth loss is higher elsewhere in the world.[94-97]

The loss of teeth is age related, with the average number of retained teeth decreasing and the prevalence of edentulism increasing as age increases.[11,92,93,98-102] Even so, U.S. adults retain more than 75% of their teeth as late as the seventh decade of life,[11,93] and even the most elderly are retaining more than half of their teeth.[11,93,99-101] Recent studies suggest that tooth loss is not associated with gender.[11,93,98-100,102]

The principal reported cause of tooth loss across all ages in the United States is caries,[103,104] which has been generally found to be the most common cause of tooth loss in other countries throughout the world.[105-114] However, studies suggest that after age 45 periodontal disease is an important cause of tooth loss,[104-107,111-114] with some studies suggesting that it becomes the most common cause of tooth loss in this age group.[106,107,113,114] Studies further suggest that tooth loss is associated with lower socioeconomic level.[91,92,102,103,115-117]

Epidemiology of oral cancer
DESCRIPTIVE FINDINGS

Approximately 30,000 new cases of oral and pharyngeal cancer are diagnosed annually in the United States,[118] the majority of which are squamous cell carcinoma, as is true in other parts of the world.[119-122] Oral and pharyngeal cancer accounts for 3% of new cancers among men and 2% of new cancers among women.[118] There are approximately 8000 deaths each year in the United States that occur as the result of oral and pharyngeal cancer, representing 2% of all cancer deaths among men (3.6 per 100,000 men during 1990-1992) and 1% of all cancer deaths among women (1.3 per 100,000 women during 1990-1992).[118] Internationally, oral and pharyngeal cancer mortality rates vary markedly. For example, during the 1990-1993 period, the age-adjusted oral cancer mortality rate in men in The Netherlands was 2.8 per 100,000, contrasted with 12.9 per 100,000 in France.[118]

The incidence of oral and pharyngeal cancers increases with age and is relatively uncommon before the age of 40.[123] Table 9-1 illustrates the variation in incidence rates for oral and pharyngeal cancer in the United States associated with anatomic site, race, and gender. Cancers of the lip and oral cavity account for about two thirds of all incident (new) oral and pharyngeal cancers, with the tongue being the most common site of incident cancers of the oral cavity. The overall incidence rate of oral

and pharyngeal cancer is higher among men compared with women. Although Caucasians have a markedly higher incidence rate for lip cancer, overall male African-Americans show the highest oral and pharyngeal cancer incidence rates, with rates markedly higher for pharyngeal sites.

Overall the 5-year survival rate for oral and pharyngeal cancers is about 50%. However, survival rates for oral and pharyngeal cancer vary considerably depending on cancer site, gender, and race. This variance is illustrated in Table 9-2, which shows that although 5-year survival rates for cancer of the lip are about

Table 9-1. Age-adjusted oral and pharyngeal cancer incidence rates (per 100,000) in the United States stratified by gender, race, and selected anatomic sites, 1983-1987

Site	White males	Black males	All males	White females	Black females	All females	All persons
Lip	3.0	0.1	2.7	0.3	0.1	0.3	1.4
Tongue	3.2	4.9	3.3	1.4	1.5	1.4	2.3
Floor of mouth	1.9	3.2	1.9	0.7	0.6	0.7	1.3
Total oral cavity	11.8	12.7	11.6	4.7	4.3	4.6	7.7
Total pharynx	5.0	11.8	5.7	1.8	2.7	1.9	3.6
TOTAL (oral cavity and pharynx)	16.8	24.5	17.3	6.5	7.0	6.5	11.3

Modified from US Department of Health and Human Services: *Cancers of the oral cavity and pharynx: a statistics review monograph 1973-1987,* Atlanta, 1991, Centers for Disease Control and Prevention.

Table 9-2. Oral cancer 5-year survival rates (percent) in the United States stratified by gender, race, and selected anatomic sites, 1981-1986

Site	White males	Black males	All males	White females	Black females	All females	All persons
Lip	91.1	*	91.1	84.5	*	83.7	90.2
Tongue	45.8	19.8	42.8	49.7	43.7	49.1	45.0
Floor of mouth	52.9	31.0	49.8	60.7	44.9	59.2	52.9
Pharynx	31.0	22.3	30.9	38.4	26.4	37.5	32.9
Total oral cavity and pharynx	52.0	26.8	49.0	56.3	42.5	54.8	50.9

Modified from US Department of Health and Human Services: *Cancers of the oral cavity and pharynx: a statistics review monograph 1973-1987,* Atlanta, 1991, Centers for Disease Control and Prevention.
*Valid survival rates could not be calculated because of the small number of cases.

90%, the survival rate for cancers of the tongue is about half that when all persons are considered together and is only about 20% among male African-Americans, who have the overall poorest oral cancer survival rates. Female subjects tend to have higher survival rates, with the exception of cancer of the lip. Although pharyngeal cancers account for only about one third of all incident oral and pharyngeal cancers, they have a relatively poor survival rate, accounting for nearly 50% of all deaths attributed to oral and pharyngeal cancer.[123] Although survival rates among female African-Americans and Caucasians have remained relatively constant during the past 20 years, the survival rate among male African-Americans may have declined.[123]

RISK FACTORS AND PROTECTIVE FACTORS

Smoking tobacco and drinking alcoholic beverages have both been shown to increase the risk of oral and pharyngeal cancer, based on consistent evidence from many studies, conducted by different researchers, across many different populations.[124-133] A dose-response relationship has also been demonstrated between both smoking and drinking and oral cancer, with a history of heavy smoking or heavy drinking over many years having been shown to convey a strong risk of oral cancer.[124-133] Importantly, many studies have demonstrated that a history of both smoking and drinking conveys an increased risk of oral cancer that is greater than the sum of the increased risks associated with either smoking or drinking alone.[124,126-129,131] At the same time studies have reported that high fruit consumption is associated with a decreased risk of oral cancer.[134]

Smoking and drinking account for 75% of the oral cancer in the United States and the world.[124,135] It is important therefore that studies have also demonstrated that when smoking is discontinued, the risk for oral cancer, adjusted for drinking, decreases over time to levels similar to that of people who have never smoked.[124,126,129,130,132] This evidence suggests that many cases of oral cancer are preventable.

More than 12 million people use smokeless tobacco in the United States, and the use of smokeless tobacco continues to increase, especially among young men.[136] Use of smokeless tobacco has also been shown to be a risk factor for oral cancer.[133,136,137] A study of U.S. female snuff dippers reported a very strong risk of cancer of the gingiva and buccal mucosa associated with this habit.[133]

Local intraoral factors such as oral hygiene, inadequate dentition, mouthwash use, and the wearing of dentures have been suspected as risk factors for oral cancer. However, studies that have investigated this question have produced inconclusive findings.[125,128,129]

Epidemiology of oral manifestations of HIV infection

The World Health Organization estimates that worldwide approximately 10 million people have been infected with the human immunodeficiency virus (HIV).[138] About half a million cases of acquired immunodeficiency syndrome (AIDS) had been diagnosed in the United States through December 1995, including about 7000 children younger than age 13.[139] Sexual contact and use of injected drugs continue to account for the majority of AIDS cases in U.S. adults,[139] whereas more than 90% of the pediatric AIDS cases in the United States have been children born to HIV-infected mothers.[140] Oral lesions are among the earliest signs of infection with HIV.[141] Oral lesions associated with HIV infection include those of fungal, bacterial, and viral origin, as well as neoplastic lesions.[142] Oral candidiasis, a fungal infection most often associated with *Candida albicans,* is highly prevalent among those infected with HIV.[141-143] Estimates of the prevalence of oral candidiasis among HIV-infected adults range between 30% and 50%, and it is the first sign of infection in about 10% of HIV-infected adults.[142] Estimates for the prevalence of oral candidiasis in HIV-infected children range between 25% and 72%.[143]

Oral hairy leukoplakia (OHL) is a white lesion found predominantly on the lateral borders of the tongue.[141] The Epstein-Barr virus has been found to be associated with the occurrence of OHL.[141,142] OHL occurs most often in HIV-infected adults and only rarely is found in uninfected individuals.[141] Although OHL is present in approximately 25% of HIV-infected adults, it is rare in HIV-infected children, with an estimated prevalence of 2%.[143]

Herpes simplex virus (HSV) infections are common in HIV-infected patients, with an estimated prevalence of between 10% and 20%.[142] Chronic recurrent herpetic lesions are the most common viral infection in HIV-infected children.[143,144] HSV infections can appear as gingivostomatitis or as vesicles that rupture to form ulcers.[143,144]

The most frequent oral malignancy associated with AIDS is Kaposi's sarcoma (KS).[145] KS is an endothelial cell multicentric neoplasm that appears as a red, blue, or purple nodule or nodules.[142] The oral cavity may be the sole site of KS in the AIDS patient.[142] However, the prevalence of KS among AIDS patients has been steadily declining and is currently seen in about 14% of adult male AIDS patients.[145] KS is rarely observed in HIV-infected women and children.[145]

Non-Hodgkin's lymphoma (NHL) is the second most common AIDS-associated malignancy.[142,145] NHL is found in approximately 3% of AIDS patients[145]; however, the prevalence has been increasing as survival times have increased.[141,145] The Epstein-Barr virus has been identified in the majority of these lesions, which appear clinically as a solitary mass or ulcer.[141,145] To date NHL has not been reported in children.[144]

Two forms of periodontal disease unique to HIV-infected patients have been described:

HIV-associated gingivitis (HIV-G) and HIV-associated periodontitis (HIV-P).[146] HIV-G is characterized by a linear band of erythema affecting the gingival margin.[147] HIV-P has been described as being characterized by pain, bleeding, soft tissue necrosis, and rapid destruction of periodontal attachment.[147] Studies of HIV-G in adults have generally estimated the prevalence between 5% and 30%.[148-150] HIV-G has also been reported in HIV-infected children.[143] The prevalence of HIV-P, if it truly exists as a distinct disease entity, is apparently rare.[146,148,149] More properly controlled studies, using unbiased representative sampling methods and rigorous scientific methodology, need to be conducted to clarify the epidemiology of periodontal disease in HIV-infected people.[151]

Epidemiology of temporomandibular disorders

Temporomandibular disorders (TMD) is a term that has been used to refer to a set of signs and symptoms associated with a broad group of underlying disorders.[152] Historically, the signs and symptoms most often related to TMD are pain, either in the temporomandibular joint (TMJ) area or in the muscles of mastication; limitation or deviations in the range of mandibular motion; or noises in the TMJ during mandibular function.[152,153] This definition is manifestational and is based on signs and symptoms only, in contrast with an etiologic definition based on underlying cause or causes. However, it is known that the signs and symptoms of TMD may be related to a host of underlying causes.[154] Therefore, although the epidemiology of these disorders have been extensively investigated,[152] the absence of a consensus on case definitions and methodology has made interpretation of findings difficult, if not impossible.[152,155,156] As recently as 1992, Dworkin and Le Resche[157] commented that diagnostic methodologies of demonstrated reliability and validity did not exist for TMD. In their meta-analysis of 51 TMD studies, DeKanter et al.[158] reported that 25% of the studies gave no case definition for TMD at all, about half of the studies failed to identify the population studied, and only 12% reported assessing the reliability of their methods. Not surprisingly, these 51 studies report a range for TMD prevalence of between 6% and 93%.[158] The limited value of these findings to elucidate the true prevalence of these disorders is self-evident and suggests that these studies have been investigating disorders of differing causes, all under the same manifestational label of TMD.[156]

It has been estimated that one in three adults will have pain in the temporomandibular region for some period of time during their lifetime.[159] A serious concern associated with this confusion over case definitions is that some patients may undergo care that is ineffective and perhaps harmful.[159] This is especially true because most articles pertaining to TMD therapy are not reports of controlled clinical trials, the standard for evaluating new therapy, and these articles have not reported findings on the outcomes from the treatments they describe.[160] Recently a new set of diagnostic criteria for research studies has been introduced entitled Research Diagnostic Criteria for Temporomandibular Disorders (RDC/TMD).[161] The RDC/TMD were developed in an attempt to rectify the lack of standardized diagnostic criteria by which the different etiologic disorders, previously all labeled simply "TMD," could be defined.[161] The RDC/TMD provides criteria by which three main groups as well as subgroups of TMD disorders can be identified. In brief, the groups identified are as follows: (1) myofacial pain, either with or without limited opening; (2) disk displacements often with associated TMJ clicking and limitation of mandibular movement; and (3) pain and tenderness in the joint capsule and/or the synovial lining of the TMJ, osteoarthritis of the TMJ, or degenerative disorder of the TMJ.[161] Ultimately, practical

standardized diagnostic methods will need to be available for use by the clinician.[155]

Epidemiology of enamel fluorosis

Enamel fluorosis is a subsurface enamel hypomineralization or porosity that occurs when a child ingests an above-optimum level of fluoride while enamel formation is occurring.[162] Clinically, the appearance of enamel fluorosis can vary from faint paper-white flecks in its mildest presentation to more noticeable snow-flaking or mottling of the enamel, sometimes with accompanying brown staining of the enamel. Enamel fluorosis is an aesthetic concern, except in the most severe cases in which pitting of the enamel or loss of enamel integrity can occur. A number of indexes have been developed to measure enamel fluorosis. Each of these indexes has particular strengths.[163] Thus the choice of the "best" index depends on its specific use.

The contribution of fluoride to the observed long-term decline in caries prevalence has been broadly accepted.[21] Paralleling this decline in caries prevalence has been an observed increase in the prevalence of enamel fluorosis.[164] Circa 1940 the prevalence of enamel fluorosis in optimally fluoridated areas was about 16%, being mostly of the very mildest forms.[164] During the same period the prevalence of enamel fluorosis in nonfluoridated areas was on average less than 1%. By conservative estimate, during the past 20 years the prevalence of fluorosis has increased on average 43% (7 percentage points) in fluoridated areas and 10-fold in nonfluoridated areas.[164] At the same time some studies have reported an increase in the severity of fluorosis that is being observed.[165,166]

Because the goal of fluoride use in dentistry has always been to achieve the maximum benefit with minimum side effects, a series of investigations with analytical epidemiologic techniques have sought to identify the specific causes or risk factors for this increase in enamel fluorosis prevalence. Enamel is at risk of developing fluorosis only during its formation. Therefore only the ingestion of fluoride during the first 6 to 8 years of life can be a risk factor for fluorosis. The use of multifactoral analyses has been important because there are numerous potential sources of ingested fluoride during early childhood.[164] Because of the inherent long follow-up required in fluorosis investigations (i.e., exposure can occur during the first year of life, but the permanent teeth do not even begin to erupt until about the age of 6), most of these studies have used a case-control design. Ultimately the criteria for a judgment of causation have been applied as decisions and recommendations have been made concerning the best future use of fluorides for the prevention of caries.

Although the studies that have been conducted have been of variable quality, some consistent patterns have emerged. The use of fluoride supplements during the first 6 to 8 years by children living in nonfluoridated areas have been consistently shown to be strongly associated with enamel fluorosis.[166-168] The use of fluoride supplements by children living in fluoridated areas, an inappropriate practice, not surprisingly has been shown to be very strongly associated with enamel fluorosis.[165] Several studies have also demonstrated an association between the use of fluoride toothpaste by preschool children and enamel fluorosis.[165,166,169-171] These findings are coherent with other research, which has indicated that preschool children tend to swallow much of the dentifrice they put into their mouths[172] and that the majority of the fluoride thus ingested is absorbed into the gastrointestinal tract.[173] Studies have further demonstrated that the use of infant formula before 1979 was also an important enamel fluorosis risk factor.[165,169,170]

The findings of these studies have led to a joint decision in 1994 by the American Dental Association and the American Academy of Pediatrics to reduce the fluoride supplement dosage schedule.[174,175] These findings have also supported the recommendation that parents supervise their preschool children during brushing to ensure that only a pea-size amount of toothpaste is used and to encourage the child to spit out the toothpaste, not swallow it. In addition, there has also been a call by some dental researchers for the introduction of a reduced-fluoride dentifrice specifically for use by preschool children.[176,177] In 1979, based on early evidence, the manufacturers of infant formula in the United States voluntarily agreed to regulate the fluoride concentration of their products at a low level.[178] The findings from a recently published investigation suggest that this action may have been sufficient to eliminate formula ingestion as an enamel fluorosis risk factor, at least in nonfluoridated areas.[166]

Acknowledgments

The author wishes to thank Dr. Ralph Katz, Dr. Douglas Morse, and Dr. Anthony Neely for their very helpful suggestions during the preparation of this manuscript.

REFERENCES

1. Black GV, McKay FS: Mottled teeth: an endemic developmental imperfection of the enamel of the teeth heretofore unknown in the literature of dentistry, *Dental Cosmos* 58:129-156, 1916.
2. MacMahon B, Pugh TF: *Epidemiology: principles and methods*, Boston, 1970, Little, Brown.
3. Henekins CH, Buring JE: *Epidemiology in medicine*, Boston, 1987, Little, Brown.
4. Monson RR: *Occupational epidemiology*, Boca Raton, Fla, 1990, CRC Press.
5. Schlesselman JJ: *Case-control studies*, New York, 1982, Oxford University Press.
6. Ast DB, Finn SB, McCaffrey I: The Newburgh-Kingston Caries Fluorine Study. I. Dental findings after three years of water fluoridation, *Am J Public Health* 40:716-724, 1950.

7. Newbrun E: *Cariology,* ed 3, Chicago, 1989, Quintessence.
8. Klein H, Palmer C, Knutson JW: Studies of dental caries. I. Dental status and dental needs of elementary school children, *Public Health Rep* 53:751-765, 1938.
9. Gruebbel AO: A meaurement of dental caries prevalence and treatment service for deciduous teeth, *J Dent Res* 23:163-168, 1994.
10. US Department of Health and Human Services: *Oral health of United States children: the National Survey of Dental Caries in U.S. School Children: 1986-1987,* National Institutes of Health Pub No. 89-2247, Washington, DC, 1989, US Government Printing Office.
11. US Department of Health and Human Services: *Oral health of United States adults: the National Survey of Oral Health in U.S. Employed Adults and Seniors: 1985-1986,* National Institutes of Health Pub No 87-2868, Washington, DC, 1987, US Government Printing Office.
12. National Center for Health Statistics: *Decayed, missing and filled teeth among persons 1-74 years: United States,* Vital and Health Statistics, series 11, No 223, DHHS Pub No (PHS) 81-1673, Washington, DC, 1981, US Government Printing Office.
13. Kaste LM et al: Coronal caries in the primary and permanent dentition of children and adolescents 1-17 years of age: United States, 1988-1991, *J Dent Res* 75(Special issue):633-641, 1996.
14. Graves RC, Stamm JW: Oral health status in the United States: prevalence of dental caries, *J Dent Educ* 49:341-351, 1985.
15. Newbrun E: Effectiveness of water fluoridation, *J Public Health Dent* 49(Special issue):279- 289, 1989.
16. Levy SM: Review of fluoride exposures and ingestion, *Commun Dent Oral Epidemiol* 22:173-180, 1994.
17. Newbrun E: Current regulations and recommendations concerning water fluoridation, fluoride supplements, and topical fluoride agents, *J Dent Res* 71:1255-1265, 1992.
18. Brunelle JA, Carlos JP: Changes in the prevalence of dental caries in U.S. schoolchildren, 1961-1980, *J Dent Res* 61:1346-1351, 1982.
19. Marthaler TM: The prevalence of dental caries in Europe 1990-1995, *Caries Res* 30:237-255, 1996.
20. Spencer AJ and others: Caries prevalence in Australasia, *Int Dent J* 44:415-423, 1994.
21. Brunelle JA, Carlos JP: Recent trends in dental caries in U.S. children and the effect of water fluoridation, *J Dent Res* 69:723-727, 1990.
22. Ripa L: Nursing caries: a comprehensive review, *Pediatr Dent* 10:268-282, 1988.
23. Winn DM and others: Coronal and root caries in the dentition of adults in the United States, 1988-1991, *J Dent Res* 75(Special issue):642-651, 1996.
24. Brown LJ, Swango PA: Trends in caries experience in U.S. employed adults from 1971-1985: cross-sectional comparisons, *Adv Dent Res* 7:52-60, 1993.
25. Downer MC: Changing trends in dental caries experience in Great Britain, *Adv Dent Res* 7:19-24, 1993.
26. DePaola PF and others: Methodological issues relative to the quantification of root surface caries, *Gerodontology* 8:3-8, 1989.
27. Aherne CA, O'Mullane D, Barrett BE: Indices of root surface caries, *J Dent Res* 69:1222-1226, 1990.
28. Beck JD: The epidemiology of root surface caries: North American studies, *Adv Dent Res* 7:42-51, 1993.
29. Banting DW: Diagnosis and prediction of root caries, *Adv Dent Res* 7:80-86, 1993.
30. Fejerskov O, Baelum V, Ostergarrd ES: Root caries in Scandinavia in the 1980s and future trends to be expected in dental caries experience in adults, *Adv Dent Res* 7:4-14, 1993.
31. Katz RV: A method for scoring and reporting root caries in epidemiologic studies, *J Dent Res* 58:389, 1979.
32. Katz RV: Prevalence and intraoral distribution of root caries in an adult population, *Caries Res* 16:265-271, 1982.
33. Lawrence HP and others: Five-year incidence rates and intraoral distribution of root caries among community-dwelling older adults, *Caries Res* 30:169-179, 1996.
34. Nordblad A: Changes in epidemiologic pattern of dental caries in cohorts of schoolchildren in Espoo, Finland, during a 3-year period, *Community Dent Oral Epidemiol* 14:126-127, 1986.
35. Winter GB: Epidemiology of dental caries, *Arch Oral Biol* 35(Suppl):1S-7S, 1990.
36. Winter GB: Prediction of high caries risk–diet, hygiene and medication, *Int Dent J* 38:227-230, 1988.
37. Grindefjord M and others: Stepwise prediction of dental caries in children up to 3.5 years of age, *Caries Res* 30:256-266, 1996.
38. Krasse B: Biological factors as indicators of future caries, *Int Dent J* 38: 1988.
39. Alaluusua S: Salivary counts of Mutans Streptococci and Lactobacilli and past caries experience in caries prediction, *Caries Res* 27(Suppl 1):68-71, 1993.
40. Holbrook WP, de Soet JJ, de Graaff J: Prediction of dental caries in pre-school children, *Caries Res* 27:424-430, 1993.
41. Thibodeau EA, O'Sullivan DM: Salivary Mutans Streptococci and incidence of caries in preschool children, *Caries Res* 29:148-153, 1995.
42. Reisine S, Litt M, Tinanoff N: A biopsychosocial model to predict caries in preschool children, *Pediatr Dent* 16:413-418, 1994.
43. van Houte J: Microbial predictors of caries risk, *Adv Dent Res* 7:87-96, 1993.

44. Demers M and others: A multivariate model to predict caries increment in Montreal children aged 5 years, *Community Dental Health* 9:273-281, 1992.

45. Stamm JW and others: The University of North Carolina assessment study: final results and some alternative modelling approaches. In Bowen WH, Tabak LA, editors: *Cariology for the Nineties*, Rochester, NY, 1993, University of Rochester Press, pp 210-234.

46. Navia JM: Carbohydrates and dental health, *Am J Clin Nutr* 59:719s-727s, 1994.

47. Hunter PB: Risk factors in dental caries, *Int Dent J* 38:211-217,1988.

48. Szpunar SM, Eklund SA, Burt BA: Sugar consumption and caries risk in schoolchildren with low caries experience, *Commun Dent Oral Epidemiol* 23:142-146, 1995.

49. Scheinin A and others: Multifactoral modeling for root caries prediction: 3-year follow-up results, *Community Dent Oral Epidemiol* 22:126-129, 1994.

50. Joshi A and others: The distribution of root caries in community-dwelling elders in New England, *J Public Health* 54:15-23, 1994.

51. Loe H: Periodontal diseases: a brief historical perspective, *Periodontology 2000* 2:7-12, 1993.

52. Jeffcoat MK: Prevention of periodontal diseases in adults: strategies for the future, *Prev Med* 23:704-708, 1994.

53. Genco RJ: Classification and clinical and radiographic features of periodontal disease. In Genco RJ, Goldman HM, Cohen DW, editors: *Contemporary periodontics*, St Louis, 1990, Mosby.

54. Ranney RR: Classification of periodontal diseases, *Periodontology 2000* 2:13-25, 1993.

55. Loe H and others: Natural history of periodontal disease in man, *J Clin Periodontol* 13:431- 440, 1986.

56. Loe H, Anerud A, Boysen H: The natural history of periodontal disease in man: prevalence, severity, and extent of gingival recession, *J Periodontol* 63:489-495, 1992.

57. Russell AL: The periodontal index, *J Periodontol* 38:585-591, 1967.

58. Ramfjord SP: The periodontal disease index, *J Periodontol* 38:602-610, 1967.

59. Loe H, Silness J: Periodontal disease in pregnancy. I. Prevalence and severity, *Acta Odontol Scan* 21:533-551, 1963.

60. Loe H: The Gingival Index, the Plaque Index and the Retention Index systems, *J Periodontol* 38:610-616, 1967.

61. Beck JD, Loe H: Epidemiological principles in studying periodontal diseases, *Periodontology 2000* 2:34-45, 1993.

62. Brown LJ, Loe H: Prevalence, extent, severity and progression of periodontal disease, *Periodontology 2000* 2:57-71, 1993.

63. Cinacio SG: Current status of indices of gingivitis, *J Clin Periodontol* 13:375-378, 1986.

64. Brown LJ, Brunelle JA, Kingman A: Periodontal status in the United States, 1988-91: prevalence, extent, and demographic variation, *J Dent Res* 75:672-683, 1996.

65. Ainamo J and others: Development of the World Health Organization (WHO) Community Periodontal Index of Treatment Needs (CPITN), *Int Dent J* 32:281-291, 1982.

66. Ainamo J, Ainamo A: Validity and relevance of the criteria of the CPITN, *Int Dent J* 4:527-532, 1994.

67. Pilot T, Miyazaki H: Global results: 15 years of CPITN epidemiology, *Int Dent J* 4:553-560, 1994.

68. Ranney RR: Differential diagnosis in clinical trials of therapy for periodontitis, *J Periodontol* 63:1052-1057, 1992.

69. Oliver RC, Brown LJ, Loe H: Variations in the prevalence and extent of periodontitis, *J Am Dent Assoc* 122:43-48, 1991.

70. Magnusson I, Walker CB: Refractory periodontitis or recurrence of disease, *J Clin Periodontol* 23:289-292, 1996.

71. Kornman KS, Karl EH: The effect of long-term low-dose tetracycline therapy on the subgingival microflora in refractory adult periodontitis, *J Periodontol* 53:604-610, 1982.

72. Kornman KS: Refractory periodontitis: critical questions in clinical management, *J Clin Periodontol* 23:293-298, 1996.

73. Committee on Research, Science and Therapy of the American Academy of Periodontology: Position paper: periodontal diseases of children and adolescents, *J Periodontol* 67:57-62, 1996.

74. Suzuki JB: Diagnosis and classification of the periodontal diseases, *Dent Clin North Am* 32:195-216, 1988.

75. Saxen L: Prevalence of juvenile periodontitis in Finland, *J Clin Periodontol* 7:177-186, 1980.

76. Saxby M: Prevalence of juvenile periodontitis in a British school population, *Commun Dent Oral Epidemiol* 12:185-187, 1984.

77. Lopez NJ and others: Prevalence of juvenile periodontitis in Chile, *J Clin Periodontol* 18:529-533, 1991.

78. Neely AL: Prevalence of juvenile periodontitis in a cirumpubertal population, *J Clin Periodontol* 19:367-372, 1992.

79. Michalowicz BS: Genetic and heritable risk factors in periodontal disease, *J Periodontol* 65:479-488, 1994.

80. Hart TC: Genetic risk factors for early-onset periodontitis, *J Periodontol* 67:355-366, 1996.

81. Page RC and others: Rapidly progressive periodontitis: a distinct clinical condition, *J Periodontol* 54:197-209, 1983.

82. Page RC: Critical issues in periodontal research, *J Dent Res* 74:1118-1128, 1995.

83. Wolff L, Dahlen G, Aeppli D: Bacteria as risk markers for periodontitis, *J Periodontol* 64:498-510, 1994.

84. Genco RJ, Loe H: The role of systemic conditions and disorders in periodontal disease, *Periodontology 2000* 2:98-116, 1993.

85. Kornman KS, Loe H: The role of local factors in the etiology of periodontal diseases, *Periodontology 2000* 2:83-97, 1993.

86. Haber J and others: Evidence for cigarette smoking as a major risk factor for periodontitis, *J Periodontol* 64:16-23, 1993.

87. Bergstrom J, Preber H: Tobacco use as a risk factor, *J Periodontol* 65:545-550, 1994.

88. Research, Science and Therapy Committee of the American Academy of Periodontology: Position paper: tobacco use and the periodontal patient, *J Periodontol* 67:51-56, 1996.

89. Beck JD: Methods of assessing risk for periodontitis and developing multifactoral models, *J Periodontol* 65:468-478, 1994.

90. Haffajee A, Oliver RC: Periodontal diseases working group: summary and recommendations. In Bader JD, editor: *Risk assessment in dentistry,* Chapel Hill, 1990, University of North Carolina Dental Ecology.

91. Weintraub JA, Burt BA: Oral health status in the United States: tooth loss and edentulism, *J Dent Educ* 49:368-376, 1985.

92. Marcus SE and others: Tooth retention and tooth loss in the permanent dentition of adults: United States, 1988-1991, *J Dent Res* 75:684-695, 1996.

93. Brown LJ: Trends in tooth loss among U.S. employed adults from 1971 to 1985, *J Am Dent Assoc* 125:533-540, 1994.

94. Ainamo J: Changes in the frequency of edentulousness and use of removeable dentures in the adult population of Finland, 1970-1980, *Community Dent Oral Epidemiol* 11:122-126, 1983.

95. Grabowski M, Bertram U: Oral health status and need of dental treatment in the elderly Danish population, *Commun Dent Oral Epidemiol* 3:108-114, 1975.

96. Swallow JN and others: A survey of edentulous individuals in a district in Amsterdam, the Netherlands, *Commun Dent Oral Epidemiol* 6:210-216, 1978.

97. Clarkson JJ, O'Mullane DM: Edentulousness in the United Kingdom and Ireland, *Commun Dent Oral Epidemiol* 11:317-320, 1983.

98. Katz RV, Gustavsen F: Tooth mortality in dental patients in a U.S. urban area, *Gerodontics* 2:104-107, 1986.

99. Hunt RJ and others: Edentulism and oral health problems among elderly rural Iowans: the Iowa 65+ rural health study, *Am J Public Health* 75:1177-1181, 1985.

100. Heft MW, Gilbert GH: Tooth loss and caries prevalence in older Floridians attending senior activity centers, *Commun Dent Oral Epidemiol* 19:228-232, 1991.

101. Douglass CW and others: Oral health status of the elderly in New England, *J Gerontol* 48:M39-M46, 1993.

102. Eklind SA, Burt BA: Risk factors for total tooth loss in the United States: longitudinal analysis of national data, *J Public Health Dent* 54:5-14, 1994.

103. Bailit HL, Braun R: Is periodontal disease the primary cause of tooth extraction in adults? *J Am Dent Assoc* 114:40-45, 1987.

104. Oliver RC, Brown LJ: Periodontal diseases and tooth loss, *Periodontology 2000* 2:117-127, 1993.

105. Corbet EF, Davies WIR: Reasons for tooth extractions in Hong Kong, *Commun Dental Health* 8:121-130, 1991.

106. Ong G: Periodontal reasons for tooth loss in an Asian population, *J Clin Periodontol* 23:307-309, 1996.

107. Klock KS, Huagejordan O: Primary reasons for extraction of permanent teeth in Norway: changes from 1968 to 1988, *Commun Dent Oral Epidemiol* 19:336-341, 1991.

108. Ekanayaka A: Tooth mortality in plantation workers and residents in Sri Lanka, *Commun Dent Oral Epidemiol* 12:128-135, 1984.

109. Bouma J, Schaub RMH, van de Poel ACM: Periodontal status and total tooth extraction in a medium-sized city in the Netherlands, *Commun Dent Oral Epidemiol* 13:323-327, 1985.

110. Baclum V, Fejershov: Tooth loss as related to dental caries and periodontal breakdown in adult Tanzanians, *Commun Dent Oral Epidemiol* 14:353-357, 1986.

111. Manji F, Baelum V, Fejerskov O: Tooth mortality in an adult rural population in Kenya, *J Dent Res* 67:496-500, 1988.

112. Johansen SB, Johansen JR: A survey of causes of permanent tooth extractions in South Australia, *Aust Dent J* 22:238-242, 1977.

113. Reich E, Hiller K-A: Reasons for tooth extraction in the eastern states of Germany, *Commun Dent Oral Epidemiol* 21:379-383, 1993.

114. Kay EJ, Blinkhorn AS: The reasons underlying the extraction of teeth in Scotland, *Br Dent J* 160:287-290, 1986.

115. Micheelis W, Baauch J: Oral health of representative samples of Germans examined in 1989 and 1992, *Commun Dent Oral Epidemiol* 24:62-67, 1996.

116. Bergman JD, Wright FAC, Hammond RH: The oral health of the elderly in Melbourne, *Aust Dent J* 36:280-285, 1991.

117. Marcus SE, Kaste LM, Brown LJ: Prevalence and demographic correlates of tooth loss among the elderly in the United States, *Spec Care Dent* 14:123-127, 1994.

118. Parker SL and others: Cancer statistics, *CA Cancer J Clin* 46 (Jan/Feb):5-28, 1996.

119. Muir C, Weiland L: Upper aerodigestive tract cancers, *Cancer* 75:147-153, 1995.

120. Ostman J and others: Malignant oral tumors in Sweden 1960-1989—an epidemiologic study, *Oral Oncol Eur J Cancer* 31B:106-112, 1995.

121. McCarten BE, Crowley M: Oral cancer in Ireland 1984-1988, *Oral Oncol Eur J Cancer* 29B:127-130, 1993.

122. Chen J, Katz RV, Krutchkoff DJ: Epidemiology of oral cancer in Connecticut 1935 to 1985, *Cancer* 66:2796-2802, 1990.

123. US Department of Health and Human Services: *Cancers of the oral cavity and pharynx: a statistics review monograph 1973-1987*, Atlanta, 1991, Centers for Disease Control and Prevention.

124. Blot WJ and others: Smoking and drinking in relation to oral and pharyngeal cancer, *Cancer Res* 48:3282-3287, 1988.

125. Marshall JR and others: Smoking, alcohol, dentition and diet in the epidemiology of oral cancer, *Oral Oncology, Eur J Cancer* 28B:9-15, 1992.

126. Mashberg A and others: Tobacco smoking, alcohol drinking, and cancer of the oral cavity and oropharynx among US veterans, *Cancer* 72:1369-1375, 1993.

127. Day GL and others: Pharyngeal cancer: alcohol, tobacco, and other determinants, *J Natl Cancer Inst* 85:465-473, 1993.

128. Graham S and others: Dentition, diet, tobacco, and alcohol in the epidemiology of oral cancer, *J Natl Cancer Inst* 59:1611-1618, 1977.

129. Kabat GC, Hebert JR, Wynder EL: Risk factors for oral cancer in women, *Cancer Res* 49:2803-2806, 1989.

130. Wynder EL, Stellman SD: Comparative epidemiology of tobacco-related cancers, *Cancer Res* 37:4608-4622, 1977.

131. Brugere J and others: Differential effects of tobacco and alcohol in cancer of the larynx, pharynx, and mouth, *Cancer* 57:391-395, 1986.

132. Kabat GC, Chang CJ, Wynder EL: The role of tobacco, alcohol use, and body mass index in oral and pharyngeal cancer, *Int J Epidemiol* 23:1137-1143, 1994.

133. Winn DM and others: Snuff diping and oral cancer among women in the southern United States, *N Engl J Med* 304:745-749, 1981.

134. Winn DM: Diet and nutrition in the etiology of oral cancer, *Am J Clin Nutr* 61:437S-445S, 1995.

135. Boyle P and others: European school of oncology advisory report to the European Commission for the Europe against cancer programme: oral carcinogenesis in Europe, *Oral Oncol Eur J Cancer* 31B:75-85, 1995.

136. US Department of Health and Human Services: *The health consequences of using smokeless tobacco: a report of the advisory committee to the surgeon general*, National Institutes of Health Pub No 86-2874, Bethesda, Md, 1986.

137. Winn DM: Smokeless tobacco and cancer: the epidemiologic evidence, *CA Cancer J Clin* 38:236-243, 1988.

138. Chin J: The global epidemiology of the HIV/AIDS pandemic and its projected demographic impact in Africa, *World Health Stat Q* 45:220-227, 1992.

139. US Department of Health and Human Services: *HIV/AIDS surveillance report* 7(2), Atlanta, Dec 1995, Centers for Disease Control and Prevention.

140. Davis SF and others: Prevalence and incidence of vertically acquired HIV infection in the United States, *JAMA* 247:952-955, 1995.

141. Greenspan D, Greenspan JS: Oral manifestations of human immunodeficiency virus infection, *Topics Oral Diagnosis* 37:21-32, 1993.

142. Itin PH and others: Oral manifestations in HIV-infected patients: diagnosis and management, *J Am Acad Dermatol* 29:749-760, 1993.

143. Chigururpati R, Raghavan SS, Studen-Pavlovich DA: Pediatric HIV infection and its oral manifestations: a review, *Am Acad Pediatric Dent* 18:106-113, 1996.

144. Leggott PJ: Oral manifestations of HIV infection in children, *Oral Surg Oral Med Oral Pathol* 73:187-192, 1992.

145. Ficara G, Eversole LE: HIV-related tumors of the oral cavity, *Crit Rev Oral Biol Med* 5:159-185, 1994.

146. Winkler JR and others: Periodontal disease in HIV-infected and uninfected homosexual and bisexual men, *AIDS* 6:1041-1042, 1992.

147. Winkler JR, Robinson PB: Periodontal disease assoicated with HIV infection, *Oral Surg Oral Med Oral Pathol* 73:145-150, 1992.

148. Masouredis CM and others: Prevalence of HIV-associated periodontitis and gingivitis in HIV-infected patients attending an AIDS clinic, *J Acquir Immune Defic Syndromes* 5:479-483, 1992.

149. Riley C, London JP, Burmeister JA: Periodontal health in 200 HIV-positive patients, *J Oral Pathol Med* 21:124-127, 1992.

150. Laskaris G and others: Gingival lesions of HIV infection in 178 Greek patients, *Oral Surg Oral Med Oral Pathol* 74:168-171, 1992.

151. Barr CE: Periodontal problems related to HIV-1 infection, *Adv Dent Res* 9:147-151, 1995.

152. Carlsson GE, LeResche L: Epidemiology of temporomandibular disorders. In Sessle BJ, Bryant PS, Dionne RA, editors: *Temporomandibular disorders and related pain conditions, progress in pain research and management*, vol 4, Seattle, 1995, IASP Press.

153. Dworkin SF and others: Epidemiology of signs and symptoms in temporomandibular disorders: clinical signs in cases and controls, *J Am Dent Assoc* 120:273-281, 1990.

154. Mosses AJ: Scientific methodology in temporomandibular disorders. I. epidemiology, *J Craniomandibular Pract* 12:114-119, 1994.

155. Clark GT, Delcanho RE, Goulet J-P: The utility and validity of current diagnostic procedures for defining temporomandibular disorder patients, *Adv Dent Res* 7:97-112, 1993.
156. Marbach JJ: Reaction paper. In Sessle BJ, Bryant PS, Dionne RA, editors: *Temporomandibular disorders and related pain,* Seattle, 1995, IASP Press.
157. Dworkin SF, LeResche L: Research diagnostic criteria for temporomandibular disorders: review, criteria, examinations and specifications, critique, *J Craniomandibular Disorders* 6:301-355, 1992.
158. De Kanter RJAM and others: Prevalence in the Dutch adult population and a meta-analysis of signs and symptoms of temporomandibular disorder, *J Dent Res* 72:1509-1518, 1993.
159. Von Korff M: Health services research and temporomandibular pain. In Sessle BJ, Bryant PS, Dionne RA, editors: *Temporomandibular disorders and related pain conditions, progress in pain research and management,* vol 4, Seattle, 1995, IASP Press.
160. Antczak-Bouckoms A: Epidemiology of research for temporomandibular disorders, *J Orofacial Pain* 9:226-234, 1995.
161. Dworkin SF, LeResche L, editors: Research diagnostic criteria for temporomandibular disorders: review, criteria, examinations and specifications, critique, *J Craniomandibular Disorders: Facial & Oral Pain* 6:301-355, 1992.
162. Fejerskov O, Thylstrup A, Larsen MJ: Clinical and structural features and possible pathogenic mechanisms of dental fluorosis, *Scand J Dent Res* 85: 510-534, 1977.
163. Rozier RG: Epidemiologic indices for measuring the clinical manifestations of dental fluorosis: overview and critique, *Adv Dent Res* 8:39-55, 1994.
164. Pendrys DG, Stamm JW: Relationship of total fluoride intake to beneficial effects and enamel fluorosis, *J Dent Res* 69(Special issue): 529-538, 1990.
165. Pendrys DG, Katz RV, Morse DE: Risk factors for enamel fluorosis in a fluoridated population, *Am J Epidemiol* 140:461-471, 1994.
166. Pendrys DG, Katz RV, Morse DE: Risk factors for enamel fluorosis in a nonfluoridated population, *Am J Epidemiol* 143 808-815, 1996.
167. Szpunar SM, Burt BA: Fluoride supplements: evaluation of appropriate use in the United States, *Commun Dent Oral Epidemiol* 20:148-154, 1992.
168. Riordan PJ: Fluoride supplements in caries prevention: a literature review and proposal for a new dosage schedule, *J Public Health Dent* 53:174-189, 1993.
169. Osuji OO and others: Risk factors for dental fluorosis in a fluoridated community, *J Dent Res* 67:1488-1492, 1988.
170. Riordan PJ: Dental fluorosis, dental caries and fluoride exposure among 7-year olds, *Caries Res* 27:71-77, 1993.
171. Pendrys DG: Risk of fluorosis in a fluoridated population: implications for the dentist and hygienist, *J Am Dent Assoc* 126:1617-1624, 1995.
172. Barnhart WE and others: Dentifrice usage and ingestion among four age groups, *J Dent Res* 53:1317-1322, 1974.
173. Ekstrand J, Ehrenebo M: Absorption of fluoride from fluoride dentifrices, *Caries Res* 14:96-102, 1980.
174. ADA Council on Access, Prevention and Interprofessional Relations: Caries diagnosis and risk assessment, *J Am Dent Assoc* 126(Special suppl), 1995.
175. Committee on Nutrition, American Academy of Pediatrics: Fluoride supplementation for children: interim policy recommendations, *Pediatrics* 95:777, 1995.
176. Beltran ED, Szpunar SM: Fluoride in toothpastes for children: suggestion for change, *Pediatr Dent* 10:185-188, 1988.
177. Horowitz HS: The need for toothpastes with lower than conventional fluoride concentrations for preschool-age children, *J Public Health Dent* 52:216-221, 1992.
178. Feigal RJ: Recent modification in the use of fluorides by children, *Northwest Dentistry* 62:19-21, 1983.

CHAPTER 10

Effective community prevention programs for oral diseases

Myron Allukian, Jr.
Alice M. Horowitz

> *An ounce of prevention is worth a pound of dental cure.*
> —Olde Dental Public Health Proverb

Oral diseases have been referred to as "the neglected epidemic" because they affect almost the total population, with many people having new diseases each year.[1] For example, at age 6 years only 5.6% of U.S. school children have had tooth decay in their permanent teeth. However, by age 17 years, 84% have had the disease with an average of eight affected tooth surfaces.[2] For vulnerable populations, such as those with low incomes, minorities, the developmentally disabled, and persons with acquired immunodeficiency syndrome (AIDS), the extent of oral disease is even greater. Yet our country has not made oral health a priority. Further, the United States does not have a national oral disease prevention program, despite a $42 billion annual dental bill.[3] Compounding the problem, a 1996 study of children eligible for Medicaid reported that only one out of five, or 20%, received dental treatment.[4] Despite the progress made in the prevention of oral diseases in the last 20 years as a result of community water fluoridation, use of other fluorides and greater emphasis on prevention in general much more remains to be done.

Prevention

Prevention of premature death, disease, disability, and suffering should be a primary goal of any society that hopes to provide a decent future and a better quality of life for its people. *Primary prevention,* or preventing a disease before it occurs, is the most effective way to improve health and control costs. *Secondary prevention* is treating or controlling the disease after it occurs, such as placing an amalgam restoration. *Tertiary prevention* is limiting a disability from a disease, or rehabilitating an individual with a disability, such as providing dentures for those who have lost all their teeth.

Prevention may be accomplished at an individual or community level. At an individual level a procedure is either provided by a professional on a one-on-one basis, for example, a dental hygienist providing a dental sealant for a child patient, or it is self-administered, that is, the patients perform the procedure themselves, such as tooth brushing. An individual procedure also may be a combination of actions of an individual patient and a dental professional, such as the prescription by a dentist of a systemic fluoride that is taken daily by a patient. Table 10-1 shows the three levels of prevention for dental caries at the individual and community level or approach.

This chapter focuses on primary preventive measures that are science based and that have been shown to be effective in preventing oral diseases with a community- or population-based approach. There are many ways to prevent oral diseases with an individual approach. A community approach, however, helps ensure a greater impact at a lower cost for a larger number of individuals, especially vulnerable populations, such as low-income and minority groups. Self-responsibility by individuals for prevention also is very important and will be discussed as an adjunct to effective community prevention programs.

Definitions

To put "effective community prevention programs" in perspective with how prevention is often considered, the following definitions are used for this chapter:

Effective—1. having an effect: producing a result; 2. producing a definite or desired result, (efficient); 3. in effect: operative, active; 4. actual, not merely potential or theoretical

Community—1. all the people living in a particular district, city, etc; 2. a group of people living together as a smaller social unit within a larger one, and having interests, work, etc., in common

Prevention—1. the act of preventing . . . prevent; 2. to keep from happening: make impossible by prior action; hinder

Program—1. orig. a) a proclamation, b) a prospectus or syllabus. . . . 2. a plan or procedure for dealing with some matter.[5]

In essence, an "effective community prevention program" is a planned procedure that prevents the onset of a disease among a group of individuals. Stated another way, effective community prevention programs are those that work for groups of individuals. A group may be as small as a school classroom or as large as a nation. Although there are many different oral diseases and conditions, this chapter focuses on methods of preventing dental caries, gingivitis, unintentional oral-facial injuries, and oral-pharyngeal cancers.

Dental caries

Dental caries, or tooth decay, is both a universal and a lifelong disease. This disease is universal in the sense that the prevalence or percent of the population affected increases with age, ultimately affecting almost the entire population. All of us are at risk for caries as long as we have our natural teeth. Thus it is lifelong and may occur as early as in the first year of life as infant caries, sometimes referred to as nursing or baby-bottle tooth decay, continue throughout childhood and young adulthood, and continue in adults as root surface caries. During adolescence, the teenage years, and into adulthood the incidence of dental caries continues depending on the level of protection, genetic influences, and dietary habits. About 99% of adults have had tooth decay by age 40 to 44 years, with an average of 30 affected tooth surfaces.[6] For adults over the age of 75, nearly 60 percent had root surface caries with 3.1 affected tooth surfaces.[7] Recurrent decay can occur at any time throughout the life cycle. Thus it is important to prevent the onset of the disease because, once a tooth has been restored, the restoration must be replaced over time and each restoration becomes larger and larger. Ultimately, costly crowns, root canals, or extractions may be needed.

Prevention of dental caries

Because dental caries is nearly ubiquitous, treating this disease is costly in terms of health, time, and money. On the basis of what we now know, dental caries can be eliminated or con-

Table 10-1. Three levels of prevention for caries by individual and community approach

| Preventive services | Levels of prevention | | | | |
| | Primary | | Secondary | Tertiary | |
	Health promotion	Specific protection	Early diagnosis and prompt treatment	Disability limitation	Rehabilitation
Individual Approach					
Services provided by individual patient (self-administered)	Diet planning; demand for preventive services; periodic visits to dental office	Appropriate use of fluoride • Ingestion of sufficient fluoridated water • Appropriate use of fluoride prescriptions • Use of fluoride dentifrice • Oral hygiene practices	Self-examination and referral; use of dental services	Use of dental services	
Individual services provided by dental professional	Patient education; plaque control program diet counseling; recall reinforcement; dental caries activity tests	Topical application of fluoride; fluoride supplement/rinse prescription; pit and fissure sealants	Complete examination; prompt treatment of incipient lesions; preventive resin restorations; simple restorative dentistry; pulp capping	Complex restorative dentistry; pulpotomy; root canal therapy; extractions	Removable and fixed prosthodontics; minor tooth movement; implants
Community Approach					
Services provided by community	Dental health education programs; promotion of research, policy, and legislation	Community or school water fluoridation; school fluoride mouthrinse program; school fluoride tablet program; school sealant program	Periodic screening and referral; provision of dental services	Provision of dental services	Provision of dental services

Modified from Dunning JM: *Principles of dental public health*, ed 4, Cambridge, Mass, 1986, Harvard University Press; Mandel I: What is preventive dentistry? *J Prev Dent*, 25, 1974; Leske GS, Ripa LW, Callanen VA: Prevention of dental diseases. In Jong AW, editor: *Community dental health*, St Louis, 1993, Mosby.

trolled when science-based, preventive measures are applied appropriately. Because caries can continue throughout life, preventive measures must be a part of the lifestyle. There are many different approaches to preventing caries. The most cost-effective method is use of a community- or population-based approach.

FLUORIDES

The use of fluorides has made a significant impact on preventing dental caries in the United States. Fluoride is a naturally occurring compound of the element fluorine, which is never found in its free state in nature. It is the thirteenth most abundant element in the earth's crust and is found at different concentrations in all water supplies and most foods. Everyone's diet contains some fluoride, but not necessarily enough to prevent dental caries. The caries preventive benefit of fluoride was first discovered by Dr. Frederick McKay, who was trying to determine the cause of "Colorado brown stain" (fluorosis, sometimes re-ferred to as mottled enamel) in the 1920s. Dr. H. Trendly Dean subsequently demonstrated the relation between dental fluorosis, the concentration of fluoride in the water, and caries prevention with his classic epidemiology studies in the 1930s. The first controlled study of adjusted fluoride level in a public water supply began on January 25, 1945, in Grand Rapids, Michigan.

Fluoride is now used in many different ways to prevent dental caries. Table 10-2 shows individual and community preventive measures that have been shown to be effective, the mode of application, and the target population. Initially it was believed that the primary anti-caries benefit from fluoride was systemic, when fluoride ion was ingested and became part of the developing tooth, before the tooth erupted in the mouth. The exact mechanisms of action of fluorides are not known. The current and most widely accepted theory is that there are some preeruptive benefits from systemic fluorides. The major impact, however, is

Table 10-2. Effective community and individual preventive measures for dental caries prevention

Measure	Mode of application	Target	Period of use
Community Programs			
Community water fluoridation	Systemic	Entire population	Lifetime
School water fluoridation	Systemic	School children	School years
School fluoride tablet program	Systemic	School children	Age 5-16 yr
School fluoride rinse program	Topical	School children	Age 5-16 yr
School sealant program (professionally applied)	Topical	School children	Age 6-8, 12-14 yr
Individual Approach			
Prescribed fluoride tablets or drops	Systemic	Children	Age 6 mo-teens
Professionally applied fluoride treatment	Topical	Individual need	High-risk populations
Over-the-counter fluoride rinse	Topical	Individual need	High-risk populations
Fluoride toothpaste	Topical	Entire population	Lifetime
Professionally applied dental sealants	Topical	Children	Age 6-8 and 12-14 yr

a result of posteruptive benefits from the fluoride levels in plaque, saliva, and gingival exudate that continuously bathe the tooth and increase the remineralization of demineralized enamel caused by acids produced by cariogenic bacteria.

COMMUNITY WATER FLUORIDATION

It has been more than 50 years since community water fluoridation was first implemented in the United States in 1945. Since then, millions of Americans have enjoyed the health and economic benefits of this prevention measure. According to *Healthy People 2000,* the national health promotion and disease prevention objectives for the United States for the year 2000 include the following: "Community water fluoridation is the single most effective and efficient means for preventing dental caries in children and adults regardless of race or income level."[8]

Community water fluoridation should be the foundation of oral disease prevention or treatment programs in communities with a central water supply. Community water fluoridation is defined as the adjustment of the concentration of fluoride of a community water supply for optimal oral health. Fluoridation is often referred to as nature's way to help prevent tooth decay. The recommended level of fluoride for a community water supply in the United States ranges from 0.7 to 1.2 parts per million (ppm) of fluoride, depending on the mean maximum daily air temperature over a 5-year period.[9] Thus, in a warm climate the fluoride level would be lower, and in a cold climate it would be higher. In the United States most communities are fluoridated at about 1 ppm, which is equivalent to 1.0 mg of fluoride per liter of water. One part per million is equivalent to 1 inch in 16 miles, 1 minute in 2 years, or 1 cent in \$10,000. At this level fluoridated water is odorless, colorless, and tasteless.

Natural fluoridation

All water contains at least trace amounts of fluoride. In the United States there are about 10

million people who live in 1924 communities with 3784 water systems that are fluoridated naturally at 0.7 ppm or higher.[10] The eight states with the most people served with natural fluoridation—6.6 million in 662 communities—are shown in Table 10-3. Texas has the highest, with almost 3 million people in 284 communities.

In contrast, there are six states and the District of Columbia in which no one is served with a naturally fluoridated water supply at the recommended level (0.7 to 1.2 ppm). These states include Alaska, Rhode Island, Maine, Tennessee, Pennsylvania, and Vermont. The next three lowest states are Massachusetts, Hawaii, and West Virginia with 659. The five states with the highest proportion of their populations having access to naturally fluoridated water are Idaho (28.5%), Texas (16.7%), Colorado (23.4%), Montana (11.6%), and New Mexico (18.2%) (see Table 10-3).

Adjusted fluoridation

In 1992, 134.6 million Americans had access to adjusted community water fluoridation in 8572 communities with 10,567 water systems.[10]

Table 10-3. Eight highest ranking states by number of persons and communities served with natural water fluoridation, 1992

State	No. of persons	No. of communities
Texas	2,955,995	284
Florida	929,105	35
Colorado	811,024	106
Illinois	442,714	127
California	414,798	29
South Carolina	386,940	2
Louisiana	359,906	31
Arizona	345,266	48
TOTAL	6,645,748	662

Fig. 10-1 shows the national fluoridation rank of states with the percentage of the population served by adjusted and natural community water fluoridation. Adjusted fluoridation is accomplished "by adding fluoride chemicals to fluoride deficient water: by blending two or more sources of water naturally containing fluoride, or partial de-fluoridating, that is removing naturally occurring excessive fluoride to obtain the recommended level."[10] There is no difference between adjusted or natural fluoridation in safety or preventive benefits. A fluoride ion is a fluoride ion, whether it occurs naturally in the water supply or whether it is placed or added by a water engineer. The three major fluoride compounds used for fluoridation with the population served and number of

water systems are given in Table 10-4. The type of compound used depends on the size and type of water facility and the preference of the water supply engineer.[11]

The United States has more people served by fluoridation than any other country in the world. Consider the following data. In 1992, 144.2 million Americans, or 62.1% of the 232 million on public water supplies, had fluoridation. This is about 56% of the total U.S. population. More than 114 million Americans did not have access to fluoridation, of whom about 26 million were not served by a public water system. It is a policy of the federal government to fluoridate the water supply on military installations. A total of 133 military installations had adjusted fluoridation, serving 1.36 million

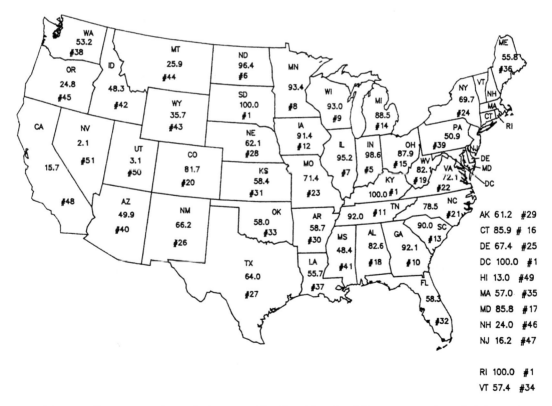

Fig. 10-1. Percentage of population served by fluoridated public water supply and state rank, 1992.

Table 10-4. Population and number of public water supply systems served by major fluoride compounds, 1992

	Populations	%	No. of water systems
Hydrofluosilic acid (fluosilic acid)	80,019,175	62.2	5,876
Sodium silicofluoride (sodium fluorosilicate)	35,084,896	28.2	1,635
Sodium fluoride	11,701,979	9.1	2,491
	127,806,050		

NOTE: Fluoride compound used was not indicated for all systems, so these data do not reflect national total.

residents with another 78,528 served by natural fluoridation.[10]

Of the 50 largest cities in the United States, all but 8 have a fluoridated water supply. These 8 cities, which have a combined population of about 7.9 million people, include: Los Angeles, Calif., Portland, Ore., San Diego, Calif., Tucson, Ariz., San Antonio, Tex., Sacramento, Calif., San Jose, Calif., and Honolulu, Hawaii. Interestingly, four of these cities are in California, which passed a statewide fluoridation law in October 1995 requiring fluoridation of all public water systems with at least 10,000 service corrections, depending on available funding. Los Angeles has already included some funds for fluoridation in the budget. Tucson voted for fluoridation in 1992, but it has yet to be implemented.

Safety

The safety of fluoridation has been well documented by numerous studies over the years.[12-15] Soon after fluoridation became known as a public health measure, beginning in the 1950s, a variety of diseases and conditions, including premature death, have been alleged to be caused by fluoridation. All have been shown to be false. The following is a partial list of some of the more common conditions falsely attributed to fluoridation: AIDS, allergies, Alzheimer's disease, bone disease, cancer, chromosomal damage, pregnancy, gastrointestinal damage, heart disease, infertility, kidney disease, mongolism (Down syndrome), pollution, and sterility.

There has been a tendency for those opposed to fluoridation for a variety of reasons to use any argument possible to capture the public interest to oppose fluoridation. The arguments range from "being a communist plot" to "causes rusty pipes" in the 1950s and 1960s to cancer, AIDS, and Alzheimer's disease in the 1970s, 1980s, and 1990s, respectively. A misuse of facts and quoting from studies lacking scientific rigor are often used to support these allegations.[16,17] The safety of fluoridation has been time-consuming and costly to document because of the range of allegations made by the opponents or "antifluoridationists" over the years. As a result, fluoridation is one of the most researched public health measures. At the same time, safety has been relatively easy to document because millions of Americans have for generations lived in communities with naturally fluoridated water. In addition, there are many communities in the United States and other countries where the fluoride level is naturally much higher than the recommended level, so that it is much easier to do studies to disprove these false allegations. The safety and effectiveness of water fluoridation as a public health measure is well established for the scientific and health communities; thus most national organizations representing these disciplines, such as the American Medical Association, the American Public Health Association, the American Association of Public Health Dentistry, and the American Dental Association, have endorsed or supported fluoridation (Table 10-5).

Effectiveness

The effectiveness of fluoridation in preventing dental caries has been well documented.[18] Early controlled studies of adjusted fluoridation demonstrated that 50% to 70% of caries was prevented in the permanent teeth of children.[19-22] Since 1980, because of the widespread use of fluorides in the United States, the measurable effectiveness of fluoridation is now about 20% to 40%.[18] This phenomenon is due, in part, to the fact that many other fluoride-containing products are now available, such as dietary fluoride supplements, rinses, toothpaste, professionally applied treatments and dilution and diffusion effects, which are described here.

A recent review of fluoridation states that fluoridation prevents caries in primary teeth by 30% to 60% for children 3 to 5 years of age, 20% to 40% for children with a mixed dentition (ages 6 to 12 years), and about 15% to 35% for adolescents and adults.[12,23] Fluoridation also helps to prevent root caries in senior adults by 17% to 35%.[23] In countries or communities where there is no widespread use of fluorides, the effectiveness would be expected to be similar to that in early studies conducted in the United States.

Dilution and diffusion effects

Water fluoridation is as effective as it ever was. Because of the widespread use of fluorides in the United States in both fluoridated and nonfluoridated communities, however, the measurable benefits of fluoridation are lower in the United States. This phenomenon is called the dilution effect. Communities without fluoridation also benefit from foods and drinks processed in communities with fluoridation and sold or used in communities without fluoridation. This factor is called the diffusion effect and it also affects the measurable benefits of fluoridation.[18] Diffusion effects also can occur when individuals who live in communities without fluoridation work or go to school in a community that has optimal fluoridation. In contrast, the effects of the increased use of bottled water and filters for tap water is not known.

Cost

Of all the preventive measures used to prevent dental caries in the United States, water fluoridation is the most economical and cost effective. In 1989 the weighted average cost of fluoridation was estimated to be $0.51 per capita per year for the United States, with a range of $0.12 to $5.41, depending on the size of the community and the complexity of the water system.[24] For larger communities the cost of fluoridation is usually less and for smaller communities it is more, as shown here[24]:

Annual cost per capita	Community population
$0.60-$5.41	<10,000
$0.18-$0.75	10,000-200,000
$0.12-$0.21	>200,000

Weighted average: $0.51

For about 85% of the population in fluoridated communities the average annual cost per capita was $0.12 to $0.75.[25] For every dollar spent on water fluoridation, an $80.00 savings in treatment cost has been estimated.[26] This is an excellent cost-benefit ratio, the highest for all the caries preventive measures used in the United States.

Practicality

Fluoridation is the most practical preventive measure in dentistry. No individual effort is

Table 10-5. National and international organizations that endorse or support water fluoridation

American Academy of Pediatrics

American Academy of Pediatric Dentistry

American Association for the Advancement of Science

American Association for Dental Research

American Association of Dental Schools

American Association of Public Health Dentistry

American College of Dentists

American Council on Science and Health

American Dental Assistants Association

American Dental Association

American Dental Hygienist's Association

American Dietetic Association

American Federation of Labor and Congress of Industrial Organizations

American Hospital Association

American Institute of Nutrition

American Medical Association

American Nurses Association

American Osteopath's Association

American Pharmaceutical Association

American Public Health Association

American Public Welfare Association

American School Health Association

American Society of Clinical Nutrition

American Society of Dentistry for Children

American Veterinary Medical Association

American Water Works Association

Association for Academic Health Centers

Association of State and Territorial Dental Directors

Association of State and Territorial Health Officials

British Dental Association

British Fluoridation Society

British Medical Association

Canadian Association of Accident and Sickness Insurers

Canadian Dental Association

Canadian Medical Association

Canadian Nurses Association

Canadian Public Health Association

Center for Science in the Public Interest

Consumer Federation of America

Department of National Health and Welfare (Canada)

Delta Dental Plans Association

European Organization for Caries Research

Federation of American Societies for Experimental Biology

Federation Dentaire Internationale

Food and Nutrition Board

Great Britain Ministry of Health

Health Insurance Association of America

Health League of Canada

International Association for Dental Research

Mayo Clinic

National Academy of Science

National Cancer Institute

National Confectioners Association

National Congress of Parents and Teachers

National Health Council

National Institute of Dental Research

National Research Council

New York Academy of Medicine

Pan American Health Organization

Royal College of Physicians (London)

Travelers Insurance Company

U.S. Department of Agriculture

U.S. Department of Defense

U.S. Environmental Protection Agency

U.S. Junior Chamber of Commerce

U.S. Public Health Service

    Centers for Disease Control and Prevention

    Food and Drug Administration

    Health Resources and Services Administration

    Indian Health Service

    National Institutes of Health

World Health Organization

needed. Everyone who lives in a community with fluoridation and consumes the water or uses it to prepare foods will receive some benefit, irrespective of age, sex, race, lifestyle, or level of education or income. Those individuals who are born in such a community and live there for their entire lives accrue maximum benefits because they receive both systemic and topical benefits for a lifetime.

The concentration of fluoride in a water supply must be monitored on a routine and systematic basis. Thus it is important for water operators to have the appropriate training in fluoridation and to maintain and monitor the concentration of fluoride as recommended.[9]

Antifluoridationists

Individuals who are against community water fluoridation are called antifluoridationists. Some of the reasons used for being against fluoridation include safety, individual rights, government mistrust, home rule, and religious freedom. None of the arguments against fluoridation have any merit based on scientific knowledge and public health experience. Further, they have no merit on the basis of state or federal laws. The U.S. Supreme Court has denied a review of fluoridation cases 13 times between 1954 and 1984.[27] The primary reasons antifluoridationists have had some limited success are mainly due to an uninformed public, weak or uninformed decision makers, and a weak or poorly organized program to promote and implement fluoridation. There have been a number of significant fluoridation battles over the years; however, with more than 50 years of health and economic benefits for millions of Americans, the arguments against fluoridation become weaker and weaker. This reality does not mean antifluoridationists have given up or ever will.

Antifluoridationists attempt to appeal to the emotions of the public and elected officials and promote fluoridation as a political issue rather than a public health program. Most communities in the United States make their decisions to fluoridate administratively on the basis of public health expertise. From 1989 to 1994, 337 communities in the United States decided to fluoridate the water supply, and 318, or 94% were decided by administrative decisions from a city council or commission.[28] Of the 32 referenda or public votes that occurred during that time 19 (61%) supported fluoridation. When the public is forced to vote on a complex public health program such as fluoridation, the antifluoridationists usually use deceptive, misleading, and incorrect information to confuse the public so that they vote for the status quo, to their own detriment. Compounding this problem is the fact that we have failed to educate the American population about how fluorides work and who benefits from their use. Numerous studies have shown that, in general, the U.S. public is not knowledgeable about fluorides and does not know that the use of fluoride is the best approach to caries prevention.[29-30] Fluoridation battles still occur in some communities; however if the political and professional will is present and the public and decision makers are well informed, the implementation of fluoridation will be successful.[31-36]

Community support

The key to achieving fluoridation in most communities is through organized community support, which is the essence of dental public health, defined by the American Board of Dental Public Health as "the science and art of preventing and controlling dental diseases and promoting dental health through organized community efforts."[37] Just as community water fluoridation should be the foundation of any caries prevention program, educating the public is the key to achieving and maintaining community water fluoridation or any other public health measure. Table 10-6 includes a list of basic concepts about fluorides that everyone should know and understand.

Table 10-6. What everyone should know about preventing oral diseases

Dental Caries	*Oral Cancers*
Fluoride	• Risk factors for oral cancers
• What fluoride and fluoridation are	• Signs and symptoms of oral cancers
• How fluorides work to protect teeth from decay	• What comprises a thorough oral cancer examination and recommended frequency
• Methods of application	
• Effectiveness of each procedure	• Need for oral cancer examination
• Who needs them	• Protective factors against oral cancers
• Recommended frequency of use and duration	*Gingivitis*
Pit and fissure sealants	• What dental plaque is
• What dental sealants are	• Role of dental plaque in oral diseases
• How they work to protect teeth from decay	• How to remove plaque
• Who needs them and when	• Frequency of plaque removal
• Monitoring and reapplication	• Recommended types of toothbrushes and floss

A planned educational program for community leaders, organizations, agencies, and institutions is important, beginning with health and human services leadership and then including all other community groups. Once there is widespread community support for fluoridation or any other type of population-based program, it is much easier to implement, support, and sustain.

As part of such an educational effort, dentists and physicians also should educate their patients, especially those who are community leaders, about the benefits of fluoridation for the community. It is beyond the scope of this chapter to detail how to organize an educational campaign for fluoridation. Many states and large cities have dental directors who have had experience with implementing and monitoring fluoridation. Further, the dental literature has many articles on fluoridation campaigns that may be helpful.[31-36,38-43]

National fluoride plan

In 1996 a national fluoride plan to promote oral health in the United States was developed by the U.S. Public Health Service.[44] The pur-

pose of this plan is to determine what needs to be done to reach the water fluoridation or fluoride-related objectives of *Healthy People 2000* and to respond to the recommendations of the U.S. Public Health Service report, *Review of Fluoride: Benefits and Risks*.[12] The plan is organized into four areas: policy, research, surveillance, and education. A status report for each area is given with recommendations for future strategies of action, which should include the following:

1. Promote and support effective coalition-building to ensure the appropriate use of fluorides and the community adoption of water fluoridation
2. Develop "on-site" field expertise and "steering committees" in states with large numbers of nonfluoridated communities
3. Encourage research in areas related to fluorides and water fluoridation
4. Provide a collateral strategy for the surveillance and quality of water fluoridation to ensure that community water systems consistently supply water with fluoride within recommended ranges, as outlined in the *CDC Engineering and Ad-*

ministrative Recommendations for Water Fluoridation, 1995

5. Promote the effective, proper, and safe use of fluorides and community water fluoridation through education, training, publications, endorsements, and broadcast, print, electronic, and visual media coverage.[45]

The National Fluoride Plan addresses the need to provide fluoridation and fluoride to the more than 100 million Americans who do not live in communities with a fluoridated water supply. In addition, the plan encourages continued studies of fluorides, especially with regard to the increase in fluorosis.

Dental fluorosis

In recent years there has been an increase in dental fluorosis in the United States in both fluoridated and nonfluoridated communities as a result of inappropriate uses of fluorides.[12] Dental fluorosis is the hypomineralization of enamel and the disruption of enamel development from excessive fluoride intake. It occurs in primary and permanent teeth, but in the United States it is less common in primary teeth. The severity of fluorosis is dependent on the amount of excess fluoride consumed over a period of time while teeth are developing, between ages 6 months to 6 years. One study suggests that the maxillary central incisors are at greatest risk for fluorosis from 15 to 24 months of age for males and from 21 to 30 months for females.[46] Once teeth have erupted, fluorosis cannot develop. Most dental fluorosis in the United States is considered a cosmetic problem, not a health problem. Very mild and mild fluorosis may occur in 10% to 15% of children reared in a community with fluoridated water.[12] In its mild form, usually only dental personnel will notice the bilateral white chalky appearance. In its more severe form, which occurs most often in communities in which the concentration of fluoride is naturally at much greater than the recommended level, there may be pitting and discoloration of teeth. Most of the increase in fluorosis in the United States is of a very mild or mild form.

The increase of fluorosis is due to the inappropriate use of dietary fluoride supplements, ingesting fluoride toothpaste, prolonged use of infant formula made from powder and mixed with fluoridated water, and the fluoride concentration of the water supply. It has been estimated that there is only a twofold increased risk of fluorosis in an optimally fluoridated community today compared with an 18-fold increase in the 1930s because of the increased risk in nonfluoridated communities.[47] Teeth with dental fluorosis are less susceptible to dental caries. In 1994 the American Dental Association's Council on Scientific Affairs recommended a new dosage schedule that reduces the dosage for dietary fluoride supplements[48] (Table 10-7). Physicians and dentists can help prevent fluorosis by prescribing dietary fluoride supplements appropriately (according to the current dosage schedule) and only for children living in communities without fluoridation. Parents should be educated by their health providers on the appropriate use of infant formula and to use only a pea-sized amount of fluoride toothpaste for children younger than six years old and to monitor their children closely to help prevent the ingestion of toothpaste.

Comparison of effective community prevention programs

Five effective community prevention programs for dental caries are used in the United States (Table 10-8). Of the five programs community water fluoridation is not only the most cost effective and practical but also the only community preventive measure that has demonstrated benefits for adults. Although salt fluoridation has been used successfully in

Table 10-7. Supplemental fluoride dosage schedule, 1994*

	Concentration of fluoride in drinking water (ppm)			
Age of child	*<0.3*	*0.3-0.6*	*>0.6*	*Preparation*
6 mo-3 yr	0.25 mg	0	0	Drops
3-6 yr	0.50 mg	0.25 mg	0	Tablets
6-16 yr	1 mg	0.50 mg	0	Tablets

*Recommended by American Dental Association, American Academy of Pediatric Dentistry, and American Academy of Pediatrics.
NOTE: Amounts represent milligrams of fluoride per day.

other countries, it has not yet been used in the United States; therefore it is not included in the list. Table 10-8 applies to the United States only because the fluoride dilution and diffusion effects decrease the measurable benefits of fluoride. In other countries where there are fewer communities with fluoridation and fewer other fluoride products the effectiveness would be comparable to the 50% to 70% reduction in caries found in the 1950s to 1970s in the United States. Table 10-8 shows the relative differences among these preventive measures. Studies are needed on effectiveness and cost because of the diffusion and dilution effects of fluoride. A thorough analysis of the literature also would be helpful to appreciate the differences in these prevention regimens.

School-based programs

When a community does not have a public or central water supply or does not yet have fluoridation for whatever reason, another approach is to use a caries preventive regimen in schools. This approach is logical in that most children in the United States attend school regularly. Preventive regimens provided in schools can be one of three types: (1) a community type, such as school water fluoridation; (2) self-applied, which refers to any health activity that is performed by an individual student, such as fluoride mouthrinse conducted in

a school setting; or (3) operator applied, which refers to any health activity that is performed by a health care provider for a student, such as the application of pit and fissure sealants in a school setting.

SCHOOL WATER FLUORIDATION

School water fluoridation was developed and tested in the United States in the 1960s for use in rural schools with an independent water supply, preferably those schools that included grades kindergarten through 12. Fluoridation of water supplies of individual schools is similar to community water fluoridation in that no direct action is required of beneficiaries other than direct consumption of or use of the water in food preparation. The major difference is that the recommended concentration for school water fluoridation is 4.5 times the concentration of fluoride recommended for community water supplies in the respective geographic area. The higher concentrations are recommended to compensate for part-time exposure because children spend only part of their time at school.[49]

Effectiveness

Studies conducted on school fluoridation have shown that a 20% to 30% reduction in caries can be expected when children have consumed school water fluoridation for 12 years.[49] Despite the higher fluoride concentra-

Table 10-8. Comparison of five effective community prevention programs for dental caries*

Program	Effectiveness (%)	Adult benefits	Cost per year	Practicality
Community fluoridation	20-40	Demonstrated	$0.51 per capita†	Excellent; most practical; no individual effort necessary
School fluoridation	20-30‡	Expected but not demonstrated	$0.85-$9.88 per child	Good; if there is no central community water supply, no individual effort necessary
School dietary fluoride daily supplement program	30	Expected but not demonstrated	$0.81-$5.40 per child§	Fair; continued school regimen required for 8-10 yr
School fluoride mouthrinse program	25-28‡	Not expected	$0.52-$1.78 per child§	Fair; continued daily or weekly school regimen required
School sealant program	51-67‖	Expected but not demonstrated	$13.07-$28.37 per child	Good; primarily done for children aged 6-8 yr and 12-14 yr

Data from Burt B: Proceedings of the workshop: Cost-Effectiveness of Caries Prevention in Dental Public Health, *J Public Health Dent*, 1989:49(5) (special issue); Allukian M: Oral diseases: the neglected epidemic. In Scutchfield FD, Keck WC, editors: *Principles and practices of public health*, Albany, NY, 1996, Delmar Publishers.

*This table is a simplified comparison of these prevention programs. A thorough analysis of the literature should be done to understand the relative merits of these programs.

†See text for range.

‡This range may now be high; no recent studies.

§Includes use of volunteer personnel.

‖First molar chewing surfaces only over 5-year period.

tion, no dental fluorosis has been produced. A primary reason for this lack of fluorosis is because of the age of children when they start school, 5 or 6 years, when dental fluorosis is less likely to occur. There are disadvantages to school water fluoridation in that there is both delayed and part-time exposure. Further, it benefits only the children attending school and the adults who work there. Finally, unlike community water fluoridation, we do not know whether there are retained benefits after a child leaves a fluoridated school environment and goes to a community in which the water is not fluoridated. In the 1980s there were approximately 600 schools in the United States whose water was fluoridated. In 1992 there were 332 schools with 117,430 children in 12 states that had access to school water fluoridation.[10] The number has diminished for several reasons. Some rural schools with an independent water supply previously using school water fluoridation have been incorporated into major, central water systems that are now optimally fluoridated, thus eliminating the need for a school water fluoridation system. One state discontinued the school water fluoridation program because state officials determined that children were receiving ample fluoride from other sources.

Cost

In 1989 school water fluoridation was estimated to cost between $0.85 to $9.88 per child per school year.[24]

Practicality

The practicality of school water fluoridation is good when a community does not have a central water supply. All the children benefit with no individual effort required on the part of the recipient. Monitoring the concentration of fluoride in the water must be conducted daily. The role and responsibility for monitoring must be worked out between the school and health and water departments. The indi-

vidual responsible for monitoring the school fluoridation equipment must be well trained.

FLUORIDE TABLETS

Another method for administering systemic fluoride in school settings is the daily use of dietary fluoride supplements in the form of tablets. Table 10-7 shows the currently recommended fluoride dosage schedule, which should be adhered to whether the supplement is used at school or home. This procedure is most often identified as one to use at home when a health care provider prescribes a fluoride supplement with or without vitamins. Because the compliance required for this regimen—daily for 16 years—may be more than most parents can achieve, this procedure often is used in schools. The usual procedure is for an adult to distribute the tablets to each participating student and then under supervision the tablet is chewed for approximately 30 seconds. The resultant solution is then swished between the teeth for another 30 seconds and then swallowed.[50] Thus this procedure provides both systemic and topical benefits. A supervising adult maintains a record of when each child takes a tablet. Supervised, self-administered use of fluoride tablets is a well-established regimen that has been used in the United States and abroad for more than 40 years.

Effectiveness

Although it is not the most popular school-based fluoride regimen used in the United States, this method is well documented with research and has been shown to be effective. Studies conducted in this country have shown that the daily use of fluoride tablets on school days will provide a 30% reduction in new caries lesions.[51]

Cost

The average cost of a school-based fluoride tablet program in 1989 was approximately $2.53 per child per school year with a range of

$0.81 to 5.40, depending on whether paid personnel or volunteers are used to supervise the procedure.[24]

Practicality

The daily consumption of fluoride tablets in school settings is an excellent method to use in areas where the water is fluoride deficient. This procedure can be supervised by a classroom teacher or volunteer with minimal training. It takes only a few minutes of classroom time and it is highly accepted by students, faculty, and parents. A major drawback to this method is that it is a daily procedure. Therefore the practicality is fair. Only children with parental consent may participate. Table 10-9 compares the advantages of using either a school-based fluoride tablet or mouthrinse regimen.

FLUORIDE MOUTHRINSE

Fluoride mouthrinse has been used in schools in the United States for nearly three decades, and it is the most popular school-based fluoride regimen in the United States.[50] Fluoride rinsing is generally supervised in classrooms by teachers or adult volunteers. In some cases health or teacher aides are responsible for this activity. For children in grades 1 and above the procedure consists of distributing a paper napkin and a paper cup with 10 ml of solution to each participating student. In unison, the students empty the contents of the cup into the mouth and rinse the solution vigorously for 60 seconds. The supervising adult times the procedure; at the end of 60 seconds students are requested to empty the contents of the mouth into the cup and to place a tissue into the cup to absorb the liquid. The materials are then collected and disposed of properly.[50] The supervising adult also maintains a record for each child who rinses.

The rinse procedure for children in kindergarten is the same as that for older students except they are advised to use only 5 ml of the solution. The rationale for this recommendation is that younger children tend to swallow some of the solution, which may contribute to fluorosis if this practice continues over time among children 6 years old or younger. Practice sessions with plain water are recommended, especially for younger children.

Table 10-9. Comparison of school-based fluoride regimens

Fluoride mouthrinse	Fluoride tablets
Safe and effective	Safe and effective
Inexpensive	Inexpensive
Easy to learn and do	Easy to learn and do
Nondental personnel can supervise	Nondental personnel can supervise
Well accepted by participants	Well accepted by participants
Little time required—5 minutes weekly	Little time required—3 minutes daily
Provides topical benefits	Provides systemic and topical benefits
	No waste materials
	Suitable for preschool children

Modified from Horowitz AM: Community-oriented preventive dentistry programs that work, *Health Values* 8(1):21-29, 1984.

Effectiveness

Numerous studies have demonstrated that dental caries can be reduced by about 25% to 28% by rinsing daily or weekly in school with dilute solutions of fluoride.[24] Because rinsing weekly with a 0.2% neutral sodium fluoride (NaF) solution requires fewer supplies and less time than daily rinsing with a 0.05% NaF solution, weekly use of school-based rinse programs are more common. Further, studies have shown that when used in school, there is little difference in caries protection between daily and weekly use.[52] Table 10-10 shows appropriate fluoride programs for use in grades 1 through 12.

Cost

The cost of this procedure in 1989 ranged between $0.52 to $1.78 depending on whether paid or volunteer adult supervisors were used.[24]

In addition, the cost varies depending on whether a unit dose (individual, premixed serving) is used or whether packets of NaF are purchased and mixed with water and dispensed into cups. The premixed unit dose is more convenient and requires less time, but the materials cost more.

Practicality

The practicality of this measure is fair because it is performed once a week. It is somewhat more practical in terms of frequency than the use of fluoride tablets, but it is less practical in that the children should not swallow the rinse thus close monitoring is required and the used products must be collected and disposed of properly.

DENTAL SEALANTS

The appropriate use of fluorides is the best approach to preventing caries. Fluoride, however, is believed to be least effective on the occlusal or chewing tooth surfaces. Most decay among school-aged children occurs on the chewing surfaces. Thus the use of fluorides and pit and fissure sealants is needed to provide nearly total caries prevention.[53] In the United States the application of dental sealants must be performed by a dentist, a dental hygienist, or a dental assistant, depending on the individual state practice act. The application procedure is relatively simple; however, it is operator dependent. Because sealant material is extremely susceptible to saliva contamination, the procedure must be done with great care.[53]

Table 10-10. Appropriate self-applied fluoride programs for use in grades 1 through 12

Fluoride in water supply (ppm)	Tablets (daily)		Mouthrinse (weekly)	Grade	Recommended procedure
<0.3	1 mg fluoride			1-8	Fluoride tablets
	1 mg fluoride	or	0.2% NaF	9-12	Fluoride tablets or fluoride mouthrinse
0.3-0.6	0.5 mg fluoride	or	0.2% NaF	1-8	Fluoride tablets or fluoride mouthrinse
>0.6	Dietary fluoride tablets should *not* be provided		0.2% NaF	1-12	Fluoride mouthrinse

A specific oral health objective in *Healthy People 2000* specifies that 50% of children should have their permanent molars sealed. Unfortunately, the most recent data show that only about 17% of U.S. children 6 through 17 years old have had this preventive procedure.[54] Unlike other countries, for example, Finland, where 85% of children have pit and fissure sealants on the permanent molars, practitioners in the United States have basically ignored this procedure. Concomitantly, the public (parents) have not been educated about the existence of and need for sealants; thus most do not have enough knowledge about them to request this preventive procedure for their children.[55]

Effectiveness

This procedure was first demonstrated to be effective in studies conducted nearly 30 years ago. Their effectiveness has been reported in the range of 51% to 67%.[24]

Cost

The 1989 estimated cost for dental sealants ranged from $13.07 to $28.37, depending on whether a dentist or dental auxiliary placed the sealant, whether they were paid or volunteer, and the type of equipment used.[24]

Practicality

Numerous states have school-based sealant programs, which, in itself, speaks for their practicality. Sealant programs focus on children 6 to 8 years old and 12 to 14 years old because the first and second permanent molars usually erupt during these years. These two molars are the teeth most often sealed in school-based programs. Some programs use mobile dental vans that are sent to schools, and children receive sealant application in the van. Other programs use portable equipment that is transported from school to school where it is set up in whatever space is available and students are brought to the designated room for the procedure. The process is well accepted by students, parents, faculty, and staff. As with all school-based caries preventive measures, parental consent is required. Table 10-6 includes concepts about dental sealants, about which parents and children should be educated.

Community-based programs used in other countries

For a variety of reasons, several different approaches to preventing dental caries are available and have supporting research but are not or rarely used in the United States. A few of these preventive approaches include salt fluoridation, fluoride varnishes, and atraumatic restorative treatment (ART).

SALT FLUORIDATION

Salt fluoridation is the controlled addition of fluoride during the manufacturing of salt for use by humans. Sodium or potassium fluoride is usually used. Adding fluoride to salt was first suggested by Wespi, who recognized the value of adding iodine to salt to prevent goiter. Recognized as an expert on iodized salt, he urged health authorities in Switzerland to add fluoride to iodized salt. Zurich was the first canton to authorize the sale of fluoridated domestic salt in 1955. By 1966 fluoridated salt accounted for 65% of the domestic salt market in Switzerland. The generally recommended concentration is roughly the equivalent of 1 ppm; however, each country would need to determine its needs on the basis of the consumption of salt and the concentration of fluoride in the local water supply.[56] Many other countries also have adopted Switzerland's innovative approach; these countries include France, Germany, Costa Rica, Jamaica, and Uruguay.

Effectiveness

Fluoridated salt has been shown to be as effective as community water fluoridation, when all domestic salt is fluoridated.[57] Domestic salt refers to that salt sold in markets and salt sold in bulk to restaurants, bakeries, hospitals, schools, and other institutions and companies that process foods. In Jamaica caries reduction among 1200 children showed an 85% reduction after 8 years of salt fluoridation. Fluorosis was negligible.[58]

Cost

Generally, salt fluoridation is as effective as community water fluoridation but costs less. It is estimated that in some South American countries the potential saving is $136.00 for each dollar invested in the regimen. On average the cost is about $0.02 to $0.04 per kilogram of salt.[58]

Practicality

Salt fluoridation provides a choice to consumers that community water fluoridation does not, sometimes a major issue in initiating this procedure. There has been some opposition to salt fluoridation by individuals who are concerned about the need to reduce salt consumption; however, this concern is not justified for several reasons. Although excess salt consumption over a lifetime is linked to higher blood pressure, it has been shown that the use of salt does not increase when fluoride is added. Further, the amount of fluoride added to salt can be adjusted. Another concern that is often cited is the question about distribution of salt in a country, state, or canton where some water has natural concentrations of fluoride that range from 0.6 to 1.2 ppm and higher. This situation, of course, is true for most countries and can be accommodated by educating the salt manufacturers and the food distributors and the public at large. In countries where fluoridated salt is sold, containers are not only labeled but are also usually color coded, a procedure also used to distinguish iodized salt from plain salt. Further, salt manufacturers ship fluoridated salt only to communities with specified lower concentrations of fluoride in the water supply. This effort does not preclude the fact that an uninformed consumer could go to a market in another community and inadvertently purchase fluoridated salt. Overall, this approach to offering a preventive regimen is one that has been given little notice in North America, where community water fluoridation is well established. However, many rural locations, for example, Native American reservations in Canada and the United States and states such as Alaska, might benefit dramatically by the use of this preventive procedure. Further, states such as Hawaii and countries such as Japan might be ripe for the use of fluoridated salt because, despite interest in community water fluoridation by a few dedicated dental public health workers, efforts to implement it have not been successful.

FLUORIDE VARNISHES

Fluoride varnishes were developed in Europe more than 30 years ago and remain in wide use there. They are operator applied, and biannual application is the usual recommendation. In Denmark varnishes are used in 92% of the community preventive programs for children.[59] Most of the clinical studies, with the exception of one Canadian trial, were conducted in Europe.[60] The original purpose for their development was to increase the uptake of fluoride by enamel, when it was thought that this factor would lead to greater caries protection. Fluoride varnishes do increase the fluoride concentration in saliva for a longer period of time than do other professionally applied fluoride products.[61] The U.S. Food and Drug Administration recently approved the marketing of DuraFlor (formally Duraphat), which has been hailed by some as a giant step forward.[62]

Effectiveness

Numerous studies have shown that there is a wide range of efficacy, between 7% and 75%.

Studies have been conducted mostly on children, but there is no reason the product could not be used on adults. This kind of fluoride may be especially useful to prevent root surface caries among the growing number of older adults who have gingival recession. In addition, fluoride varnishes may be especially attractive for use with disabled children and bedbound patients who still have their own teeth. More recently, fluoride varnishes have been used on an experimental basis to help prevent infant or early childhood caries among children in some Women, Infant and Children (WIC) and Head Start programs.

Practicality

The use of fluoride varnishes is as practical as any operator-applied fluoride treatments.

ATRAUMATIC RESTORATIVE TREATMENT

In recent years research has provided an increased understanding of the process of dental caries, how to prevent it, and better approaches to treating the disease. Keeping a tooth healthy and intact through appropriate use of fluorides and pit and fissure sealants helps ensure against costly repairs.[63] In many developing countries and, for some populations within highly industrialized countries, dental caries is a widespread problem and treatment often is available only for the affluent. When the caries process is left untreated, the only choice of treatment often is extraction of the tooth. A new method for treating caries is "atraumatic restorative treatment" (ART).[64] ART is a secondary preventive measure. This procedure offers treatment to disadvantaged populations and consists of caries removal with use of hand instruments only and then the application of adhesive restorative material. No electricity, water, drill, or expensive dental equipment is necessary. This procedure is being used in 25 countries, including Zimbabwe, China, Thailand, and Cambodia. Further, the World Health

Organization endorses its use. Although there is a growing body of research to support the use of this procedure, additional studies are needed and many are underway.[64]

Practicality

ART is extremely practical in that only hand instruments are used along with an adhesive dental material. Thus the equipment and materials are easy to pack, carry, or mail. This procedure may have applicability for bed-bound patients and others who are physically challenged. Although ART has yet to be used in the United States, the procedure could be beneficial for the disadvantaged, especially children, who have no way to finance dental treatment. ART is closely related to the application of pit and fissure sealant material in that similar dental material is used and both are minimal intervention methods. The major difference, of course, is that sealants are used to *prevent* caries, whereas ART is used to treat the disease.

Periodontal disease prevention

Periodontal diseases consist of a variety of inflammatory and degenerative conditions of the supporting structures of the teeth. The two most common types are gingivitis and periodontitis. There is ample evidence to demonstrate the relationship between the presence of bacterial plaque and gingivitis. These diseases are insidious and can affect children and adults, although more severe types are more likely to be found among adults. Gingivitis—inflammation of the soft tissue surrounding teeth—can be prevented or controlled by thoroughly removing dental plaque periodically.[65]

Although there are no studies that clearly define the necessary frequency of thorough plaque removal to prevent gingivitis, it is generally recommended that plaque should be removed at least daily. Generally, thorough plaque removal is accomplished mechanically with a toothbrush and dental floss or tape.[65]

Dental plaque also can be controlled with the use of antimicrobial products such as chlorhexidine.[66] In community-based programs, however, only mechanical plaque removal has been used. At one time, school-based plaque removal regimens were very popular. These toothbrushing drills often did not include the use of a fluoride dentifrice, thus severely limiting their value. Today, toothbrushing in classrooms is not used as much as it was two decades ago. Instead, children often are shown in school how to remove plaque with a toothbrush and sometimes dental floss or tape. These procedures may or may not include actual use of the implements. In either case, a toothbrush and floss are sometimes sent home with instructions to use them on a routine basis. If toothbrushing is to take place in a school environment, a fluoride dentifrice should be used so that both dental caries and gingivitis prevention are addressed. Dental floss or tape should be used only after proper instructions, so that the gingival tissues are not injured. All students should be taught the concepts listed in Table 10-6 regarding the prevention of gingivitis.

EFFECTIVENESS

Studies conducted in the 1970s and early 1980s showed that regular, thorough plaque removal under supervision could reduce gingivitis among school children.[67] In one study, however, where examinations were conducted at the beginning and at the end of each school year, it was observed that much of the gain achieved in reducing gingivitis over the school year disappeared or at least was reduced over the summer when plaque removal was not supervised.[67]

COST

An estimate for this procedure is not known, but it is relatively expensive because of the expense of toothbrushes, dentifrice, floss (if used), and various paper products if a sink is not used. In addition, teachers' time must be taken into consideration.

PRACTICALITY

Although toothbrushing in classrooms is possible, most public school teachers are less than enthusiastic about its practice. Much of this reluctance is understandable in that the procedure is invariably messy when dealing with younger children. Further, not all classrooms have sinks, thus making it necessary to use multiple types of paper products including paper cups, towels, or napkins. Moreover, the toothbrushes must be stored in a place where they can be kept clean and the waste products must be properly disposed of.

Brushing in school-based programs is found more frequently in Head Start classes where teachers appear to be more accepting of spills and the need to clean up than in public schools. The purpose is to teach the children how to brush, to help instill the need for routine toothbrushing and the feel of a "clean, fresh mouth," and, in some cases, to provide the only toothbrush the child has owned.

High-risk or vulnerable populations

There are some groups of individuals who are more vulnerable, more susceptible, or at higher risk for oral diseases and conditions than others, because of their knowledge, attitudes, behavior, education, income, occupation, sex, age, health status, residency location, race, ethnicity, culture, or minority status.[8,37,68-70] These individuals who share these common attributes have been called high-risk, vulnerable, underserved, special needs, or disadvantaged populations. Effective community prevention programs for dental caries are either for the whole community, such as fluoridation, or a specific age group, such as school prevention programs. However, a school prevention program such as dental sealants may be targeted to higher risk children, maximizing limited services.[71] Also, a school dental program may be targeted for those schools, where there are children at either higher risk for disease or at higher risk for being unable to obtain treatment. Effective community prevention programs for dental caries can also be supplemented with an individual approach for children who are at high risk, such as use of home fluoride gels or rinses for individuals undergoing orthodontic treatment or taking medications that decrease salivary flow.[48] Populations also may be at "high risk" because of beliefs, behavior, or cultural patterns. Infant caries may be high in groups of children whose mothers or other care givers put sugar or juices in their baby bottles, and oral cancer is high among persons who smoke and drink alcohol excessively.

When a community prevention program is being planned, the needs of high-risk populations must be considered. A high-risk group in one culture, neighborhood, or community may not be at high risk in another. For example, low income children in the United States usually are at high risk for dental caries. However, low income children in a developing country, especially in rural areas, usually are at low risk for dental caries because they do not have access to candies and other sweets.[68] Examples of some high-risk or vulnerable populations are as follows: bed bound, chemically dependent, cultural minorities, dentally indigent, developmentally disabled, elderly, ethnic minorities, children in Head Start programs, homebound, homeless, institutionalized, linguistic minorities, medically compromised, migrants, Native Americans, persons with AIDS/human immunodeficiency virus, rural populations, and teenagers.

The diversity of high-risk populations requires an understanding and appreciation of their needs, attitudes, knowledge, and behavior to develop an effective prevention program. These high-risk populations often have the greatest dental needs, the least resources and access to care, and the least knowledge about preventing diseases, and few or no fact-finding skills, making primary prevention of disease even more important.

Unintentional oral-facial injuries

Oral-facial injuries may be intentional or unintentional. Intentional oral injuries may occur from abuse, domestic violence, self-mutilation, or violence in general. Dental personnel have a role in and responsibility for early detection, treatment, and referral for these patients. This section will discuss the prevention of unintentional injuries that usually occur from contact sports, recreational activities, motor vehicles, and daily living.

Unintentional injuries result in about 100,000 deaths a year, making them the fourth leading cause of death in the United States.[8] About half these deaths are from motor vehicles, followed by falls, poisoning, drowning, and residential fires. More lives are lost from unintentional injuries the first 40 years of life than from infectious or chronic diseases. Nonfatal injuries result in high medical costs and lost productivity, accounting for 1 in 6 hospital days and 1 in 10 hospital discharges.[8] Unintentional oral-facial injuries may result in broken and avulsed teeth, facial bone fractures, concussion, permanent brain injury, temporomandibular joint dysfunction, blinding eye injuries, and even death.[72] Although there are no national data on the extent of oral-facial injuries, the following is known:

- About 25% of the U.S. population, aged 6 to 50 years, have had incisal tooth trauma.[73]
- Almost half of abused children have oral-facial trauma.[74]
- About 25 million children in the United States participate in competitive school sports and about 20 million play in organized sports outside of school.[75]

Prevention of unintentional oral-facial injuries

There is no single mechanism or program to prevent all the different types of unintentional injuries. An organized community effort is needed that includes many different disciplines, such as health, education, transportation, law, engineering, architecture, and safety services.[8] Although not directly related to dentistry, support by the dental profession of the following injury prevention programs on community and individual levels may result in fewer oral-facial injuries:

- Increased use of mass transit
- Drunk driving prevention programs
- Seat belt and child safety seat laws and programs
- Improved pedestrian safety
- Motorcycle and bicycle helmet laws and programs
- Safe playground equipment
- Protective bars on upper story windows
- Home fire safety measures
- Protective mouthguards and headgear for sports

Table 10-11. Estimated number and percentages of children who played organized sports in United States, 1991

Sport	No. of children	%
Baseball/softball	9,338,980	24.4
Soccer	4,906,134	12.8
Football	3,824,708	10.0
Karate/judo	977,180	2.6
Wrestling	960,763	2.5
Field/ice hockey	603,008	1.6
Lacrosse	141,480	0.4
Boxing	144,380	0.4
Rugby	52,686	0.1

Data from Nowjack-Raymer RE, Gift HC: Use of mouthguards and headgear in organized sports by school-aged children, *Public Health Rep* 111:82-86, 1996.

- Home environment modifications
- Timely emergency medical services

Although no national data for the various causes of oral-facial injuries exist, sports appear to account for a significant proportion, with some estimates as high as 33%.[76,77] More than 14 million of the 20 million school-age children in the United States who participate in sports do so in at least one sport listed in Table 10-11, which does not include basketball. More than 25% of these children participate in two sports.[72] Baseball and softball are the most popular sports, played by 24% of school-aged children, followed by 12.8% of children for soccer and 10% for football.[72] The highest number of unintentional injuries from product-associated sports treated in emergency departments in 1995 were from basketball, followed by bicycles, football, baseball, soccer, and softball (Table 10-12).[78]

Protective headgear and mouthguards have been demonstrated to prevent unintentional injuries in sports. About 50% of all high school football injuries were to the face and mouth before 1962, when protective oral-facial devices became required by the National Alliance Football Rules Committee.[79] One in 10 players had a chance of receiving such an injury during the playing season.[79] With the use of face guards and mouth protectors, there has been a dramatic reduction in oral-facial injuries in football since 1962.[79] Currently, only five amateur sports require mouthguards during games and practice: boxing, football, ice hockey, lacrosse, and women's field hockey.[80]

Mouth protection is needed in other sports. One statewide study showed that nearly 31% of high school basketball players sustained an oral-facial injury during the varsity basketball season, and 22% of these injuries required professional attention.[81] Only 4% of these players wore mouth protectors, and the injury rate for those without mouth protection was nearly seven times greater. In a study in another state of high school athletes, 9% of all players had some form of injury and 3% reported loss of consciousness.[82] About 40% of the injuries were in baseball and basketball, with 75% occurring in players not wearing mouth protection. There also were fewer concussions in those athletes wearing mouth protection. In a national study of high school students who played baseball or softball, only 35% wore headgear and 7% mouthguards all or most of the time.[72] About 40% of the males wore headgear compared with 25% of the females. About 12% of these ball players wore mouthguards compared with 7% of soccer players and 72% of football players.[72] Table 10-13 shows the comparison of headgear and mouthguard use for baseball and football by gender, grade level, race, ethnicity, and socioeconomic level.

Studies also show that more children are injured in sports outside of school (60%) than when in school, and more injuries occur during practice (60%) than when in games.[75,83] Protective sportswear usually is used much less often in sports outside of school and in practice. In *Healthy People 2000* one of the national prevention objectives is to "Extend requirements of the use of effective head, face, eye, and mouth protection to all organizations, agencies, and institutions sponsoring sporting and recreation events that pose risk of injury."[8]

Promotion of regulations, requirements, and guidelines for the use of effective protection in sports should include the mouth. Custom-fitted mouthguards allow for easier breathing and better speech; therefore compliance is much better than with stock mouthguards. Referees, coaches, parents, school officials, the dental profession, athletic organizations, and local and state health departments should all play a role in protecting the health and safety of children and athletes.[84-86]

Prevention and early detection of oral-pharyngeal cancers

Annually nearly 30,000 Americans are diagnosed with oral cancers, which translates into the fact that one person dies each hour, approximately 8000 annually, as a result of these cancers. More Americans die from oral cancers than from cervical cancer or melanoma.[87] Oral cancers can occur in all sites of the oral cavity including the tongue, the floor of the mouth, the soft palate, the tonsils, the salivary glands, the back of the throat, and the lips. Of these, the floor of mouth and the tongue are the primary sites. Ninety percent of all oral cancers are squamous cell carcinoma.[88] In the United States, oral cancer is more prevalent among males than females and it is most often diagnosed among persons aged 45 years and older.

Table 10-12. Estimated number of sports injuries treated in U.S. hospital emergency departments by age, 1995

		Percent by age (yr)		
	No. of cases	*0-4*	*5-14*	*15-24*
Basketball	692,386	0.3	30.5	48.0
Bicycles	549,988	7.4	56.3	15.1
Football	389,463	0.3	45.9	43.5
Baseball	210,395	4.0	50.3	23.2
Soccer	156,960	0.3	44.9	38.6
Softball	155,669	0.9	23.0	27.5

Data from National Safe Kids Campaign, *Sports Injury Fact Sheet*, Washington, DC, 1996.

Table 10-13. Percentages of children who wear headgear and mouthguards while playing baseball or football by selected variables

| | Baseball | | Football | |
	Headgear	Mouthguards	Headgear	Mouthguards
Total	*35%*	*7%*	*72%*	*72%*
Gender				
Male	40	8	77	77
Female	25	5	15	15
Grade level				
Elementary	35	6	52	52
Middle	36	9	80	79
High school	35	12	88	88
Race				
Black	33	17	74	71
White	35	6	72	72
Ethnicity				
Hispanic	33	11	46	52
Non-Hispanic	36	7	77	75
Poverty level				
Below	24	11	54	54
At/above	36	6	77	75
Parent's education				
<HS/HS	34	8	68	69
>HS	36	6	78	75

From Nowjack-Raymer RE, Gift HC: Use of mouthguards and headgear in organized sports by school-aged children, *Public Health Rep* 111:82-86, 1996.

Oral cancers in advanced stages cause pain, loss of function, and frequently disfiguring impairment that cause social isolation. The 5-year survival rate for oral cancers for advanced cases is 16% compared with 75% for localized lesions. Oral cancers have one of the lowest 5-year survival rates of 11 major cancer sites.[89] When oral cancers are detected early, prognosis for survival is much better than for most other cancers.

Primary risk factors for oral cancers in the United States are use of tobacco and alcohol products and, for lip cancers, unprotected exposure to the sun. Tobacco and alcohol use account for 75% of all oral and pharyngeal cancers.[88-90] Other dietary factors also may play a role. Similar to other cancers such as colorectal cancer, eating fruits and vegetables that contain essential vitamins (A,C,E) and other nutrients may provide protection against the development of oral cancers.[91] Betel nut, which is used in many other countries, has been found to be a risk factor for oral cancers.

Despite available knowledge about risk factors for and signs and symptoms of oral cancers, the American public is ill informed about these matters.[92,93] Further, recent data show that only 14% of U.S. adults have ever had an oral cancer examination.[93] Additionally, preliminary data suggest that dentists and physicians are not as knowledgeable as they might be.[94] Complicating the problem is the fact that about 25% of U.S. dental schools use health history forms that are deficient in determining a patient's high-risk behaviors related to oral cancers—use of tobacco and alcohol products.[95] It is apparent that comprehensive educational interventions directed at all health care providers and the public at large need to be implemented.[95] Table 10-6 contains basic information that everyone should know and understand for the prevention and early detection of oral cancers.

In addition to well-planned educational interventions, community-based supports such as policy, legislation, and ordinances are critically needed for prevention and early detection of oral cancers.[95] In the United States there is a trend to use public policy to help decrease or prevent behaviors that contribute to diseases. For example, no smoking policies in schools, hospitals, worksites, and restaurants help curtail smoking and make it socially unacceptable. These policies may be especially influential among youth who are the ones most likely to get hooked on the use of tobacco products. Further, *enforced* ordinances and laws making it more difficult for underaged youths to purchase tobacco or alcohol products also represent strong support for decreasing the initiation of their use. Concomitantly, enforcing fines and other disciplinary actions against individuals who sell or give these products to youths are equally necessary.

Other policies might be directed at health care providers. For example, dental and dental hygiene schools could require students to have exit competence in oral cancer examinations.[95] No state or regional dental board currently requires applicants to demonstrate competence in providing an oral cancer examination. Thus dental examining boards could require that applicants perform an oral cancer examination for licensure. Further, relicensure could require that applicants take a refresher course in oral

cancer prevention and early detection—a strategy used in other content areas.[95]

School-based drug interventions frequently begin in primary grades and often focus on developing self-esteem, building skills to resist peer pressure, and urging children to remain free of tobacco, alcohol, and other drugs. These school-based efforts often are implemented in conjunction with other community-based activities aimed at preventing children and youths from starting the habit and urging users to stop. Unfortunately, these kinds of educational interventions often do not identify tobacco products as risk factors for oral cancers. Similarly, efforts focusing on alcohol use as a risk factor for fetal alcohol syndrome, cirrhosis of the liver, and liver cancer usually do not identify alcohol as a risk factor for oral cancers.[95]

Need for health promotion in oral disease prevention

Today, we know how to prevent or control most oral diseases. With the appropriate use of fluorides and pit and fissure sealants, dental caries can be nearly eliminated. Also, with thorough and frequent plaque removal by an individual and periodic appointments with a dental care provider, most periodontal diseases can be prevented. Further, and most important, risk factors for and signs and symptoms of oral cancers have been established and there is an oral cancer screening examination for early detection. The knowledge resulting from scientific studies, however, is superfluous if it is not applied by appropriate lay and professional users. No matter how effective a preventive measure may be, the public cannot benefit if the procedure is unknown and not used appropriately. There are enormous gaps between what we know about preventing oral diseases and what we do.[96] It is now accepted that health promotion influences knowledge and behaviors at all levels of social organization. Health promotion helps bridge the gap between the knowledge generated by scientific studies and its appropriate application.[97]

Over the past 25 years interest in health promotion and disease prevention has increased significantly. At least three factors are responsible for this trend. First, ever-increasing expenditures for health care, most of which pay for the treatment of diseases or conditions, have taken an ever larger proportion of the U.S. gross national product. Second, a growing body of data has confirmed that many chronic diseases result from lifestyles that, theoretically, could be changed. Third, and very important, a body of scientific literature in health education and promotion has accumulated. Today, health promotion is recognized as a viable approach to preventing diseases and disorders and promoting health. To better understand health promotion, health education must be addressed.

HEALTH EDUCATION

Health education is "any combination of learning experiences designed to facilitate voluntary actions conducive to health."[98] These actions or behaviors may be on the part of individuals, families, institutions, or communities. Thus the scope of health education may include educational interventions for children, parents, policy makers, or health care providers. Education is necessary at all stages of designing, implementing, evaluating and continuing appropriate oral health programs. Education of all relevant groups is a critical factor in the process to gain acceptance and use of preventive measures, although education alone cannot function as a method to prevent disease. Knowledge is an important aspect of empowerment.[98-101] Without appropriate knowledge, individuals can neither make nor be expected to make intelligent decisions about their oral health or, in the case of decision makers, for the oral health of their constituents. Table 10-6 shows a list of content areas that all relevant publics need to know to attain

and maintain optimal oral health. Figs. 10-2 through 10-4 are examples of printed materials that might be used. It must be understood, however, that simply handing out a brochure on water fluoridation or a poster about the evils of tobacco use does not constitute a comprehensive educational program. It is clear that simply having information or knowledge does not automatically mean that appropriate actions or behaviors will follow. Thus education is necessary, but not sufficient to prevent oral diseases and conditions. However, without such information, the likelihood of taking appropriate actions is severely diminished.

HEALTH PROMOTION

Health promotion is "any planned combination of educational, political, regulatory, and organizational supports for actions and conditions of living conducive to the health of individuals, groups or communities."[98] Supports are intended to either alter a person's environments in a way that will improve health in the absence of individual actions (water fluoridation) or will enable the individual to take advantage of preventive procedures by removing barriers to their use. An example is making dental sealants available to children, especially those in low-income groups or in school settings. Health promotion is the processes used to transfer research results to appropriate users to improve health.[101]

Summary

Oral diseases are considered a "neglected epidemic" because they affect almost the total population, with millions of people having new disease each year. By age 17 years 84% of youths have had tooth decay, with an average of eight affected tooth surfaces, and, by age 40 to 44 years, 99% of adults have had tooth decay with an average of 30 affected tooth surfaces. For vulnerable populations, including low-income persons, minorities, the develop-

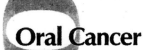

Oral Cancer

Early Detection Saves Lives

It's important to find oral cancer EARLY—before it has time to spread. The survival rate is much better for those whose cancer has not spread to other parts of the body.

Possible Signs and Symptoms

- a white or red patch in the mouth

- a sore, irritation, lump, or thickening in the mouth

- hoarseness, or a feeling that something is caught in the throat

- difficulty chewing or swallowing

- difficulty moving the jaw or tongue

- numbness of the tongue or other areas of the mouth

- swelling of the jaw that causes dentures to fit poorly or become uncomfortable

See your dentist or physician if any of the above symptoms last for more than two weeks.

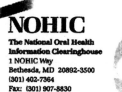

over

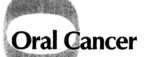

Oral Cancer

Lower Your Risk

- Do not use tobacco products—cigarettes, chew or snuff, pipes, or cigars

- If you drink alcohol, do so only in moderation

- Eat a diet rich in fruits and vegetables (research suggests this might lower the risk of oral cancer)

Have an Exam

A head and neck exam should be a routine part of your dental visit. Ask your dentist or physician to do the exam at least once a year.

Remember:
Early detection saves lives!

A message from the
National Oral Health Information Clearinghouse,
a service of the National Institute of Dental Research,
National Institutes of Health

For more information on oral cancer, contact:

NOHIC

**The National Oral Health
Information Clearinghouse**
1 NOHIC Way
Bethesda, MD 20892-3500
(301) 402-7364
Fax: (301) 907-8830
e-mail nidr@aerie.com

Fig. 10-2. Oral cancer information. (*Available from The National Oral Health Information Clearinghouse.*)

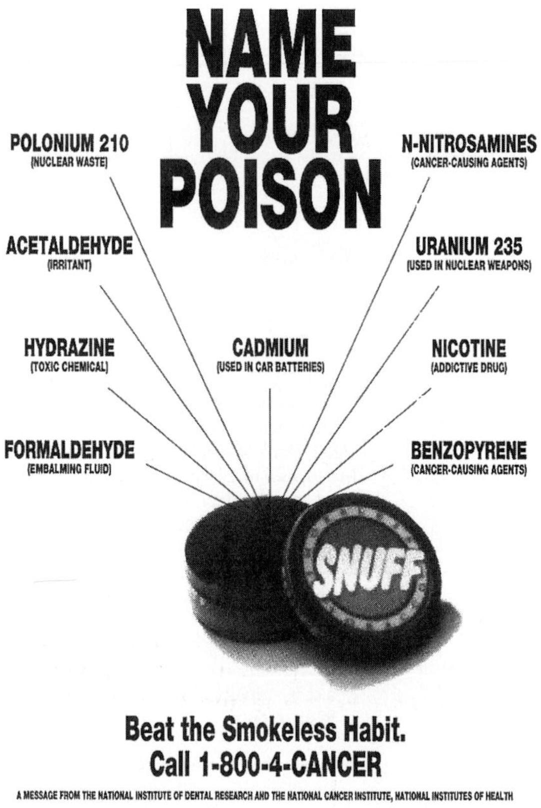

NAME YOUR POISON

POLONIUM 210
(NUCLEAR WASTE)

N-NITROSAMINES
(CANCER-CAUSING AGENTS)

ACETALDEHYDE
(IRRITANT)

URANIUM 235
(USED IN NUCLEAR WEAPONS)

HYDRAZINE
(TOXIC CHEMICAL)

CADMIUM
(USED IN CAR BATTERIES)

NICOTINE
(ADDICTIVE DRUG)

FORMALDEHYDE
(EMBALMING FLUID)

BENZOPYRENE
(CANCER-CAUSING AGENTS)

SNUFF

Beat the Smokeless Habit.
Call 1-800-4-CANCER

A MESSAGE FROM THE NATIONAL INSTITUTE OF DENTAL RESEARCH AND THE NATIONAL CANCER INSTITUTE, NATIONAL INSTITUTES OF HEALTH

Fig. 10-3. "Name Your Poison" poster. (*Available from The National Oral Health Information Clearinghouse.*)

Community Water Fluoridation

THE #1 WAY TO PREVENT DENTAL DECAY

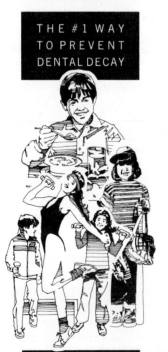

Fig. 10-4. Fluoridation leaflet. (*Available from American Association of Public Health Dentistry, 10619 Jousting Lane, Richmond, VA 23235-3838.*)

mentally disabled, the homebound, and those with AIDS, the extent of the problem is even greater. Although $42 million is spent every year in the United States for dental care, only one of five children receiving Medicaid, or 20%, receive dental care. Unfortunately, oral health is not a priority in this country, and we do not have a national oral disease prevention program.

Prevention of disease, disability, and suffering should be a primary goal of any society that hopes to provide a decent quality of life for its people. Primary prevention is the most effective way to keep people healthy and to control costs because the disease is prevented before it occurs. Secondary prevention treats the disease after it occurs and tertiary prevention limits or rehabilitates a disability from disease. Prevention on the community or population-based level is the most cost-effective approach and has the greatest impact on a community, whether it is a school, neighborhood, or nation. Community prevention programs should be used only when they have been shown to be effective by well-designed clinical studies. The use of fluorides, the thirteenth most abundant element in the earth's crust, has made a significant impact on preventing caries in the United States.

Community water fluoridation should be the foundation of oral disease prevention and treatment programs. Fluoridation is the most cost-effective prevention measure in dentistry. At 1 ppm fluoridation prevented tooth decay by 50% to 70% in the early controlled studies, and now, as a result of the widespread use of fluoridation and other fluoride products in the United States, it prevents caries in primary teeth by 30% to 60% and in mixed dentition by 20% to 40%, and 15% to 35% for adolescents and adults, respectively. It also prevents root caries in older adults by up to 35%.

In 1992 more than 144 million Americans, or 62% of the 232 million people on public water supplies, had fluoridation, nearly 56% of the total population. About 10 million of these Americans live in communities that are naturally fluoridated at the recommended level. The safety and legality of fluoridation has been well documented since the first controlled studies in 1945. A well-planned educational program for community leaders and decision makers is important to help them understand all the benefits of this public health measure. This education must continue over time. A well-educated community is the best weapon against antifluoridation activities.

School-based fluoride programs are an alternative when community water fluoridation is not available. These programs may include school water fluoridation, dietary fluoride supplements, or fluoride rinses. School dental sealant programs are effective on the occlusal surfaces of the teeth of children ages 6 to 8 and 12 to 14 years of age when the first and second molars erupt.

Periodontal disease (gingivitis) prevention programs on a community level have been shown to be effective when supervised, but they are not very practical. Everyone, however, needs to practice proper oral hygiene and have a prophylaxis or mechanical plaque removal periodically.

Unintentional oral-facial injuries may result in broken teeth, facial fractures, concussions, and temporomandibular dysfunction. More than 25 million U.S. children participate in competitive school sports and 20 million in organized sports outside school. Protective headgear and mouthguards have reduced dramatically the number of oral-facial injuries in football. Other sports such as basketball, baseball, and soccer need to have regulations and promotion for effective head, face, eye, and mouth protection.

About 30,000 Americans are diagnosed with oral cancer each year. More Americans die from oral cancers than from cervical cancer or melanoma, about 8000 persons yearly. Oral cancer has one of the lowest 5-year survival rates of 11 major cancer sites because of late detection. Tobacco and alcohol account for 75% of all oral and pharyngeal cancers. Community-based incentives for policy, legislation, and ordinances to prevent and control tobacco use are important. Dentists, physicians, and other primary care providers can play a significant role in oral cancer prevention and early detection.[102]

Health promotion, which includes health education, is pivotal to implementing primary effective community prevention programs. Effective community prevention programs for oral diseases must be the foundation for responding to this neglected epidemic if we are to have a healthy society.

REFERENCES

1. Allukian M: The neglected American epidemic, *Nation's Health*, 20(5):2, May-June, 1990.
2. National Institute of Dental Research: *Oral health of United States children: The National Survey of Dental Caries in U.S. School Children: 1986-1987*, DHHS pub, NIH 89-2247, Bethesda, Md, 1989, US Department of Health and Human Services.
3. National Center for Health Statistics: *Health United States, 1995*, Hyattsville, Md, 1996, US Public Health Service, US Department of Health and Human Services.
4. Office of Inspector General, Children's Dental Services Under Medicaid: *Access and utilization*, OBI-09-93-00240, Washington, DC, 1996, US Department of Health and Human Services.
5. *Webster's new world dictionary of American English,* ed 3, New York, 1993, Prentice Hall/MacMillan.
6. National Institute of Dental Research: *Oral health of United States adults: The National Survey of Oral Health in US Employed Adults and Seniors: 1985-1986*, DHHS pub, NIH 87-2868 Bethesda, Md, 1987, U.S. Department of Health and Human Services.
7. Winn DM et al: Coronal and root caries in the dentition of adults in the United States, 1988-1991, *J Dent Res* 75 (special iss): 642-651, 1996.
8. *Healthy people 2000,* PHS pub no 91-50212, Washington, DC, 1990, US Public Health Service, US Department of Health and Human Services.
9. Centers for Disease Control and Prevention: Engineering and administrative recommendations for water fluoridation, *MMWR Morbid Mortal Wkly Rep* 44:RR-13, 1-40, Sept 29, 1995.
10. Centers for Disease Control and Prevention: *Fluoridation census: 1992*, Atlanta, 1993, US Public Health Service, US Department of Health and Human Services.
11. Reeves TG: Technical aspects of water fluoridation in the United States and an overview of fluoridation engineering worldwide, *Commun Dent Health* 13:(Suppl 2):21-26, 1996.
12. *Review of fluoride: benefits and risks,* Washington, DC, 1991, US Public Health Service.
13. Kaminsky LS, et al: Fluoride: benefits and risk of exposure, *Crit Rev Oral Biol Med* 1(4):261-281, 1990.
14. National Research Council: *Health effects of ingested fluoride,* Washington, DC, 1993, National Academy Press.
15. Fluoridation facts, Chicago, 1993, American Dental Association.
16. Wolf CA et al: *Abuse of the scientific literature in an antifluoridation pamphlet,* Baltimore, 1985, American Oral Health Institute.
17. Hunt J et al: Putting Yiamounyannis into perspective, *Br Dent J* 179:121-123, 1995.
18. Ripa LW: A half-century of community water fluoridation in the United States: review and commentary, *J Public Health Dent* 53:17-44, 1993.
19. Arnold FA Jr et al: Fifteenth year of Grand Rapids fluoridation study, *J Am Dent Assoc* 65:780-785, 1962.
20. Hillboe HE et al: Newburg-Kingston caries-fluorine study: final report, *J Am Dent Assoc* 52:290-325, 1956.
21. Blayney JR, Hill IN: Fluorine and dental caries, *J Am Dent Assoc* 74:(special issue) 233-302, 1967.
22. Brown HK, Poplove M: The Brantford-Sarnia-Stratford fluoridation caries study: final survey, 1963, *Can J Public Health* 56(80):319-324, 1965.
23. Newbrun E: Effectiveness of water fluoridation, *J Public Health Dent* 49(special issue):279-289, 1989.
24. Burt B: Proceedings of the workshop: Cost-Effectiveness of Caries Prevention in Dental Public Health, *J Public Health Dent* 49(special issue):250-344, 1989.
25. Centers for Disease Control and Prevention: *Fluoridation census 1989: summary*, Atlanta, 1991, US Public Health Service, US Department of Health and Human Services.
26. Centers for Disease Control and Prevention: Public health focus: fluoridation of community water systems, *MMWR Morbid Mortal Wkly Rep* 41(2):372-375, 381, 1992.
27. Block LE: Antifluoridationists persist: the constitutional basis for fluoridation, *J Public Health Dent* 46:188-197, 1986.
28. Neenan ME: Obstacles to extending fluoridation in the United States, *Commun Dent Health* 13(Suppl 2):10-20, 1996.
29. Gift HC, Corbin SB, Nowjack-Raymer RE: Public knowledge about prevention of dental caries and symptoms of gum disease—1990 NHIS, *Public Health Rep* 109:397-404,1990.
30. O'Neill HW: Opinion study comparing attitudes about dental health, *J Am Dent Assoc* 109:910-915, 1984.

31. Allukian M, Steinhurst J, Dunning JM: Community organization and a regional approach to fluoridation of the greater Boston area, *J Am Dent Assoc* 104:491-493, 1981.

32. Allukian M, Ackerman J, Steinhurst J: Factors that influence the attitudes of first-term Massachusetts legislators toward fluoridation, *J Am Dent Assoc* 104:494-496, 1981.

33. Boriskin JM, Fine JI: Fluoridation election victory: a case study for dentistry in effective political action, *J Am Dent Assoc* 102:486-491, 1981.

34. Easley MW: The new antifluoridationists: who are they and how do they operate? *J Public Health Dent* 45:133-141, 1985.

35. Smith KG, Christen KA: A fluoridation campaign: the Phoenix experience, *J Public Health Dent* 50:319-322, 1990.

36. Frazier PJ: Priorities to preserve fluoride uses: rationales and strategies, *J Public Health Dent* 45:149-165,1985.

37. Executive summary: application for continued recognition of dental public health as a dental specialty, *J Public Health Dent* 46:35-37,1986.

38. Allukian M: Fluoridation—a continual struggle in Massachusetts, *Harvard Dent Alum Bull* 28:77-80, 84, 1968.

39. Collier DR: The statewide fluoridation program of Tennessee through the voluntary process, *J Am Dent Assoc* 93:837-838, 1976.

40. Clark DC, Hann HJ: A win for fluoridation in Squamish, British Columbia, *J Public Health Dent* 49:170-171, 1989.

41. Faine RC et al: The 1980 fluoridation campaigns: a discussion of results, *J Public Health Dent* 41:138-142, 1981.

42. Jones RB, Mormann DN, Durtsche TB: Fluoridation referendum in La Crosse, Wisconsin: contributing factors to success, *Am J Public Health* 79:1405-1407, 1989.

43. Horowitz AM, Frazier PJ: Promoting the use of fluorides in a community. In Newbrun E, editor: *Fluorides and dental caries*, ed 3, Springfield, Ill, 1986, Charles C Thomas.

44. Oral Health Coordinating Committee: *National fluoride plan to promote oral health*, Washington, DC, 1996, U.S. Department of Health and Human Services, US Public Health Service.

45. Oral Health Coordinating Committee: *Nation fluoride plan to promote oral health, executive summary*, Washington, DC, 1996, US Department of Health and Human Services, US Public Health Service.

46. Evans AW, Darvell BW: Refining the estimate of the critical period for susceptibility to enamel fluorosis in human maxillary central incisors, *J Public Health Dent* 55:238-249, 1995.

47. Pendrys DG, Stamm JW: Relationships of total fluoride intake to beneficial effects and enamel fluorosis, *J Dent Res* 69(special issue):529-538,1990.

48. American Dental Association, Council on Access, Prevention and Interprofessional Relations: Caries diagnosis and risk assessment: a review of preventive strategies and management, *J Am Dent Assoc Spec Suppl* 126:1-24, 1995.

49. Heifetz SB, Horowitz HS, Brunelle JA: Effect of school water fluoridation on dental caries: results in Seagrove, NC, after 12 years, *J Am Dent Assoc* 106:334-337, 1983.

50. Horowitz AM, Horowitz HS: School-based fluoride programs: a critique, *J Prevent Dent* 6:89-94, 1980.

51. Stephen KW: Systemic fluorides: drops and tablets, *Caries Res* 27(suppl 1):9-15, 1993.

52. Driscoll WS et al: Caries-preventive effects of daily and weekly fluoride mouthrinsing in a fluoridated community: final results after 30 months, *J Am Dent Assoc* 105:1010-1013, 1982.

53. Ripa LW: Sealants revisited: an update of the effectiveness of pit-and-fissure sealants, *Caries Res* 27(suppl 1):367-380, 1993.

54. Selwitz RH et al: The prevalence of dental sealants in the US population: findings from NHSNES III, 1988-91, *J Dent Res* 75(special issue):652-660, 1996.

55. Mertz-Fairhurst EJ: Pit-and-fissure sealants: a global lack of science transfer [Guest editorial], *J Dent Res* 71:1543-1544, 1992.

56. Kunzel W: Systemic use of fluoride and other methods: salt, sugar, milk, etc., *Caries Res* 27(suppl 1):16-22, 1993.

57. Marthaler TM et al: DMF teeth in school children after 18 years of collective salt fluoridation, *Caries Res* 23:428, 1989.

58. Estupinan-Day S, Baez R, editors: *Impact of salt fluoridation in preventing caries in Jamaica*, Washington, DC, 1996, Pan American Health Organization.

59. Seppa L: Studies of fluoride varnishes in Finland, *Proc Finn Dent Soc* 87:541-547,1991.

60. Clark DC et al: Results of a 32-month fluoride varnish study in Sherbrooke and La-Megantic, Canada, *J Am Dent Assoc* 111:949-53,1985.

61. Horowitz HS, Ismail AI: Topical fluorides in caries prevention. In Fejereskov O, Ekstrand J, Burt BA, editors: *Fluoride in dentistry*, ed 2, Copenhagen, 1996, Munksgaard.

62. Mandel ID: Fluoride varnishes—a welcome addition, *J Public Health Dent* 54:67,1994.

63. Anusavice KJ: Treatment regimens in preventive and restorative dentistry, *J Am Dent Assoc* 126:727-740, 1995.

64. Proceedings of the IADR symposium minimal intervention technique for dental caries, *J Public Health Dent* 56:129-166, 1996.

65. Frandsen A: Mechanical oral hygiene practices. In Loe H, Kleinman DV, editors: *Dental plaque control measures and oral hygiene practices,* Washington, DC, 1986, IRL Press.

66. Mandel ID: Antimicrobial mouthrinses: overview and update, *J Am Dent Assoc* 125:2-S–10-S, 1994.

67. Horowitz AM et al: Effects of supervised daily dental plaque removal by children after 3 years, *Oral Epidemiol Commun Dent* 8:171-176, 1980.

68. Chen MS: Oral health of disadvantaged populations. In Cohen LK, Gift HC, editors: *Disease prevention and oral health promotion,* Copenhagen, 1995, Munksgaard.

69. Bolden AJ, Henry JL, Allukian M: Implications of access, utilization and need for oral health care by low income groups and minorities on the dental delivery system, *J Dent Educ* 57: 888-900, 1993.

70. Allukian M: Oral health—an essential service for the homeless (editorial), *J Public Health Dent* 55:8-9, 1995.

71. Heller KH et al: Longitudinal evaluation of sealing molars with and without incipient dental caries in a public health program, *J Public Health Dent* 55:148-153, 1995.

72. Nowjack-Raynor RE, Gift HC: Use of mouthguards and headgear in organized sports by school-aged children, *Public Health Rep* 111:82-86, 1996.

73. Kaste LM et al: Prevalence of incisor trauma in persons 6 to 50 years of age: United States, 1966-1991, *J Dent Res* 75(special issue):696-705, 1996.

74. Becker DB, Needleman HL, Kotelchuck M: Child abuse and dentistry: oralfacial trauma and its recognition by dentists, *J Am Dent Assoc* 97:24-28, 1978.

75. National Safe Kids Campaign: Sports injury fact sheet, Washington, DC, 1996.

76. Lephart SM, Fu FH: Emergency treatment of athletic injuries, *Dent Clin North Am* 35:707-717, 1991.

77. Meadow D, Lidner G, Needleman H: Oral trauma in children, *Pediatr Dent* 6:248-251, 1984.

78. National Injury Information Clearinghouse: *Estimates for sports injuries,* Washington DC, 1995, U.S. Consumer Project Safety Commission.

79. Heintz WD: Mouth protection: a progress report, Report of Councils and Bureaus, *J Am Dent Assoc* 77:632-636, 1968.

80. Ranalli DN, Lancaster DM: Attitudes of college football officials regarding NCAA mouthguard regulations and player compliance, *J Public Health Dent* 53:96-100, 1993.

81. Maestrello-deMoya MG, Primosch RE: Orofacial trauma mouth protector wear among high school varsity basketball players, *J Dent Child* 56(1):33-39, 1989.

82. McNutt T et al: Oral trauma in adolescent athletes: a study of mouth protectors, *Pediatr Dent* 11:209-213, 1989.

83. Soporowski NJ, Tesini DA, Weiss AI: Survey of oralfacial sports-related injuries, *J Mass Dent Soc* 43:16-20, 1994.

84. Elliott MA: Professional responsibility in sports dentistry, *Dent Clin North Am* 35(4):831-840, 1991.

85. Ranalli DR, Lancaster DM: Attitudes of college football coaches regarding NCAA mouthguard regulation and player compliance, *J Public Health Dent* 55:139-142, 1995.

86. Winters JE: Sports dentistry: the profession's role in athletics, *J Am Dent Assoc* 127:810-811, 1996.

87. Boring CC et al: Cancer statistics, 1994, *CA Cancer J Clin* 44:7-26, 1994.

88. Silverman S Jr, Shillitoe EJ: Etiology and predisposing factors. In Silverman S Jr, editor: *Oral cancer,* ed 3, Atlanta, 1990, American Cancer Society.

89. Murphy GP, Lawrence W Jr, Lenhard RE Jr, editors: *Textbook of clinical oncology,* ed 2, Atlanta, 1995, American Cancer Society.

90. Mecklenburg RE et al: Tobacco effects in the mouth: a National Cancer Institute and National Institute of Dental Research Guide for Health Professionals, Bethesda, Md, 1992, National Cancer Institute, US Department of Health and Human Services, US Public Health Service, NIH pub no 92-3330.

91. Winn DM: Diet and nutrition in the etiology of oral cancer, *Am J Clin Nutr* 61: (Suppl):437S, 1995.

92. Horowitz AM, Nourjah P, Gift HG: US adult knowledge of risk factors for and signs of oral cancers: 1990, *J Am Dent Assoc* 126:39-45, 1995.

93. Horowitz AM, Nourjah PA: Patterns of screening for oral cancers among US adults, *J Public Health Dent* 56:333-335, 1996.

94. Yellowitz JA, Goodman HS: Physicians' and dentists' oral cancer knowledge, opinions and practice, *J Am Dent Assoc* 126:53-60, 1995.

95. Yellowitz JA et al: Assessment of alcohol and tobacco use in dental schools health history forms, *J Dent Educ* 59:1091-1096, 1995.

96. Horowitz AM et al: The need for health promotion in oral cancer prevention and early detection, *J Public Health Dent* 56:319-330, 1996.

97. Horowitz AM: The public's oral health: the gaps between what we know and what we do, *Adv Dent Science* 9:91-95, 1995.

98. Frazier PJ, Horowitz AM: Prevention: a public health perspective. In Cohen LK, Gift HC, editors: *Disease prevention and oral health promotion,* Copenhagen, 1995, Munksgaard.

99. Green LW, Kreuter MW: Health promotion planning: an educational and environmental approach, ed 2, Mountain View, Calif, 1991, Mayfield.

100. Glanz K, Lewis FM, Rimer BK, editors: Health behavior and health education theory research and practice, San Francisco, 1990, Jossey-Bass.

101. Frazier PJ, Horowitz AM: Oral health education and promotion in maternal and child health: a position paper, *J Public Health Dent* 50:390-395, 1990.

102. Centers for Disease Control and Prevention: *Proceedings: National Strategic Planning Conference for the Prevention and Control of Oral and Pharyngeal Cancer,* August 7-9, 1996, Atlanta. Bethesda, MD, 1997, US Department of Health and Human Services, US Public Health Service.

CHAPTER 11

Dental health education

Marianne B. DeSouza
Nancy R. Kressin

Why is dental health education still important?

Results from a recent survey of the nation's oral health indicate that, although caries rates have decreased in recent years, 45% of children and adolescents still have evidence of the disease. The survey also found that 10% of adults are completely edentulous, and only one third have all 28 teeth. Periodontal disease indicators showed that a third of individuals 25 to 34 years old had moderate attachment loss, as did 63% of 45 to 54 year olds and 80% of people more than 65 years old. More severe periodontal disease was found in 15% of those surveyed.[1] These data indicate that oral disease remains a public health problem for Americans; one way this problem can be addressed is through dental health education.

Although the American Dental Association (ADA) recommends that individuals brush and floss their teeth at least once a day in addition to having regular dental examinations,[2] research suggests that many individuals do not adhere to this recommendation. Lang, Ronis, and Farghaly[3] found in a recent survey of Detroit area residents that although more than 96% of the individuals surveyed did brush at

least once a day, only 84% demonstrated adherence to their definition of "acceptable" brushing technique (e.g., brushing all teeth, including those that do not show when smiling). In the same study only 33% of individuals reported flossing daily, and only 22% demonstrated "acceptable" flossing technique (e.g., flossing all teeth). Because these data suggest a need for improvement in individuals' oral self-care, the need for effective dental health education remains clear.

What is dental health education?

Dental health education for the community is a process that informs, motivates, and helps persons to adopt and maintain health practices and lifestyles; advocates environmental changes as needed to facilitate this goal; and conducts professional training and research to the same end.*[4-8] Health education is any com-

*Modified from the definition of consumer health education adopted by the 1975 National Institutes of Health Fogarty International Center and American College of Preventive Medicine Task Force on Consumer Health Education.

bination of learning opportunities designed to facilitate voluntary adaptations of behavior that are conducive to health.[9] Health education programs are not isolated events but educational aspects of any curative, preventive, or promotional health activity. Comprehension of the multifactorial variables in dental disease and their interaction has increased the emphasis now placed on the educational process to assist in achieving desired health outcomes.

It has been well documented in dentistry and other health areas that correct health information or knowledge alone does not necessarily lead to desirable health behaviors.[10] However, knowledge gained may serve as a tool to empower population groups with accurate information about health and health care technologies, enabling them to take action to protect their health.[11] Both internal and external variables influence whether an individual or community will comply with recommended disease prevention, health maintenance, or health promotion procedures. Health promotion is any combination of educational, organizational, economic, political, and environmental supports for behavior conducive to health.[9] Health promotion refers to actions that are intended either to alter the living environment of persons to improve their health, despite individual actions such as community water fluoridation, or to enable and empower individuals to take advantage of preventive procedures or services by reducing or eliminating access barriers. Other actions might include making available—or removing financial barriers to—procedures such as the appropriate use of fluoride supplements, use of dental sealants, supervised removal of dental plaque, and effective referral and follow-up services for children and women who need treatment.[12] "Education" and "promotion"' are intertwined to achieve long-term improved health for maternal and child focus populations and for other populations within American society.

Procedures implemented through promotion can prevent a given disease or condition, but only education can foster informed decision making and maintenance of needed programs, services or behaviors. Health education and promotion processes permeate all levels of individuals and groups, and may include working with patients, parents, legislators, industry, and all other levels of influential policy makers, including health care providers.[12]

The dental health educator must be cognizant of available resources and demographic changes affecting social, economic, and health services environments. In addition, the educator must weigh internal and external variables in relation to clinical and behavioral research findings when designing a community program that will be effective in achieving long-term results.

Knowledge of program planning and community organization is essential, and skill development in these areas warrants inclusion in the professional preparation of the dentist and dental hygienist. To date, however, development of these skills has received little attention. The ADA and the American Dental Hygienists' Association (ADHA) have responded to the expanding role of the dentist and the dental hygienist as health educators in the clinical practice setting and in the community by developing a variety of educational resources. Professional development products include guides, brochures, posters, flyers, and videos, many of which are available in English and in Spanish for individual or group education during community presentations. The ADA catalog for 1996 to 1997, "Materials You Need for Your Effective Practice," includes the following general topics: Educating Patients, Managing Your Practice, Controlling Infection, Posters & Plaques, and Videos that Teach. The ADA has developed a new two-part teaching guide called "Smile Magic" with lesson plans, activities, and activity sheets for preschool to grade 2 and grades 3 through 5. The ADA also offers a National Children's Dental Health Month

Planning Guide, Starter Kit, and Supplemental Materials to promote a successful annual February observance.[13]

The ADHA has developed an audiocassette self-study continuing education program of courses and other professional development products that present the latest in theories and techniques intrinsic to successful dental hygiene practice. The ADHA also offers an array of practical guides for helping career-minded individuals and active program planners achieve success in community outreach programs and public relations and legislative action skill development.[14]

Most professional training revolves around learning specific technical procedures and working with patients on a one-to-one basis. In this situation individual patient motivation is the primary objective of dental health education and unfortunately constitutes only a small component of the overall treatment plan.[15] Ideally, this relationship allows the dental practitioner to tailor the preventive prescription to each individual patient's needs, and patients can identify their own short- and long-term dental health goals. Through this process the dental professional is able to help those patients amenable to prevention to internalize the value of good oral health and to practice preventive measures. Chambers,[4] however, has concluded that strong evidence suggests that only a limited number of Americans are amenable to an at-home program of controlling plaque. A principal factor suppressing this number is that healthy habits of living are not supported by deep-seated cultural values. The role of the health educator becomes an essential component in the management of dental disease and in helping patients assume responsibility for their own oral health maintenance.

In most cases the same skills that were developed in working with patients on a one-to-one basis are carried over to the community setting. As a result, community dental health programs are usually conducted in much the same manner as individual patient education. Specific educational efforts focus on presenting dental health information and on trying to change an individual's attitudes and behaviors with regard to oral hygiene habits and diet rather than on emphasizing an organized community approach to prevention and control of disease. Emphasis is placed on correct brushing and flossing techniques to help prevent, or at least control, periodontal disease and on nutritional counseling, sealants, fluoride therapy for caries control, use of mouthguards in contact sports, and antismoking and anti-smokeless-tobacco education.

Success of these primary health promotion endeavors relies on the individual's development of specific skills and their incorporation into the person's lifestyle to reduce the prevalence of caries, periodontal disease, oral injuries, and oral cancer. Although popular, when it is used alone, this approach to disease prevention has had limited success in reducing oral disease and may not be an appropriate focus for public health education.[12,16,17,18] Behavioral theories applicable on an individual level may not be directly transferable to solving group and community level health problems—theories of public health and epidemiology may be more relevant for societal change.[11,19] In each case the health educator needs to choose the framework most appropriate for addressing the problem.[20] Given Winslow's definition of dental public health—the science and art of preventing and controlling dental disease and promoting dental health through organized community efforts—an alternative approach focusing on individual behavior change would be to target health education efforts to community leaders, as suggested by Frazier.[21] This approach would redirect the educational processes to the selection of prevention and control programs that operate at the community level and do not require daily compliance on the part of the individual. Further,

Frazier and Horowitz[11] suggest that focusing health education and promotion efforts with a broader range of children and parent subpopulations produces a positive potential for a major impact on the oral health of future generations of families in different socioeconomic groups. All mothers and infant caretakers—whether male or female, young or old—need to know how to prevent oral diseases. By imparting that knowledge to the children in their care and by reinforcing good daily oral health habits the oral health of future generations could improve dramatically. School-based health education and promotion activities are viable ways of reinforcing healthy behaviors.

The purpose of this chapter is to present an overview of the current issues and concepts in dental health education and to discuss the transition in educational activities from the traditional approach to current and suggested approaches. By examining continuing community programs and examples of other organized community efforts, the student should be able to determine which program goals are appropriate for public health education and possible ways to accomplish those goals. In addition, areas of recent and recommended educational research will be highlighted. We hope that previously held beliefs will be challenged and that the extent, complexity, and importance of community dental health education will be better understood.

Key issues in dental health education

Although much progress has been made in the state of the nation's oral health through dental health education efforts in the past, a number of important dental public health problems remain, and existing programs can benefit from giving special consideration to the unique needs of a variety of populations that may need such education. Many issues still need to be addressed by future dental health

education efforts. A few of these are mentioned here to provide the reader with a general understanding of the types of problems that future dental health education should address.

WATER FLUORIDATION

The appropriate use of fluorides is the best method available to prevent the onset of dental caries. Interventions that used fluoride have been successful in both preventing dental caries, averting pain and discomfort, and saving money. The most cost-effective method to provide protection against dental caries for the community is community water fluoridation.[22] It is a challenge for all health care providers to reach the entire population with preventive interventions at the community level. The Centers for Disease Control and Prevention estimates the per-person cost for community water fluoridation at $0.50 per year, or approximately $40 for a lifetime. Yet only 135 million people, or 61% of the population on community water supplies, are receiving this preventive measure. Nonfluoridated community water supplies are predominantly in cities in the northeastern and western United States.[23] Dental health educational efforts are needed to continue to inform community residents and legislators about the beneficial effects of fluoridation.

ORAL SELF-CARE BEHAVIORS

Oral self-care behaviors by individuals are still not at recommended levels.[2,3] Educational efforts aimed at individuals and communities are still needed to increase the prevalence of such behaviors to improve their oral health status.

ORAL SCREENING AND RISK FACTORS FOR ORAL CANCER

A 1993 report from the American Cancer Society relative to the incidence of and mortality rates resulting from cancers of the oral pharnyx and the oral cavity are sobering and fortify the need for routine oral cancer screening at each dental visit. In 1993 20,900 people in the United States were diagnosed with oral cancers, and 7700 deaths were attributed to these cancers. Oral cancers are more common than leukemia, melanoma, and cancers of the brain, liver, kidney, thyroid, stomach, ovary, or cervix. Possible sites include tongue, lips, floor of the mouth, soft palate, tonsils, salivary glands, and the nasopharynx.[24] Risk factors include use of tobacco products and alcohol, exposure to the sun (lip cancer), dietary factors, and exposure to carcinogens in the workplace.[25] Use of tobacco products has also been identified as a major risk factor for periodontal diseases relative to increased susceptibility, onset in young adults, severity and extent of disease, disease progression, and treatment failure.[26] According to the American Cancer Society, 70% of adults who have smoked began before the age of 18 years.[24] To reduce mortality from oral cancers in accordance with the *Healthy People 2000* initiative, oral care providers need to ask patients about lifestyles and risk-taking behaviors, especially preteens and teens. Resources are available to assist health professionals in improving the health of their patients and students by implementing smoking and tobacco education and prevention and cessation programs in their practices and in the school curriculum.[27] Several health organizations have taken action to institute tobacco control programs and recommendations. In 1995 the ADA established a new clinical service code, #01320, "Tobacco counseling for the control and prevention of dental disease." The Institute of Medicine took action to protect children and youth by adopting policy recommendations for communities, states, and the federal government.[28] In 1996 the Agency for Health Care Policy and Research published clinical practice guidelines for smoking prevention and cessation.[29] Readers are encouraged to review the tobacco use prevention and cessation resource list published in the March-April 1995 issue of the *Journal of Dental Hygiene*. Tobacco use remains at epidemic levels, and young people still begin to smoke and use smokeless tobacco at alarming rates.[30] Dental health education efforts by dental care practitioners, other health care professionals of all types, classroom teachers, and community health educators can help decrease these trends by emphasizing how tobacco causes oral disease and many physical health problems.

BABY-BOTTLE TOOTH DECAY

Baby-bottle tooth decay is a growing problem in the United States, increasingly affecting affluent members of the population in addition to the racial and linguistic minority groups that have previously been known to be affected.[31] Dental health education efforts need to be targeted to a wide range of the population, pediatric and family practice physicians, pediatric nurse practitioners, nurses, and physician assistants, parents and caregivers, so that a broad-based understanding of the causes, effects, and methods of preventing this devastating condition can be effectively communicated.

ORAL HEALTH EFFECTS OF ANOREXIA NERVOSA AND BULIMIA

The oral health effects of anorexia nervosa and bulimia may assist in the clinical diagnosis of these disorders. Health care professionals need to be aware of the oral manifestations so that they can make appropriate referrals for dental treatment. These are serious psychologic disorders that may lead to death as a result of physical complications or suicide. The National Association for Anorexia Nervosa and Associated Disorders in Highland Park, Illinois, reports that at least 8 million people in the United States suffer from eating disorders that last from 1 to 15 years with only half of those diagnosed with long-term disorders are ever cured.[32]

Dental professionals may play a significant role in identifying patients with eating disorders on the basis of specific oral symptoms (enamel erosion, caries, periodontal disease, changes in oral mucosae [i.e., contusions or lacerations of soft palate associated with induced vomiting, dehydration, erythema, angular cheilitis, and swollen salivary glands]).[33,34] It is the responsibility of dental professionals to be familiar with the diagnostic criteria for eating disorders. Providing appropriate treatment in a supportive environment, information, and referrals for pyschologic and medical help and follow-up could save a life.

ORAL HEALTH EFFECTS OF HIV/AIDS

The oral health effects of human immunodeficiency virus (HIV) and acquired immunodeficiency syndrome (AIDS) need to be recognized and addressed by health care professionals. Dental health educators should play a part in communicating information about the effects of the disease on oral health. Dental professionals, especially dental hygienists, should be familiar with the primary manifestations of HIV and AIDS: candidiasis (thrush), hairy leukoplakia, recurrent aphthous ulcers and herpetic lesions, Kaposi's sarcoma, linear gingival erythema (formerly HIV-G), and HIV periodontitis.[35] The initial diagnosis of AIDS or HIV may be made on the basis of oral lesions and symptoms.[35] Although there is no documentation of HIV transmission from patient to dental care providers or from patient to patient, providers struggle with fears of HIV transmission. Passage of the Americans with Disabilities Act in 1990 has led to a number of lawsuits against dentists for refusal to treat patients with HIV. Federal courts have ruled consistently that people with HIV can be treated safely in private dental offices with universal precautions as recommended by the Centers for Disease Control and Prevention, the ADHA, and the ADA.[36] Ideally, the hygienist and the dentist are members of a comprehensive care team working closely with the patient's physician in the medical and support group caring for people with AIDS. These is-

sues are discussed in greater detail in Chapters 4 and 17.

CULTURAL ISSUES INHERENT IN DENTAL HEALTH EDUCATION

Because dental health education must take place within a cultural context, sensitivity to such cultural issues may increase the efficacy of such efforts. Oral self-care practices, attitudes, and knowledge vary across cultural groups, and these differences are important to understand before educational interventions are designed.[37] For example, if a particular cultural group has a fatalistic view that says that health can't be influenced by any actions taken by the individual, then the suggestion to brush or floss the teeth to improve oral health might go against this deeply held cultural assumption. Kiyak has suggested that there may be several general factors that may affect a particular group's health care practices; these include "cultural values, the socioeconomic status of a given ethnic group, language differences, misinterpretations of verbal and behavioral cues in the health care encounter, and the previous medical experiences of a given ethnic group."[38]

It is also important to recognize that socioeconomic status is frequently intertwined with racial and cultural factors. In the United States members of racial minority groups frequently have lower incomes and less education than whites do. Although these socioeconomic differences are associated with different racial groups, it is important to understand that the effects of race are not the same as the effects of socioeconomic factors. For example, a recent study comparing oral self-care behaviors of blacks and whites found significant differences in the frequency of dental visits of the two racial groups, but when socioeconomic status was taken into account, these differences were reduced.[39] Additional information concerning cultural issues is presented in Chapter 6.

DENTAL HEALTH EDUCATION FOR OLDER ADULTS

The importance of preventive oral self-care behaviors may increase in later life with the advent of age-related comorbidities or medication usage that affects oral health (causing, for example, xerostomia). Declines in oral health may result in inadequate dentition, potentially leading to nutritional declines, speech problems, or threats to social interaction because of related functional impairments or cosmetic factors. Given the declines in physical health and physical activities that some elderly people face, activities involving the oral cavity (e.g., eating, talking) may assume increased importance at this stage of life. The maintenance or preservation of oral health may therefore be more important in late life than at any other life stage. Thus the promotion of oral self-care behaviors and the assurance of their performance by elders are key issues in gerontologic health and must be addressed by dental health educators (see Chapter 7 for more detailed information about the dental needs of older adults).

DENTAL HEALTH EDUCATION FOR SPECIAL NEEDS POPULATIONS

With more than 53 million U.S. citizens physically or mentally impaired, dental professionals need the training to meet the challenge of accommodating and appropriately treating the special needs of patients with or without disabilities. Since the Americans with Disabilities Act was signed into law in 1990, many dental offices have been structurally modified to accommodate the disabled, yet little has been done to understand the psychologic needs of special patients. By eliminating discrimination against those with disabilities and impairments, standards of performance have been established that dental professionals may not be adequately trained to meet. The Americans with Disabilities Act affects our employment, the architectural design of our workplace, and the delivery of dental services.

Casamassimo notes that more disabled people are seeking care and that this trend is likely to continue into the next century as the population ages and as health care reforms bring capitation, portability of benefits, and extended coverage to many more people.[40] Many people in this segment of the population continue to experience difficulty in accessing dental services. For many, the attainment of adequate oral hygiene is difficult or impossible unless a care giver is available to assist in daily care for the prevention of oral disease.

Preventive methods are available to meet the unique requirements of the person with special needs and may include the use of adaptive aids and chemotherapeutic agents that eliminate or control microbial organisms associated with caries, gingivitis, and periodontal and other oral diseases. These measures are particularly suited for persons for whom the usual mechanical hygiene procedures of brushing and flossing present difficulties. The oral health care of special patients is intimately linked with medicine and the larger health care delivery system. Appropriate oral care is an integral part of maintaining the health and well-being of people with disabilities.

Under the leadership of dental professionals, effective oral care programs in the many special care settings in which persons with disabilities are situated can be instituted with innovative approaches to staffing and the delegation of oral care tasks. Steifel states that "for no other group is the achievement of good oral health as important as for those with severe disability."[41] For many, the mouth takes on critical importance in terms of psychologic significance and physical function; it may be the only part of the body over which the individual retains voluntary control. In the event that the dentition is lost, the disabled person may be unable to wear a denture to aid in eating or to assist in verbal or device-activated communication. Also, the disabled person may often face negative consequences in appearance, self-esteem, social acceptability, and employability. In addition, dental disease and its consequences can place the individual at serious medical risk. A comprehensive team approach that includes a continuing program of education involving patients and their families, allied health professionals and direct care staff, administrators, and dental practitioners is necessary to improve the oral health of persons with disabilities.[41] In January 1994 the National Institute of Dental Research, one of the federal National Institutes of Health, initiated a new information clearinghouse (NOHIC) that focuses on the oral health concerns of special care patients. Readers are encouraged to contact NOHIC at (301) 402-7364.[42]

DOMESTIC VIOLENCE IDENTIFICATION AND REFERRAL

An ethical obligation of oral care providers is domestic violence identification and referral, a situation that may be difficult for some providers to encounter. Domestic violence has been termed a "horrifying epidemic" and declared a "public emergency" that occurs more often than any other crime.[43] Domestic violence has been defined as "the repeated subjection of a woman to forceful physical, social and psychological behavior to coerce her without regard to her rights."[43] In January 1992 the Joint Commission of Healthcare Organizations (JCAHO)required all nationally accredited hospital emergency departments and ambulatory care facilities to implement a protocol to identify, treat, and refer victims of domestic violence to appropriate services.[44] On March 21, 1995, President Clinton introduced the Violence Against Women Act to prevent domestic violence and assist victims. Oral care providers should become familiar with the physical signs of domestic violence, especially because 68% of battered women's injuries involve the face, 45% the eyes, and 12% the neck.[45] Dental professionals have an ethical duty to learn what patients may exhibit as evidence of domestic violence or sexual assault. It is also important

to be aware of the possibility of child or elder abuse. When abuse is suspected, skills in counseling and referring victims are necessary. For dental care providers to obtain such skills, there is a need to expand the educational curricula and continuing education to include strategies for dental professionals to address issues of family violence. Readers are encouraged to review the list of Domestic Violence National Information Centers and the suggested readings compiled by Gibson-Howell.[46]

Basic concepts of dental health education

The content and method of health education are derived from the fields of medicine and public health and from the physical, biologic, social, and behavioral sciences. Certain concepts and theories developed in these fields have influenced the efforts and practices of health educators. In the area of dental health education, many of the proven theories of behavioral scientists have been either neglected, forgotten, or unaccepted. Given that the goal of dental health education is the prevention and control of dental disease, organized efforts aimed at achieving this goal should adhere to the proven theories and concepts relevant to health education activities. Current theories of health education that research has proved effective are reviewed below so that future dental education efforts can incorporate them.

Research has shown that a fundamental error in many dental health education activities is the assumption that increasing a patient's dental health knowledge will help change dental care behavior. This approach, based on a solely cognitive model, assumes the following sequence:

Knowledge → Attitude → Behavior change

If this relationship were true, every dental health education program that increased the participants' level of dental knowledge would have resulted in a behavioral change that improved the oral health status over a long period of time. To date, no evaluation of a dental health education program has produced such results.[4-8]

An error commonly made with this cognitive approach occurs when the educator fails to assess the learners' level of knowledge before the educational encounter and treats the individuals as if they were void of any knowledge or past experiences at all. As Yacovone[7] notes, it is important to realize "that the person is already 'behaving' when we encounter him—maybe not as we would like him to, but 'behaving.'" To influence a person's behavior through health education activities, an understanding of the dynamics of behavior is paramount.

A person's behavior is the result of both internal and external forces. Beliefs, attitudes, interests, values, needs, motives, personality, expectations, perceptions, and biologic factors, plus the influence of family, peer groups, and mass economic factors such as occupation, education, and media, shape and affect actions.[47] Sociodemographic factors such as age, race or culture, sex, occupation, education, and income have also been shown to have a strong influence on dental health practices and should be considered in designing and implementing health education strategies. The interaction of these forces has been illustrated in a model il-

lustrated by Kressin (Box 11-1). Considering this model, it becomes evident that a straight-line relationship between the educator's efforts and the learner's behavior usually does not exist. To develop an effective dental health education program, the educator must be aware of the interaction of all the forces on the learner. The educator must first assess the learner or learners to develop and implement a rational educational program that will result in a sustained behavior change.

SOCIAL COGNITIVE THEORY

This perspective on health behavior says that an individual's behaviors are motivated by both beliefs (cognitive factors) and the factors in the social environment (such as one's community, friends, and family).[48] The specific beliefs that are viewed as most important are concerned with an individual's perceptions of *self-efficacy*, that is, beliefs that the individual can perform a particular behavior effectively and with good results. Aspects of the social environment important in this theory include learning how to perform a specific behavior by watching others do so and receiving support or reinforcement from others in the environment for practicing certain behaviors.

A number of studies conducted by Tedesco and associates[49,50] have demonstrated that as-

---

BOX 11-1

FACTORS INFLUENCING THE DENTAL EDUCATION PROCESS

Aspects of the *learner(s)* to consider when designing dental education programs
- Sociodemographic factors (e.g., age, sex, race/culture, income)
- Values, attitudes, beliefs
- Readiness to change behaviors
- Education

Aspects of the *social environment* to consider when designing dental education programs
- Cultural norms (e.g., how much of the population smokes, how many people floss their teeth)
- How supportive the environment is for behavioral change
- Possible ways in which education/information can be offered

Courtesy N. Kressin, 1996.

pects of social cognitive theory are important in the development and maintenance of oral self-care behaviors such as brushing and flossing. Individuals participating in the educational programs designed by Tedesco brushed and flossed for a longer period of time when they learned about these behaviors by practicing them as part of the educational process and when they received support and reinforcement from the dental educators about their capability to perform the behaviors. The findings from this research highlight the importance of actually practicing new behaviors as part of an educational intervention and of receiving positive feedback from dental educators for practicing the behavior correctly. Together, these factors increased the participants' self-efficacy—their beliefs that they could successfully improve their oral self-care.

THEORY OF REASONED ACTION

The theory of reasoned action states that individual's behaviors are primarily determined by intentions to perform the behavior.[51] In turn, the individual's intentions are determined by attitudes and beliefs about the behavior. Specifically, attitudes about what will result from performing a certain behavior (for example, that flossing will prevent periodontal disease and that retaining natural teeth is important) are thought to influence the likelihood that the individual intends and actually performs a certain behavior. Also important to understanding attitudes are beliefs about how others will respond to the behavior (for example, that others will notice and approve of cleaner-looking teeth and gums).

Dental health education efforts based on this theory should be directed toward increasing individuals' intentions to care for their oral health by (1) emphasizing the importance and value of maintaining oral health and retaining the natural teeth, (2) educating and reassuring people that they can indeed effectively care for their oral health and prevent oral disease, and (3) changing community and societal norms so that more individuals are motivated to care for

their own oral health and to support their friends and family in doing so.

HEALTH BELIEF MODEL

Developed by Rosenstock[52] the health belief model considers a variety of factors thought to influence individuals' health behaviors. The first factor is an individual's *readiness to act*. Without this readiness, a person is unlikely to change a particular behavior, whether it involves quitting smoking or starting to floss the teeth daily. This readiness is considered a function of two things: the individual's perceptions about the *severity* of the disease and the person's *susceptibility* to it. If an individual does not think he or she is likely to get oral or lung cancer as a result of smoking or periodontal disease if he or she does not floss, then the individual is less likely to stop smoking or start flossing.

The second factor that the health belief model considers is an individual's consideration of the *perceived costs and benefits* of performing a certain behavior. If a person perceives a lot of difficulty withdrawing from nicotine and perhaps gains weight as a result of quitting, he or she may conclude that the costs of quitting smoking are too great. Similarly, if a person feels that the time and energy required to floss daily are more than can be handled, that person might be less likely to do so. Alternatively, if a person's views of the benefits of quitting smoking are strong and highlight the money saved, being able to breathe easier, and decreasing risks to physical and oral health, then these perceptions might make it more likely that such individuals will quit smoking.

The last set of factors that the health belief model considers are referred to as *cues to action*. These cues prompt individuals to act by reminding them of the need to change their behaviors. These stimuli may be internal (such as pain or discomfort) or external (such as advertising campaigns reminding people of the harm done by smoking or a physician telling someone how much smoking hurts health).

From the perspective of the health belief model, a major obstacle to preventing dental disease through preventive behaviors may be the perception that the consequences of dental disease are not serious. In most cases dental disease is not life-threatening, and a large portion of the population functions without their natural teeth. In a survey conducted by Opinion Research Corporation for the ADA, the public's chief barrier to prevention of dental disease was identified as the low value many Americans place on regular preventive dental care.[53] Educational efforts designed with the health belief model in mind will emphasize the fact that most individuals are vulnerable to the development of oral disease if they do not care for their teeth and that such disease may result in losing the natural teeth and that oral functions such as smiling and chewing are easier with natural teeth (emphasizing the severity of the disease and the individual's susceptibility). Further, such educational efforts should emphasize that caring for the dentition through regular flossing, brushing, and preventive care will have the long-term benefit of retaining the teeth (emphasizing the perceived benefits) and that such efforts are relatively easy and require just a few minutes of time each day (emphasizing the ease with which perceived barriers can be overcome). Finally, dental health education based on the health belief model will provide cues to action that remind people about the need to take care of their oral health.

STAGES OF CHANGE MODEL

The stages of change model of behavioral change describes common stages of change through which individuals go when trying to change health-related behaviors.[54] The first stage is *precontemplation,* which represents a time during which an individual is not actively thinking of changing a particular behavior. The next stage, *contemplation,* is when the individual begins to think about behavioral change. During this time he or she may think, read, or talk to others about changing a behavior and may become open to health education, in preparation for taking actual steps to change behaviors. The *action* stage is when an individual actually takes steps to change the behavior. Individuals are in particular need of support for their changed behaviors during this time, which may include specific training or education and social support from family and friends. Assuming that successful actions are taken, the individual moves into the *maintenance* stage, where he or she attempts to continue the behavioral change. At this time it is helpful to identify factors that may tempt a person to relapse, so as to prevent, avoid, or learn how to deal with these factors. *Relapse* occurs when the individual is unable to continue to maintain the changed behavior; relapse is extremely common. The model and process is circular, however, so an individual can move on to another stage when ready to try again to change behavior.

Dental health education efforts should be mindful of the various stages of change that individuals can be in because these affect receptivity to educational efforts and the subsequent efficacy of the education. On the basis of this model, it is important to offer education to individuals who are ready to hear it (i.e., those in the contemplation, action, or maintenance stages). However, in community-based efforts where attendance is voluntary it is likely that only individuals in these stages would attend educational programs.

CONTEMPORARY COMMUNITY HEALTH MODEL

The fourth and most current approach is the contemporary community health (or public health) model of health education, which takes into account social, cultural, economic, and other environmental factors that influence health. Rather than "blaming the victim" for noncompliant behavior and subsequent illnesses, the need for changes in influential variables such as the social, political, economic, and industrial environments is recognized. The community health model emphasizes the important role of public involvement in identifying individual and community health problems, setting priorities, and developing solutions to these problems and it empowers population groups with accurate information about health and health care technologies. The utility of broad approaches to health education and promotion at the community level has been demonstrated in studies of other health areas.[16,55-57] However, with few exceptions, many of the community-level methods used in these demonstrations have not yet been accepted by dental professionals. The World Health Organization[58,59] has clearly stated the need for using sound community organization and community development principles of working with focus populations, such as sharing in decision making.

The objective of community organization is to create awareness, interest, and desire to solve a problem while working with others to solve the problem. By involving people in making decisions about regimens or programs to improve their own health, people will tend to unite and maintain the level of commitment to and motivation for carrying out necessary actions to solve the problems.[11,12] Students are encouraged to review the Stanford Five City Project,[55] which describes the communication-change framework; social marketing; the application of formative research in designing, modifying, and distributing printed educational materials; the use of mass media education; program planning; and evaluation. The Stanford Five City Project is an evaluation of a community-wide approach to the control of cardiovascular disease through healthy changes in behavior. This approach may be generalizable to dental disease prevention efforts as we continue to learn to unite a variety of medical, behavioral, communication, and social science theories with demonstrated applications to solve health problems.[16]

Media influence

Silversin and Kornacki[60] have stated that the media has a role in promoting behavioral change: "Media-based campaigns to promote dental health have been shown to be more effective if they continue over long periods of time, appeal to multiple motives, are coupled with social support, and provide training in requisite skills." In addition, product advertising may influence public opinion and behavior.

Organizations such as Action for Children's Television (ACT),[61] the Center for Science in the Public Interest (CSPI),[62] the National Congress of Parents and Teachers (National PTA),[63] and the American Academy of Pediatrics (AAP)[64,65] have expressed concern about the marketing of relatively nonnutritious foods to children. A nonprofit consumer-advocacy group based in Washington, D.C., CSPI[66] has focused on nutrition and food safety issues since its founding in 1971.

In 1992 the Children's Television Act took effect, setting limits on the number of advertisements allowed during children's shows and mandating that all broadcasters carry children's educational or instructional programming as a condition for license renewal by the Federal Communications Commission (FCC). However, the FCC has concluded that this requirement can be met by citing public service announcements or short vignettes in fulfillment of the programming requirement. The academy emphasizes that local oversight is necessary to monitor how stations meet these guidelines. The academy urged parents to take an active role in educating their children to become responsible and informed consumers and noted that media literacy should be taught to children in schools and in a variety of other settings.[64,65]

The increased frequency of violence in programming and the increased use of tobacco products (smoking cigarettes and cigars and using chewing tobacco) in films and on commercial television is a cause for concern. Despite the tobacco industry's agreement with the FCC to voluntarily remove tobacco advertising from television in 1969, the tobacco industry pays stage and screen actors to smoke while acting, claiming that smoking is essential to the character or situation. In reality, performers who may serve as significant role models for our youth may by their actions be promoting dangerous and often deadly lifestyle behaviors for personal gain and tobacco industry profits. In a nation where an estimated 3000 youngsters begin smoking each day, the print, film, and advertising media are effectively influencing the actions and ultimately the health of our children. Recent surveys conducted by the Centers for Disease Control and Prevention indicate that brand choices of adolescent smokers were heavily concentrated on those brands with the largest advertising budgets.[67,68] Further, a 1991 survey in the *Journal of the American Medical Association* found that Joe Camel is as recognizable as Mickey Mouse to 6-year-olds. It is not surprising that, as a result of R.J.Reynolds's Camel campaign, which was backed by a company research program, Camel's share of the youth market jumped from roughly 3% in 1988 to 13% in 1993.[69] Cigarette advertising is an important influence on the smoking behavior of the young, with advertising sensitivity being about three times larger among teenagers than among adults. Cigarette advertising puts children at greater risk by influencing and distorting their perceptions of the pervasiveness, image, and function of smoking within society.[70]

Dr. David Kessler, former Commissioner of the Food and Drug Administration (FDA) has referred to smoking as a "pediatric disease" because the average smoker begins by age 15 years, and is a daily smoker by age 18 years. Although smoking levels among adults have been declining, smoking is on the rise among those under 19 years. Kids who start smoking every day end up as statistics a few decades later. According to Michelle Bloch of the American Medical Woman's Association, "Fully half of all long-term smokers, especially those who begin in their teenage years, will be killed by tobacco. Of those half will die early in middle age."[69]

In August 1995 President Clinton announced that the FDA proposed to regulate nicotine in tobacco as a drug, despite the tobacco industry's 100-year-old claim that tobacco is neither food, drug, nor cosmetic. The FDA launched a major initiative to strictly limit tobacco advertising to youth and other measures intended to curb youth access to tobacco products. The FDA's goal is to reduce the number of children and adolescents who use tobacco products by 50% within the next seven years. It is hoped that by putting restrictions on the sale and distribution of nicotine-containing cigarettes and smokeless tobacco products this rule will limit minors' access to these highly addictive products. The ADHA has stood strongly in support of public policy and legislative efforts to curb underage smoking.[71]

On August 23, 1996, President Clinton signed an executive order that passed the final version of regulations proposed a year earlier. The FDA plans to phase them in over a period of 6 months to 2 years. The tobacco industry, the advertising industry, and the wholesale and farm communities have three lawsuits pending, however, attempting to block the implementation of the rules. The rules focus on reducing easy access by children, reducing appeal to children, and implementing a public education campaign.[72]

Budgets for promoting preventive dental health interventions cannot compete with budgets for promoting products that are pushed and pulled into the marketplace with huge sums of money (i.e., tobacco, automobiles, cosmetics). The success of product advertising is based on linking personal satisfaction or enhanced self-esteem with the use of a product. Thus far, dental health promotion has not succeeded in linking preventive dental behaviors with motives other than health.[60]

Parents and school programs

Rubinson[73] has identified parents as the most pervasive intervening variable in school dental health programs. Frequently program developers and evaluators do not consider enlisting the cooperation of parents. Rubinson further states that "the parents will certainly have a direct influence on dental health habits and should be involved with programmatic efforts."[73] The evaluation of dental health programs should be redirected to focus on efforts stressing skill acquisition and reduction of behavioral risk factors through an evaluation plan that is both plausible and realistic in the school setting. Perry and associates[57] have demonstrated the effectiveness of combined school, parent, and community approaches to child health behavior in the Minnesota Home Team Project. This case demonstrated how sharing responsibility can be accomplished and it established the superior impact of shared responsibility between the school and the home on children's knowledge, skills, and practices with respect to dietary intake of more healthful foods.[16]

The School Health Education Evaluation (SHEE), conducted in collaboration with the Centers for Disease Control and Prevention,[74] from 1982 through 1984 suggests that exposure to health education curricula in schools can result in substantial changes in students' knowledge, attitudes, and self-reported practices.

The SHEE has provided evidence that school health education curricula can effect changes in health-related knowledge, practices, and attitudes and that such changes increase with the amount of instruction. The potential impact of these changes is significant.[74] In response to this study, many school systems are reevaluating their health curricula and considering increased integration of health messages throughout the curriculum. Teachers will require additional training to develop greater competency on health issues. In view of budget limitations, teachers will continue to be the primary source for the dissemination of health education in our schools, with the assistance of health professionals in the community. Students are encouraged to review the 10 basic elements that constitute comprehensive school health education as defined in the SHEE study.[75]

The complexity of the variables that must be taken into account in designing a dental health education program to motivate behavioral change for an individual has been briefly discussed. Greater detail and step-by-step procedures can be found in books devoted solely to the techniques of behavior modification and to the social sciences in dentistry.[10,76,77]

Health education in transition

Dental health education programs for the community have gone through, and will continue to undergo, periods of transition as further study reveals educational methods that will produce desired preventive practices. Research has shown that behavior is not transmitted; behavior is learned. In health care learning requires active participation on the part of the learner. For this reason the primary objective of most dental health education programs is to motivate individual students to seek the goal of disease prevention and tooth conservation.

Historically, dental health education for children has been a priority for the dental profession because of the high prevalence of dental caries in this age group. As a result, the school system has emerged as the most logical and practical setting to implement large-scale dental health education programs.[78] The school-based dental health program provides an opportunity to reach the largest number of children during early stages of development when habit patterns can more easily be modified or changed. The school setting also provides an environment conducive to learning and reinforcement for a considerable period of time and allows the teachers to use various strategies for inducing children to participate in appropriate preventive dental health actions.[79]

Early school-based dental health programs based on the cognitive learning model primarily consisted of dental professionals and students participating in short-term projects such as National Children's Dental Health Week, high school career days, and one-time visits to elementary and secondary school classrooms. These projects did not seek to incorporate dental health into the school curriculum; they were (and are where they still exist) seen as an "add-on" activity. Administratively, one-time visits present little difficulty and are often welcomed by the teacher and administration; however, reinforcement or evaluation of the dental health lesson is not usually part of the activity. Most reports on dental health education in the classroom agree that the most effective situation is when the classroom teacher works closely with the dental professional. So, regardless of who actually makes the presentation, the teacher can augment and reinforce oral health concepts and practices. The most significant behavior for the teacher is to be an effective role model of good oral health practices.[80] Although public interest may be aroused and dentistry's image enhanced, the early school programs, passive and cognitive in nature, were not found to motivate changes in oral health attitudes and behavior.[4,78,80] According to Raynor and Cohen,[81] research in the dental health area suggests that

There must be something more than motivation per se to establish oral hygiene behavior as a habit. Learning oral hygiene must involve the acquisition of a value, or a change in a value. . . . For adults, this involves change in cognitive structure, but for children, cognitive learning is secondary to motivational learning.

As a consequence of this realization, the "show and tell" approach has now evolved into programs of "show and do."

A survey of state school health programs by the American School Health Association revealed that only seven states mandate the teaching of dental health and oral hygiene.[82] Unfortunately, even in those seven states requiring instruction on specific health content areas, dental health is given a low priority on the list of required subjects. If dental health education is more than rhetoric and teachers are expected to include it in the curriculum, then adequate teacher training programs are prerequisite.[83] Dental health professionals in the community can serve as valuable resources to the school. Dental health education should be an integral component of all school health education curricula. Regrettably, the majority of dental health education programs were supported through grant funds, and many were terminated when funding expired.[84] Unless a strong constituency supports dental health programs, continued efforts may be stunted as a result of budgeting constraints.

An interesting byproduct of school-based dental health education programs may be the "spread effect"[85] or the "ripple effect."[86] These terms have been used to describe the impact of school-based health education programs on parents. Croucher and associates[85] conducted an investigation to assess the possible indirect influence of "Natural Noshers" (a school-based dental health education program that emphasizes home activities for skill development) on the dental behavior and knowledge of other family members. "Natural Noshers" contains two distinct dental health messages, one relating to the prevention of gum disease and the other to dental decay. Take-home literature and supplies emphasize these messages. The results of this study indicate that the parents of children who had been taught "Natural Noshers" had reported new dental information more often than the parents in the control group.[85]

In another project a group of health educators at the University of Maine at Farmington developed a series of health-related games, the "Healthway Arcade."[86] The games were used primarily for an audience of kindergarten through third grade and were structured to address several health issues. "Floss Is the Boss" was a popular follow-along story that used repetition, funny sounds, and a variety of motions to cleverly state the importance of flossing the teeth. Parental feedback indicated that this live arts format was well received and that many youngsters insisted on reciting parts of the story at home for the family. This ripple effect is another way of getting a message into the home and community.[86]

Some factors may enhance the success of dental health programs in schools: (1) determining who will be responsible for dental health education, (2) involving parents who can provide reinforcement of dental health practices at home, (3) identifying and using community health resources that can contribute expertise or materials to support dental health education efforts, and (4) evaluating the results of the program.[87]

Two large-scale teaching programs in Texas and North Carolina, based on both the social-cognitive and the health belief learning models, are next described in terms of program development, philosophy and goals, implementation, and evaluation. In addition, a number of innovative community educational outreach programs are also featured. A third program, Special Athletes/Special Smiles, based on the contemporary community health model will also be described. Findings of formal research investigations as reported in the literature are also presented for review. The student is asked to keep in mind the desired properties of a good oral public health measure and the planning and implementation strategy and criteria for the prevention of dental diseases when critiquing each program in terms of public health planning. Although all details for each program have not been presented, all major concepts have been included.

Current approaches
TEXAS STATEWIDE PREVENTIVE DENTISTRY PROGRAM: "TATTLETOOTH II, A NEW GENERATION"
Development

The Tattletooth Program was first developed in 1974 to 1976 as a cooperative effort between Texas dental health professional organizations, the Texas Education Agency, and the Texas Department of Health through a grant from the Department of Health and Human Services to the Bureau of Dental Health. In its original format this program was used by approximately 500,000 children in Texas per year before the new program was completed in 1989.[88]

In 1985 the Texas legislature mandated that the essential elements for comprehensive health education curricula identified in the School Health Education Evaluation Project[75,89] be incorporated into the curriculum statewide and be taught to the state's more than 3 million schoolchildren. Dental health is one of the required elements. This legislative action stimulated a need for the Tattletooth Program statewide.[87,88,90]

In 1989 the Bureau of Dental Health developed a mostly new program, Tattletooth II, A New Generation for Grades K-6, so named because the characters in the artwork for grades Kindergarten through grade 2 were from the old curriculum. This new curriculum was modified to reflect recommendations obtained from the formative evaluation process. Also, name recognition by the users of the prior program was considered a valuable asset. Separate lesson plans were developed for each grade. In October 1993 a preschool program titled "SuperBrush" was completed. The preschool curriculum was designed for use with personnel in Headstart programs, public and private child care centers, public school programs, and family day homes. A systems approach was used to develop all educational material.[90,91]

Program philosophy and goals

In Texas dental health education has long been the primary prevention effort of both the private and public dental sectors.[90]

The basic goal of the program is to reduce dental disease and to develop positive dental habits to last a lifetime in participants. The major thrust of the Tattletooth Program is to convince students that preventing dental disease is important and that they can do it.[88,90,91]

Tattletooth Program lessons are correlated with the health and science essential elements. The material in the lesson is often integrated into other subject areas, such as language arts. Both share mutual elements and may fulfill the requirements of the essential elements of both subjects. Some teachers integrate subject matter. References to cultural differences are made throughout each unit, and lessons are currently being translated into Spanish (in response to the cultural and linguistic needs of the growing Hispanic population).

To satisfy the legislative requirement that student performance be assessed, the Texas Education Agency requires that the Texas Assessment of Academic Skills (TAAS) be given to students in grades 3, 5, 7, 9, and 11. The Tattletooth program is correlated with the objectives and instructional targets of TAAS, thus providing students an opportunity to practice meeting those objectives before testing.

The Tattletooth lessons incorporate all the items that could be written into lessons. A scope and sequence chart shows the teacher what is to be taught and what the teacher in the previous grade level should have taught. It also tells the teacher what the students are to learn the next year.

The Tattletooth II Program embraces the six elements of effective lesson design: anticipatory set, setting the objective, input modeling, checking for understanding, guided practice, and independent practice. It emphasizes the important aspects of planning in successful teaching. Teaching decisions fall into three categories:

1. What content to teach next
2. What the student will do to learn
3. What the student will do to prove that learning has occurred.

Program implementation

The Texas Department of Health is divided into eight public health regions and employs 20 dental hygienists and dental assistants in the regions who implement the Tattletooth Program statewide. The hygienists instruct teachers with videotapes designed for teacher training and provide them with a copy of the curriculum. In some instances the hygienists are training lead teachers who, in turn, provide training for teachers in their schools.

Each grade level has five core lessons and two enrichment lessons. Background information for the teacher is provided at the beginning of each lesson. Educational strategies are suggested for integrating dental topics into other subject areas, such as language arts, mathematics, and science. Health promotion activities are encouraged and publicized within the school community. Teachers are encouraged to invite a dental professional to demonstrate brushing and flossing in the classroom. A field trip to a dental office is strongly recommended for kindergarten children. Each unit has a brief introduction that summarizes and gives a theme to the unit. Some units have planning notes that remind the teacher of the need for advance preparations. A unit test is provided so that the teacher will not have to write one. It can also be used as a pretest for diagnostic purposes.

Other resources include bulletin board suggestions, a book list, films, and videotapes available on a free loan for appropriate grade levels, a list of companies providing supplementary classroom resources, and a comprehensive glossary of vocabulary words that are used in all grade levels written for the teacher in English and Spanish.

Topics covered in the curriculum include correct brushing and flossing techniques, awareness of the importance of safety, and factual information relating to dental disease and its causes and preventive techniques.

Cost of program

The Texas Department of Health has no tangible studies to support the cost effectiveness of the Tattletooth II Program in all eight public health regions. In 1990 the regional dental director for Public Health Region Six assessed the cost for program implementation at $289.25 per workshop. Because an average of 953 children benefit from each workshop, the cost per child was estimated at $0.60.

Program evaluation

In the spring of 1988 Tattletooth II underwent formative evaluation by teachers who were selected equally from each of the eight public health regions in Texas.

In 1989 a statewide summative evaluation of the seven levels of the Tattletooth II curriculum was conducted. The results of the evaluation were positive, with teachers and students praising the teacher-student interaction that was present as a result of the format. About half the teachers responding had used the previous program, and half the teachers were new to the program. Approximately 94% of the teachers felt that teaching oral health can have a positive effect on children's dental health habits. Most teachers (90%) taught dental health once per year, and the average number of hours in which dental health was taught was 4.2. The bureau states that, given teaching requirements, the fact that 88.7% of the teachers spent 45 minutes to 6.5 hours teaching "Tattletooth II, A New Generation" is an indication that the curriculum was well received.

The curriculum materials were successful in teaching dental information and in increasing awareness of dental health practices. However, results indicate that the majority of teachers did not provide students with the opportunity to practice the skills of brushing and flossing. Toothbrushes and floss are not readily avail-

able because they are no longer provided by the dental program. Although teachers demonstrate dental hygiene skills, students will not master skills unless they are given an opportunity to practice them. Greater efforts need to be made to provide all classroom teachers with an adequate quantity of toothbrushes and dental floss to establish and maintain daily oral care programs.

TATTLETOOTH II, A NEW GENERATION: "SUPERBRUSH" PRESCHOOL CURRICULUM

The SuperBrush curriculum is intended for teachers and caregivers who work with children 3 and 4 years old in such settings as Head Start programs, prekindergarten, or public and private child care centers. The oral health curriculum consists of seven units, and the primary purpose is to teach basic toothbrushing skills and to establish toothbrushing as a daily routine in schools or day homes. The curriculum contains (1) children-directed activities that children do largely on their own and (2) teacher-directed activities that teachers do with children in large or small groups. All learning activities are developmentally appropriate for preschool children. The curriculum includes songs, games, stories, art projects, a resource list, and videotapes to show parents. The curriculum is available in English and Spanish. The curriculum is free to teachers and care givers who participate in the health department's training sessions on how to use the materials.

In June 1993 a summative evaluation report of the SuperBrush curriculum was completed. The report included an evaluation of the in-service training and recommendations for revisions to the curriculum before final production and an assessment of the potential impact of the curriculum.

Approximately 200 preschool teachers were invited to participate in the pilot test, which was conducted from April to May 1993. Overall, the preschool dental health curriculum was received enthusiastically by teachers and children alike. Teachers reported that it was fun and easy to use and that it provided many options that allowed them to tailor it to the needs of the classroom and to the resources they had available. The selection of activities implemented during the pilot test appears to have been determined primarily by time constraints or personal preference rather than by the merits of individual activities. Most teachers reported satisfaction with the in-service training and the level of technical support and reported that they would use the curriculum the following year. It also appears that, by introducing the curriculum early in the year as opposed to late in the year, many teachers may have more time to prepare and incorporate more of the suggested activities.

As of June 1993 approximately 10,000 preschool settings existed in Texas. Of the preschools that participated in the pilot test, the number of classrooms that received dental health instruction during the spring of 1993 increased by 21% for independent school districts, 5% for Head Start centers, and 33% for day care centers. Widespread availability of the program to preschool programs throughout Texas would help to increase the amount and quality of dental instruction provided to children between the ages of 3 and 6 years. It is well recognized that the preschool setting provides an important opportunity to build a foundation for healthy mental, physical, and emotional development. There lies the potential to instill in young children the importance and practice of dental health habits that will last a lifetime.[91]

Other major components of the program include a parent program; a senior citizen program; a prenatal and postnatal program; a nursing home oral health program; a pregnancy, education, and parenting (PEP) program; and a dental health manual for school nurses. Additionally, the Texas Department of Health maintains the Office of Smoking and Health, whose educational efforts are geared toward tobacco education, prevention, and cessation.*[4]

NORTH CAROLINA STATEWIDE DENTAL PUBLIC HEALTH PROGRAM
Development

North Carolina has a long history of involvement in dental public health and school dental health education. The need for a school dental health education program was realized as early as 1918 when the first scientific paper addressing this subject was presented to the North Carolina Dental Society. Since then many supportive actions have been initiated, including fluoridation of community water supplies and comprehensive state surveys of the dental disease problems.[92] In 1970 the North Carolina Dental Society passed resolutions advocating a strong preventive dental disease program embracing school and community fluoridation, fluoride treatments for school children, continuing education on prevention for dental professionals, and plaque-control education in schools and communities. From a modest beginning in 1973 through continuation and expansion, the North Carolina Preventive Dentistry Program for Children (NCPDPC) became the first statewide program of its magnitude and remains the largest and most comprehensive of all state public health dental programs.

Program philosophy and goals

The North Carolina Dental Public Health Program is a unique public and private partnership dedicated to the mission of ensuring conditions in which North Carolina citizens can achieve optimal oral health. Dental health is considered an important part of general health and can be achieved through the coordinated efforts of individuals, professionals, and community members.[92-96]

*For additional information on school-based and community outreach dental programs, contact Ms. Sandra Tesch, Texas Department of Health, Bureau of Dental Health, 1100 W. 49th, Austin, TX 78756.

The Division of Dental Health's programs are based on prevention and education. The division is organized to provide as many direct services to the citizens of North Carolina as possible. The majority of the staff, public health dentists and dental hygienists, are located in the counties to provide services through local health departments. Primary prevention and education are considered to be the most effective means of decreasing dental disease and promoting dental health. All program activities include educational components to modify the behavior patterns of individuals to improve their oral health habits through dietary change, toothbrushing, and flossing. Young children are the primary focus for education because the earlier a child is reached, the greater the potential for positively affecting the child's attitudes, values, and behaviors. Fluoride is recognized as the most effective public health measure for preventing dental caries.

Objectives that will facilitate attainment of the goals of the division include (1) appropriate use of fluoride, (2) health education in schools and communities, and (3) availability of public health dental staff in all counties.

Program implementation

Dental surveys provide epidemiologic and sociodemographic data useful for program planning, implementation, and evaluation. Dental public health program decisions in North Carolina are founded on statewide, population-based oral health surveys conducted by the Division of Dental Health and the University of North Carolina School of Public Health.[97,98] In the dental health status report presented in 1973, dental disease was found to affect 95% of the total population.[98] Rozier in 1982 stated that the teenage population is at greater risk of developing dental caries than any other age group and that 45% of children and adolescents show evidence of periodontal disease, almost all of which is reversible. According to the 1986 to 1987 North Carolina School Oral Health Survey, 53% of children 5 to 17 years old have never had a cavity in the permanent teeth.[99]

Disease levels have been going steadily downward since the 1960s. This trend is true for all races and for both the younger and older age groups, but in different degrees of magnitude. There has been a continuing increase in dental care for all children.

The epidemiologic and sociodemographic data from surveys provide needed information for planning, implementing, and evaluating a community-based program. The comprehensive nature of the problem's definition is reflected in the uniqueness of the program, which is designed to reach several segments of the population: young children, parents, teachers, dental professionals, and community leaders. The fiscal year 1995 to 1996 services delivered through the program included weekly fluoride mouthrinse for almost 280,000 targeted elementary children in 665 schools and screening and referral for about 270,000 targeted children. Almost 16,000 dental sealants were applied by dental public health staff, with staff emphasis on promotion. Dental health education was presented to more than 272,000 children and almost 38,000 adults in addition to the development, printing, and distribution of more than 600,000 pieces of educational materials. More than 61,000 people attended and received information through the 100 plus point-of-contact dental health education exhibits. With 10 varied topics, the exhibit promotion was used by 54 individuals representing state and local health care professionals.[93]

The coordinated efforts of the staff of dentists, dental hygienists, and health educators is extremely important in program implementation. The activities of the central office consultant staff (made available to all public health dentists and hygienists in the state) provide for continuity in program planning and implementation. With 49 public health dental hygienists and 14 public health dentists working in local programs, it is important that consultation services necessary for program growth be available to them.[99] Also, the consultants serve in a capacity that helps coordinate the individual county programs and needs of staff through statewide conferences, in this way retaining and promoting the philosophy of the statewide preventive dental health program.To reach children, public health dental staff provide training and consultation to those who work with preschool and school-aged children and maternal and child health programs, for example, elementary school teachers, health department staff, and parents. Teachers are believed to be the key in the educational program; to improve their capability for teaching and reinforcement of sound dental principles, they receive preservice, in-service, and follow-up training to cover dental health concepts, practice oral hygiene skills, and integrate dental health into the curriculum.

Table 11-1 provides an overview of the total program integrating the three components: education, prevention, and dental care. It also illustrates the focus of education for parents, dental professionals, and community leaders.

North Carolinians believe that one reason their community dental health program has been so successful is the support of the North Carolina Dental Society, which in 1972 went before the legislature to seek funding for the statewide program.

The Division of Dental Health's State and local public health staff traditionally screen elementary school children each year for caries. The screening is useful for identifying and referring those children who need dental care to privately practicing dentists. Although the dental screening is useful for case finding to refer children in need of care, it cannot be used for surveillance because screeners have not calibrated their techniques and information is collected at a level too crude for program planning. Results cannot be used to track changes within the county over time or compare one county with another.

In the 1996 to 1997 school year the North Carolina Division of Dental Health implemented a technique to modify and standardize dental screenings to give a new "assessment" process. This assessment gives a simple measurement of decayed and filled teeth, which could be added to the public health dental hygienists' annual screenings to give an indication of the prevalence of dental disease by county. Intense training and calibration increased the comparability and accuracy, and therefore the usefulness, of the dental data so that they can be better used by the counties. This assessment technique will be used annually for all kindergarten and fifth-grade children in North Carolina. These data will allow county and state health personnel to use this information to develop better county profiles for program planning and funding requests, to monitor dental disease levels over time, to compare disease in one county with another, and to provide accountability for expenditure of funds for public health programs.

Program evaluation

Evaluation has been and will continue to be a necessary continuing process to measure the effectiveness of the dental health program. Some of the evaluations that have been conducted include the following[93-96;100,101]:

1. The results of a 1968 survey of school children at the Happy Valley School in Caldwell County, North Carolina, where the school water supply had been fluoridated for 8 years, indicated a 34% reduction in decayed, missing, and filled permanent teeth for children who had 8 years' experience drinking fluoridated water at school.
2. A 1976 survey of school children in Asheville, North Carolina, where the community's water supply had been fluoridated for 10 years, revealed a 53% reduction in decayed, missing, and filled

Table 11-1. Schematic presentation of preventive dental health program in North Carolina

Agencies involved	Target audiences	Approaches
North Carolina Department of Public Instruction	1. Teachers and staff of preschool programs and elementary schools	In-service training for teachers
		Preservice training in teacher-training institutions
North Carolina Department of Environment, Health, and Natural Resources, Division of Dental Health		Public health dental consultation
		Provision of educational materials
North Carolina Dental Society	2. Students in preschool and elementary grades	Fluoridation of community water supplies
University of North Carolina School of Dentistry and School of Public Health		Fluoride mouthrinse and other programs
North Carolina Dental Hygienist's Association		Educational programs and materials for schools
North Carolina Dental Assistant's Association		Preventive dental services for eligible children
North Carolina Association of Local Health Directors	3. Parents of students	Parent education
		Education such as agricultural extension clubs, 4-H, civic and community groups
		Use of mass media for education
		Partnership with public health personnel such as health educators, nurses, and public health programs such as Maternal and Child Health
	4. Dentists and auxiliaries including students	Representation on advocacy committees for dental public health
	5. Community leaders, official and lay	Professional education

From North Carolina Department of Environment, Health, and Natural Resources Division of Dental Health, Raleigh, NC.

permanent teeth for children who had had 10 years' experience drinking fluoridated water.

3. A 1984 survey on the use of sealants in public health dental programs demonstrated an 86% total retention rate after 4 years on permanent teeth.

4. In 1994 a study was conducted to look at the effectiveness of the North Carolina school-based fluoride programs: fluoride mouthrinse and school water fluoridation. The Division collaborated with faculty at the University of North Carolina Schools of Public Health and Dentistry and the North Carolina Dental Society. The study showed that the fluoride mouthrinse was more effective in reducing caries than the school water fluoridators were. As the programs have operated in North Carolina, the fluoride mouthrinse program was also more efficient at about one sixth the cost per person of the school water fluoridation program. School selection for the school water fluoridators was always limited and was becoming more difficult because of techni-

Items in dental public health program	Sources of funds
1. Fluoridation of community water supplies 2. Appropriate use of fluorides such as mouthrinse programs	Primarily state appropriations for salaries, clinical supplies, office supplies, and educational materials
3. Dental health education in preschools and elementary schools, including preservice and in-service training for teachers and staff 4. Dental education for consumers to include parents and community leaders via agencies such as agricultural extension, industry, civic clubs, and mass media	Salaries for central office staff include 3 public health dentists, 5 dental health educators, 1 dental hygiene consultant, and other administrative staff to work with 47 field-based public health hygienists and 11 public health dentists as team for educational and clinical services and other services such as statistical assistance for research, artwork, photography, film rental or purchase

5. Support services such as
  a. Provision of public health dental staff, health educators, maintenance staff
  b. Provision of supplies and equipment for dental staff
  c. Production and distribution of educational training aids
	Six of 100 counties in North Carolina provide local funding for dental public health programs, including the salaries and supplies for dentists, dental hygienists, and dental assistants; several other counties fund salaries of dental hygienists and dental assistants; 61 staff are employed full-time by county health departments

6. Coordinated planning among agencies such as North Carolina Dental Society, North Carolina Committee for Dental Health, and Division of Dental Health	Federal funds augment state funds in fluoridation of community water supplies for equipment and training

cal and logistic problems. Therefore, on the basis of the results of this analysis, the school water fluoridation program, started in 1968, was discontinued state-wide. Fluoride mouthrinse continues to be provided to targeted children.

5. The division continuously evaluates its sealant initiative for effectiveness in reaching the healthy Carolinians sealant goal for the year 2000 to have half of all children with sealants (1986 baseline for North Carolina: 12%). In the 1994 to 1995 school year staff initiated screening for and reporting of the presence of dental sealants in fifth and sixth graders as part of routine school screenings. These data give annual, county-specific information on the proportion of children with sealants and shows overall progress toward the goal.

In addition to these surveys, the effectiveness of the education program in changing knowledge, attitudes, values, and practices of students is evaluated. Effects of the educational program may not become evident for 15 to 20 years; however, the results are expected to be positive (Table 11-2).

Table 11-2. Summary of dental health education programs in terms of development, program philosophy and goals, implementation, costs, and evaluation

Name of program	Characteristics of program	
	Development	*Philosophy and goals*
Texas Department of Health, Tattletooth II program (Pre-K thru 6th), parent program, senior citizen program, PEP, nursing home program, school nurse training program	Texas Department of Health	Goal—reduce dental caries and develop positive dental habits to last a lifetime Program tries to convince students that preventing dental caries is important and they can do it Program focuses on dental health as part of total health
North Carolina dental public health program	North Carolina Division of Dental Health, dental organizations, Department of Public Instruction, University of North Carolina School of Dentistry and School of Public Health, plus support of general assembly Based on documented needs assessment of North Carolina citizens	Prevention and education: prevention and education are most effective methods to significantly change prevalence and incidence of dental disease and to promote, protect, and ensure oral health for citizens Priority—children Mission: ensure conditions in which North Carolina citizens can achieve optimal oral health Long-range plan for continuing use of dental health materials in competency-based curriculum "Framework for Dental Health Education"—emphasizes role of classroom elementary teacher for integrating dental health education into curriculum
Special Athletes/Special Smiles	Partnership formed between Boston University School of Dental Medicine, Oral Health America, Academy of Dentistry For Persons with Disabilities, and Special Olympics International	Provide unique opportunity to open door to dental health and fuller health for people with special needs in unconventional environment Priority—Special Olympians Mission: sensitize, educate, and encourage dental professionals to assist people with special needs in obtaining dental services, enjoyment of oral health and improved quality of life; increase access to care and pool of skilled professionals to treat population

	Characteristics of program	
Name of program	Development	Philosophy and goals
Dental hygienists serve as technical consultants for school districts and promote dental education for expectant women, parents, and senior citizens		
Supportive materials are available for teachers and program hygienists		
Statewide implementation plan	Estimated at $0.60 per child; state-legislated budget	Field testing
Teachers are trained to present dental health information for school-aged population		Statewide continuous monitoring of material use
Priorities are community water fluoridation; fluoride mouthrinse programs and sealants	State budget includes salaries	Comprehensive survey of dental disease in 1976 and 1986-1987 funded by Kate B. Reynolds Health Care Trust
Public health dental staff provides training and consultative services to teachers, parents, professionals, and community		Survey to assess sealant retention in 1984
Media campaign promoting sealants		Survey of schoolchildren after 10 years of community water fluoridation and 8 years of rural school water fluoridation
Several teaching adjuncts are available: curriculum videotapes, guides, and exhibits		After 26 years of school water fluoridation in rural communities, 1994 study finds fluoride mouthrinse more effective, more efficient, and less costly in reducing dental caries than school water fluoridation is
		Survey of fifth and sixth graders to assess presence of dental sealants
Volunteer dentists, hygienists, assistants and students facilitate oral screenings, referrals, and oral health education services	Primary sponsorship provided by: Colgate-Palmolive and its subsidiary Colgate Oral Pharmaceuticals; other partners: Boston University, Oral Health America, and other corporations and foundations	Oral screenings for >10,000 athletes at 11 regional events and Special Olympics World Summer Games, which attracted athletes from 143 countries in 1995
Priorities are to provide services for people with special needs (i.e., mental retardation and developmental disabilities) raise public and professional awareness of severity of oral health needs; offer continuing education course for Special Athletes/Special Smiles volunteers; increase access to care; data collection to better assess oral health conditions of population		Pilot testing of continuing education course at four locations in 1996
		Pilot testing oral health survey instrument 1996, revisions and further testing planned in cooperation with Centers for Disease Control and Prevention

EDUCATION/PROMOTION INITIATIVES
Sealant initiative

The sealant initiative is designed to help the state meet the dental objective in "Healthy Carolinians, Health Objectives for the Year 2000" by increasing the number of children who have dental sealants. The primary goal of the health education/health promotions component is for every person in the state to have heard or read about dental sealants by the year 2000. This initiative has five major parts:

- School-based sealant demonstration projects are targeted to children, parents, and personnel in the school setting.
- As a continuing effort, copies of North Carolina's interactive health promotion exhibit "Common Sense and Sealants" are strategically placed across the state and used by dental public health staff in parent meetings, mall exhibitions, and health fairs targeted for middle-income parents to encourage them to ask the family dentist about sealants.
- Sealant promotion in private offices is a public/private partnership where privately practicing dentists use their facilities to place sealants on eligible children at no cost.
- A health care provider media campaign is underway targeting practicing dentists, pediatricians, and pharmacists, using flyer distribution and strategically located posters, to reach middle-income parents and stimulate interest in dental sealants.
- A statewide media campaign using public service announcements distrubuted to radio, television, and cable access stations across the state was designed to encourage parents to request sealants for their children's teeth when they visit the dentist.*

*For additional information on school-based and community outreach dental programs, contact Edna R. Hensey, M.P.H., Chief, Office of Dental Health Education, North Carolina Department of Environment, Health and Natural Resources, North Carolina Division of Dental Health, P.O. Box 29598, Raleigh, NC 27626-0598.

SPECIAL ATHLETES/SPECIAL SMILES—AN EXPANDING EFFORT TO REACH OUT TO PEOPLE WITH SPECIAL NEEDS IN A NONTRADITIONAL SETTING
Development

For people with mental retardation and other developmental disabilities, dental care often takes a back seat to more pressing medical issues. In fact, oral health is one of the most serious concerns facing these individuals and those who care for them.

For the majority of people with mental retardation, access to dental care is severely limited, or in many cases, completely denied. Many dentists and hygienists feel they are inadequately trained in special patient care. Because employees of group homes and other care settings are often inexperienced, underpaid, and poorly trained, oral care is not a priority. The side effects of medications and other physical and mental concerns create or complicate dental problems.

Perhaps the most significant cause for poor access to care is lack of financing. Health care for persons with mental retardation is provided by Medicaid, which offers dental care only until a child becomes an adult. Beyond that threshold, in most states even the most basic preventive care is not offered. Currently 43 states do not offer adult dental services through Medicaid. In the 7 states that do, however, the reimbursement levels are so low that most practitioners are reluctant to participate.

In 1993 Special Athletes/Special Smiles (SASS) was founded as a national oral health screening, education, and referral initiative for the athletes of Special Olympics International (SOI) through the efforts of Dr. Steven Perlman, assistant professor of pediatric dentistry at Boston University, and Eunice Kennedy Shriver, founder and honorary chairman of SOI. SASS was developed collaboratively among Boston University, SOI, Oral Health America (formerly the American Fund for Dental Health), and the Academy of Dentistry for Persons with Disabilities. SASS has become one of the largest oral health programs serving the special needs population, with the help of many organizations and through the primary sponsorship of Colgate-Palmolive and its subsidiary Colgate Oral Pharmaceuticals.[102]

Program philosophy and goals

In 1993 a mission statement and program goals were adopted. SASS is an oral health initiative designed to improve access to dental care for people with special needs and to raise the public's and the dental community's awareness of the oral health problems many of those with special needs face. This will be accomplished by working with SOI, its state chapters, and its national programs in a caring and supportive environment and with the firm conviction that oral health is vital to overall health.[103]

There are 10 program goals:

1. Conduct dental screening and educational programs at Special Olympics events around the United States and at all world winter and summer games.
2. Increase dental professionals' awareness of the particular oral health concerns that people with special needs face. This will be accomplished, in part, through participation in the Special Olympics programs.
3. Provide lists of regional dental professionals who care for people with special needs to all athletes who participate in the Special Olympics dental programs.
4. Develop and implement dental education programs for dental professionals, dental schools, community residences, institutional facilities, and Special Olympics athletes. This will also serve to promote Special Olympics as a recreation program and reach populations that are difficult to access (particularly persons with profound retardation or severe physical handicaps).
5. Serve as advocates on standards and equality of care issues.
6. By working with Special Olympics medical consultants, ensure that athletes who participate in Special Olympics dental programs have access to the most current information on medical issues.
7. Establish a sports injury prevention program for Special Olympics athletes.
8. Develop and promote nutritional guidelines and programs for Special Olympics athletes.
9. Help develop adaptive devices and orofacial sports programs for quadriplegics.
10. Work with established programs to help dental professionals recognize and report suspected physical and sexual abuse in patients with special needs.[104]

Program implementation

Since 1994 SASS has offered screening events, many in inner-city neighborhoods, at Special Olympics games around the country. Dental practitioners, dental students, and dental hygiene students participate in this community oral health experience. Students have an opportunity to become acquainted with the special needs population, become sensitized to the needs of the population, and enjoy personal gratification in providing a valuable community service for an underserved population. Each SASS event includes one-on-one instruction with the athletes on proper brushing techniques and a noninvasive screening of oral health conditions. The athletes receive copies of the screening review, a list of local dentists who treat patients with special needs, and a souvenir bag with tee shirt, cap, toothbrush, toothpaste, and educational booklet. In 1995 the program was offered at 11 regional Special Olympics games nationwide at sites in Miami, San Antonio, Kansas City, Philadelphia, New York, Boston, Los Angeles, New Orleans, Chicago, Atlanta, New London, Washington, DC, and the international summer world games in New Haven, Connecticut.[104] Nutritional counseling has also been provided to athletes at selective sites. A mouthguard program for injury prevention was introduced at the world games in New Haven in July 1995 and resulted in the fabrication of 2000 mouth-guards for special athletes.[102]

In 1996 a continuing education course was developed for program volunteers of SASS. The course was piloted in four locations. Plans are to offer the course at every SASS event in 1997, and Dr. Perlman plans to explore other venues as well, such as inclusion of nutritional counseling for athletes and a mouthguard program for sports injury prevention at all sites. He also has plans to work closely with the Centers for Disease Control and Prevention to begin extensive data collection in 1997, so that a significant body of knowledge about the particular oral health problems of people with special needs can be developed.[102]

"Special Smiles, A Guide to Good Oral Health for Persons with Special Needs" was also developed as an educational tool in association with SASS to help in establishing personal oral hygiene programs for persons with disabilities.[105]

There are plans for future expansion of the screening events, not only in the United States but in other countries as well.[102]

Cost of program

Funding is provided by Colgate-Palmolive, its subsidiary Colgate Oral Pharmaceuticals, Boston University, Oral Health America, and from other corporate and foundation contributions. Other community partners include local dental and dental hygiene schools, state and national dental hygiene societies and associations, national oral health associations, the Centers for Disease Control and Prevention, and dental and dental hygiene practitioners from across the country who volunteer their services. No information concerning cost per athlete is currently available.[102]

Program evaluation

In 1995 SASS succeeded in partnering with 14 dental schools and 5 state and national dental associations. A total of 2500 dentists, hygienists, and students turned out to participate at the events. More than 10,000 athletes were screened at regional and world games from 143 countries. According to SOI, for each athlete participating in the program at least four more people were touched by the experience. Therefore approximately 40,000 family members, care givers, coaches, and volunteers were reached through SASS participation.

SASS, the Georgia Dental Association, the Georgia Dental Society, and the Centers for Disease Control and Prevention made great strides in quantifying the oral health problems facing this population by test piloting on-site data collection to compare the oral health conditions of special-needs patients with those of the general population. Every athlete screened in SASS at the Atlanta state games was included in the study. The Centers for Disease Control and Prevention is currently developing a comprehensive data collection system with plans to expand 1997 data collection to five sites. Plans to monitor athlete treatment referrals and follow-up are under development.

SASS's effective use of the media was reflected in its comprehensive market-by-market media relations campaign, which successfully generated preevent, on-site, and postevent publicity for the event.*[106]

Suggested approaches

Each of the community dental health education programs that has been described was chosen for three reasons: (1) they are some of the most widely known and reported in the lit-

---

*For more information about Special Athletes/Special Smiles, contact Glenn Kaufhold, Executive Director, Boston University Goldman School of Dental Medicine, 560 Harrison Ave., Suite 402, Boston, MA 02118.

erature, (2) they represent a variety of approaches to dental health education, and (3) they illustrate the range of success that can be expected to be achieved, given their programmatic structure and goals. With the criteria that are presented in Chapters 10, 12, and 13, several issues for discussion should become apparent. For instance, if we assume that the goal for a dental health education program for the community is to reduce the prevalence of dental caries, which of the programs, if any, is using the most cost-effective and clinically proved preventive measures? Which of the programs is using evaluation criteria that will measure caries experience? Which of the programs has determined its priorities on the basis of the collection of data gathered through a formal needs assessment? Which programs are easily implemented and administered?

Answers to these questions begin to identify the inherent weaknesses in the majority of the programs, which to a large extent have lost sight of the goals of disease prevention and tooth conservation. In these cases the primary objectives emphasize motivating a group of students to practice positive health behaviors as if they were individual patients. Success is based on long-term behavior change, which is difficult to obtain and may not be practical for dental public health.[4,19,107,108] As concluded at a 1973 conference on prevention and oral health sponsored by the Fogarty International Center for Advanced Study in Health Sciences and the National Institute of Dental Research, "mechanical procedures for plaque prevention do not offer a promising solution to the problem of control of dental diseases for the population at large."[109] In addition, a clear-cut cause-and-effect relationship between dental plaque and caries has not been clinically proved in human populations. The Research Committee of the American Association of Public Health Dentists in their report "Programs for the Mass Control of Plaque: An Appraisal" states "On theoretical grounds, it may appear evident that

the daily, thorough removal of plaque should have a marked effect on reducing the increment of new carious lesions. As this report attempts to point out, however, this supposition cannot be supported with clinical evidence."[107]

Yacavone[7] has also noted, "Some authorities in community health feel that prevention will only be successful when individual behavior is eliminated." If this is the case, then community educational efforts must focus on those disease-prevention strategies that require the least compliance on the part of the individual. This would require a reorientation to health education and its goal and redirecting the educational efforts to community leaders in an attempt to improve the oral health status through organized community efforts.[21]

This is not to say that school-based educational programs should be eliminated or are not valuable; it does, however, indicate the need for further behavioral research and the need for communities to decide which of the preventive programs and the strategies or measures now used in each program should take priority. If community leaders are expected to make these decisions, then they must be given the tools to do so. This would necessitate a new role or new responsibilities for the community dental health educator. Frazier[21] states that the appropriate educational methods for this target group are those designed to (1) provide accurate information about the relative merits of various disease prevention and control measures and (2) stimulate group decision making and action regarding the adoption of effective organized programs.

If these new responsibilities are to be assumed, we must know whether community dental health educators are prepared and willing to adopt this new role. Environmental change and societal needs and expectations will necessitate that we expand functions and responsibilities to care for community health, practice prevention, and promote healthy lifestyles. In the oral health care field, dental hygienists are the preventive health education specialists and as such must prepare for new and challenging roles, both in and out of the traditional dental office, without reliance on the direct supervision of a dentist in alternative practice settings (i.e., nursing homes, school-based dental programs, health centers, etc.).[110]

In 1995 the Institute of Medicine released its latest report "Dental Education at the Crossroads: Challenges and Change," which examined dental education and proposed 22 recommendations for future dental education. The committee recommends the "more productive use of allied dental personnel in the provision of services to underserved populations." The study further recognizes the need for "new and challenging roles for dental hygienists" and for "more rather than less education." This recommendation supports ADHA's objective to expand access to care for consumers, enhance career opportunities for dental hygienists, and increase the number of types of settings in which dental hygienists practice.[111,112]

Although students generally participate in school-based community programs, other types of organized community efforts should serve as viable field experience alternatives. Following are several issues that require professional support and involvement and are currently receiving national attention:

1. Water fluoridation
2. Appropriate use of fluoride mouthrinses, supplements, and topical applications
3. Oral cancer prevention
4. Baby-bottle tooth decay
5. Sealants
6. Frequency of use, types of product used, patterns of use, and knowledge about the harmful effects of smokeless tobacco
7. Efforts by consumer interest and child advocacy groups to monitor and restrict advertising of cariogenic, high-cholesterol, nonnutritious foods and tobacco advertising and violence in programming directed at children
8. Infection-control measures
9. Access to care for special needs populations
10. Domestic violence identification and referral
11. Issues of cultural and linguistic diversity
12. *Healthy People 2000* national health promotion and disease prevention objectives[113]

The need for active participation in these areas cannot be overemphasized.

One of the objectives in *Healthy People 2000* is the proposed increase to at least 75% the proportion of people served by community water systems providing optimal levels of fluoride. This would require that approximately 30 million people gain access to the benefits of fluoride through the addition of community water fluoridation to the public water supply systems.[114] Visible support and action in the community, for instance, can make the difference in whether a referendum for water fluoridation is passed.[114-118]

In the 1990s community water fluoridation continues to be both a legal and political issue. Statewide ballots to prohibit fluoridation have surfaced in Oregon, Washington, and Utah. There have also been attempts by antifluoridationists to rescind fluoridation in communities where the water supply is currently fluoridated by promoting legislation to allow local option (home rule) for fluoridation in the eight states that currently mandate fluoridation—Connecticut, Georgia, Illinois, Michigan, Minnesota, Nebraska, Ohio, and South Dakota.[114]

Although there is broad support for water fluoridation among scientists, health professionals, and the courts as safe, cost effective, practical, equitable, and in accord with individual rights guaranteed by the U.S. constitution, opponents have been successful in defeating fluoridation efforts by creating an illusion of controversy and inciting fear.[114]

Two examples illustrating this point are the defeat of the referendum to continue water fluoridation in Flagstaff, Arizona, in March 1978 and the passage of the referendum in Seattle, Washington, in 1973.

Fluoridation in each of these cases and in most cases has proved to be a highly emotionally charged issue. In Flagstaff organized opponents to water fluoridation, namely, the National Health Federation (NHF), held public forums and disseminated large amounts of propaganda. The usual tactic was to link fluoridation to cancer. Other arguments—that fluoridation is unconstitutional, fluoridation is a form of medication, and fluoridation is contrary to the right of "free choice of health care"—were also cited.[119] To combat these unscientific charges and the emotional fervor with which they are made, it is incumbent on all dental professionals in the community and students during their training to familiarize themselves with the strategies of the NHF and other antifluoridation groups and with the documented evidence refuting their claims. It is also a professional responsibility to educate voters, community leaders, and agencies regarding the benefits of fluoridation and regarding movements opposed to fluoridation, which pose a danger to the oral health of the community.

In the Flagstaff, Arizona, case an initial survey indicated that the referendum would pass 2 to 1; however, the NHF was able to reverse this prediction by creating an illusion of scientific controversy. Fortunately, in Seattle, Washington, the opposition was not as active or as successful. Here the dental profession focused on building a broad base of community support; it educated people to understand the workings of the ballot and on how to vote. Fifteen days before voters went to the poll, dental and dental hygiene students along with community volunteers actively campaigned door to door for fluoridation. This successful strategy should be examined by communities where fluoridation is an issue. Success at one point does not mean that at some future date the decision could not be reversed, as it was in Flagstaff. In 1980, 41 fluoridation referenda were held in the United States; of those, only 8 approved fluoridation. Between 1977 and 1982, about 25% of the ballot measures on fluoridation were approved. Dental professionals must continue to be visible in the community to reinforce the benefits of fluoridation and the decision made by the voters. Dental health education must be provided on a continuous basis if it is to serve as a means for health promotion.[114]

Student activities and the degree of involvement in each of the listed areas may vary from state to state. An examination of existing legislation and accreditation standards for primary and secondary schools can provide students with "ammunition" to assist communities in improving oral health. Action taken by the Alabama Dental Association to eliminate the sale of sweets in local schools led to their discovery of the Southern Association of Schools' accreditation standard, which prohibits the sale of sweets in schools, and resulted in its enforcement. The standard was not being enforced by the Accrediting Division of the Department of Education because it did not have a working definition of the word *confection.* The Alabama Dental Association and the Alabama Nutrition Council were able to provide the needed definition and a list of acceptable snack foods. This effort should serve as an example of what can be accomplished, and it identifies activities in which students can certainly become involved.[11]

As the oral health preventive education specialist, the dental hygienist is uniquely qualified to instruct patients on preventive self-examination, implement the Smoking Cessation Clinical Practice Guidelines, and implement the National Cancer Institute's "How to Help Your Patients Stop Using Tobacco" program in a variety of practice settings.[120] Knowledge of addiction, the effects of nicotine on the human body, and options for nicotine replacement therapies and cessation programs are necessary, as well as a professional/practice commitment to implement a sound tobacco intervention system. Health educators can actively promote and support legislative action on the local, state, and national level to address the issues of youth access to tobacco and smoking in public places, restaurants, and the workplace.

Dental professionals can also take an active role in developing school-based dental sealant programs in their communities by use of a new resource manual developed by the American Association of Community Dental Programs. *Seal America: The Prevention Invention* includes a 10-minute video and manual that covers the following topics: selecting a target population, winning community support, program budget, funding, implementation, and evaluation.*[121]

Educational experiences in these areas will afford students the opportunity to begin developing necessary organizational and planning skills. Only through working with dental and other professional societies, state and local agencies, and community leaders and decision makers can an organized community effort be effective in preventing and controlling dental disease. Efforts to increase levels of knowledge of the public and the dental profession about oral disease prevention are required to achieve national objectives for oral health.[122]

Research

Oral diseases continue to be among the most prevalent problems in our society, despite the importance of oral health to personal overall

*Produced with financial support from the U.S. Public Health Service, Maternal and Child Health Bureau of the Ohio Department of Health and the Centers for Disease Control and Prevention. The manual is available free of charge. To obtain a copy, contact Dr. William Hall, National School-Based Oral Health/Dental Sealant Resource Center (M/C 922), University of Illinois, School of Public Health, 2121 W. Taylor St., Chicago, IL 60612-7260.

health and well-being.[122] The most promising avenue to improving oral health lies in the prevention of dental disease.

The National Institute of Dental Research (NIDR) National Caries Program conducted an 11-year study beginning in 1972 to determine the long-term effects of the combination of student-applied fluoride agents (fluoride mouthrinse, fluoride tablets, and fluoride toothpaste) among school children living in a rural area with low concentrations of fluoride in the drinking water. In school participating students ingested a 1 mg fluoride tablet and rinsed weekly with a 0.2% sodium fluoride solution. The children also received fluoride dentifrice and toothbrushes for home use throughout the calendar year. In 1983 dental examinations of study participants aged 6 to 17 years, who had continuously participated in the program for 1 to 11 years depending on school grade, showed a mean prevalence of 3.12 decayed missing filled surfaces (DMFS), which was 65% lower than the corresponding score of 9.02 DMFS for children of the same ages at the baseline examinations. The preventive program inhibited decay in all types of surfaces: 54% in occlusal surfaces, 59% in buccolingual surfaces, and 90% in mesiodistal surfaces.[123]

The National Preventive Dentistry Demonstration Program (NPDDP), carried out between 1976 and 1983, was the largest, most comprehensive school-based preventive dentistry program ever conducted anywhere. Its purpose was to determine the costs and effectiveness of several types and combinations of generally accepted school-based preventive dental procedures to provide the database for developing the most effective modern school-based preventive dental program. The preventive procedures selected included five general categories: (1) fluorides (topical and systemic), (2) sealants, (3) diet regulation, (4) plaque control, and (5) classroom health education. The major findings from this program include the following:

1. There was a sharp decline in the prevalence of dental caries from the later 1970s to the early 1980s.
2. The application of dental sealants was the most effective preventive measure of those used in the program.
3. Community water fluoridation was effective in reducing dental caries.
4. Classroom-based preventive measures were ineffective.[124,125]

The study was reviewed and critiqued by a review committee of the American Public Health Association. Although the committee had reservations as to the specific design of the study and the analytic methods applied, their consensus was that the first three findings of the study appear to be correct. The fourth finding is considered questionable because of possible flaws in the study design. Niessen[126] forecasts that health education programs will continue to be an important component of the dental public health program.

The NPDDP suggests several elements of dental research that need improvement or greater emphasis. The profession should adopt a more conservative attitude when projecting the expected benefits from the practical application of preventive measures whose merit is supported by only a few clinical trials conducted by a limited number of investigators. Many clinical trials conducted by totally independent investigators should be mandated before any preventive measure is regarded as safe, effective, and efficient.

It is imprudent to neglect basic research while pushing ahead with practical application. The lack of basic research on the mechanism of fluoride action in the prevention of dental decay and in the production of enamel fluorosis was evident from this study. Several of the modes of application of the agent may have been duplicating rather than reinforcing each other.

Greater attention should be given to monitoring the prevalence of dental diseases so that up-to-date indices are available that will further delineate characteristics of populations to be studied. There is a need for maintenance of an established pool of skilled clinical investigators who would be available to take part in large-scale national clinical trials. Also, there is a need to foster new research leading to improved clinical trial methods, reduced cost, and possibly reduction in the size of groups to be studied.

As a result of this study, two additional areas of research have been identified: (1) there is a definite need to develop and apply better outcome measures for the evaluation of the effectiveness of school dental health education programs and (2) more research is needed to identify the significant characteristics of groups susceptible to dental diseases.[125]

In 1986 to 1987 the National Institute of Dental Research (NIDR)[127] conducted the National Survey of Dental Caries in U.S. School Children, which revealed that 53% of children aged 6 to 8 years and 78% of 15-year-olds had caries. Further, the proportion of black and Hispanic adolescents with untreated decay was approximately 65% higher than for the total population. Periodontal disease was also quite prevalent. Results from the North Carolina School Oral Health Survey of 1986 to 1987 referenced earlier parallel much of the data from the NIDR survey.[101]

From 1988 to 1994 NIDR conducted the National Health and Nutrition Examination Survey (NHANES III).[1] In 1996 data from phase I (1988 to 1991) were released, and data from phase II are expected to be released in late 1996. These data will assist oral health providers in assessing which age and ethnic groups are in greatest need.

Some of the most noteworthy survey results follow. Tooth decay in children and adolescents continues to decline, with 55% of children and adolescents with caries-free permanent teeth. Black children had the highest caries-free rate of 61%, followed by white children at 55% and Mexican American children at 51%. Only 33%

of 12- to 17-year-olds were caries free in their permanent dentitions. Although 80% of the caries in the permanent teeth of children and adolescents had been treated, black children had more than twice as much untreated decay as white children did. Among 2- to 9-year-olds 62% had no caries in the primary teeth. Among 2- to 4-year-olds 87% of white children were caries free in the primary dentition compared with 78% of black children and 68% for Mexican American children. Dental caries in the primary teeth of 2- to 9-year-old children were left untreated in 47% of the study subjects, with Mexican American children having the highest rate of untreated teeth, 62%, followed by 59% for black children and 41% for white children. Since 1986 to 1987 dental sealant use has more than doubled but still remains low with only 22% of white children, 8% of black children, and only 7% of Mexican American children benefiting from this effective preventive treatment.

Survey results relative to tooth decay and tooth loss in adults revealed that 94% of people aged 18 years and over have had either untreated decay or fillings in the crowns of their teeth. On average, American adults had 22 decayed, missing, or filled coronal surfaces. Females had more caries than males (24 surfaces versus 21) but had less untreated decay. White adults had the highest rate of coronal caries (24 surfaces), followed by Mexican Americans (14 surfaces) and black adults (12 surfaces). Root caries was noted in 23% of adults. Only 10% of adults are missing all their teeth. For adults 75 or older, 44% were missing all their teeth. Among adults aged 18 to 74 years, roughly 20% wore removable dentures with 60% reporting problems with their appliances.

In terms of periodontal disease in adolescents and adults, it was found that women had better periodontal health than men; white adolescents and adults had fewer periodontal problems than did blacks and Mexican Americans. Moderate attachment loss of 3 to 4 mm was noted in 30% of 25- to 34-year-olds, 63% of

45- to 54-year-olds, and 80% of people more than 65 years old, whereas 15% of those surveyed exhibited more severe loss of attachment of 5 mm or greater. The highest prevalence of bleeding gums was among adolescents (13 to 17 years old) with three fourths of those surveyed bleeding on gentle probing.

NHANES III included an assessment of tooth trauma and occlusal problems, which found that 25% of Americans between the ages of 6 and 50 years had sustained injury to the incisors. It was also found that one fourth of children and adults aged 8 to 50 years had perfect alignment of the front teeth. Both malocclusion and orthodontic treatment were more common in whites than in blacks or Mexican Americans. Eighteen percent of children and adolescents and 20% of adults had undergone orthodontic treatment.[1,128]

Survey statistics suggest several challenges face future oral health care professionals. Harold Slavkin, NIDR Director, has identified the top three challenges. First is the changing patterns of disease. Birth rates are up—4.2 million live births per year, which reflects an increase of a half a million more than in 1992 to 1993. Population projections for the year 2010 suggest that one in five Americans will be aged 65 years or older and that pressing oral health issues will likely focus on conditions such as chronic facial pain, temporomandibular disorders, xerostomia, and implants. These demographic changes point to access to care and managed health care as the other two top challenges. Slavkin also sees managed health care as having a direct impact on the nation's oral health primarily because of issues of quality of life and access to care, especially for children born in abject poverty and for senior citizens who are homebound or have special needs. Further, Slavkin notes that "one-third of the U.S. population has no access to oral healthcare. By either state and/or federal legislation and the goodwill of managed healthcare companies, we must meet the special challenge to get these people access to care."[129]

Given that fluoridation is highly cost effective and requires no behavior change on the part of the individual to produce its effects, future research should explore strategies for increasing its acceptance.[60] In fluoridated areas surveys should be conducted to determine whether families are consuming fluoridated tap water versus purchased bottled water, which may lack the appropriate fluoride content. Perhaps targeting groups at high risk may be a more effective way to reach individuals affected with caries.[126]

Further details about each of the previously mentioned research projects can be obtained from the organizations involved.

Summary

An analysis of the information presented in this chapter leads to several conclusions regarding the status of and future for community dental health education programs. We have seen that the traditional educational activities based on either the cognitive or behavioral models of learning alone cannot be effective in achieving the goal of disease prevention and control. Techniques developed and refined for educating an individual patient differ from those that should be applied to the community. Behavioral research and expert opinions agree that educational methods are now available that can be successfully applied to the community at large, as demonstrated by the Stanford Five City Project and the Minnesota Home Team.

Are dental public health professionals ready and willing to use the public health model for contemporary health education and for fostering community involvement in decision making? The challenge remains for health care professionals in the private and the public sectors, for school programs, and for the news media to develop and implement a variety of relevant, culturally sensitive, and effective approaches to enhance public knowledge of the appropriate use of fluorides and dental sealants, control of gingival conditions, and the value of community water fluoridation, specifically for adults in their roles as eligible voters or parents.[122] Will such community involvement change the perception of dental disease so that persons will seek early detection and treatment for problems? Will financial barriers continue to alienate many subgroups within American society from obtaining desired or needed dental treatment? Are we fostering public- and private-sector partnerships to advance health education and health promotion in a managed-care environment? Are we continuing to build a strong network of support for dental public health by forming coalitions with other health care professionals, industry, legislators, parents, patients, and health advocacy organizations? Are we prepared to leave politics behind to create high-performance teams of dental professionals with expanded functions, responsibilities, and shared benefits that are highly productive, efficient and cost-effective to meet societal needs and expectations? Are we as health professionals monitoring children's television programming and advertising to ensure that broadcasters carry children's educational or instructional programming that promotes health and well-being? Are we participating in efforts on the state and local community levels to achieve *Healthy People 2000* national health promotion and disease prevention objectives?

Gift, Corbin, and Nowjack-Raymer[122] offer the following strategies to further the public's oral health: (1) changing guidelines for regulations and legislation to provide an oral disease prevention program in each state public health department and federally sponsored health center, (2) permitting efficient and cost-effective delivery of services by oral health personnel, and (3) making policy, regulatory, or institutional changes to ensure adequate reimbursement in the public and private sectors for age-appropriate oral disease prevention strategies.

Dental health education programs for the community should be applicable to all segments of the population and should be developed through appropriate program planning and implementation criteria to facilitate education of the public and health care providers to increase knowledge, understanding, and practices that foster improved oral health for the individual and the community.[122] A needs assessment should be conducted to define the extent of the problem and serve as baseline data and to determine program objectives and priorities, alternative solutions, and evaluation guidelines. Formative and summative evaluation must be a continuing, integral component of the plan; it must focus on measuring the program's effectiveness in terms of disease reduction, not merely increased knowledge or an improved performance level. Longitudinal behavioral studies should be conducted to validate the cost-benefit and cost-effectiveness ratios of each program. Existing curricula and field experiences for dental, dental hygiene, and dental assisting students must be reexamined and revised in light of the new responsibilities these professionals must assume in the community setting. Students should be educated in community organization, group dynamics, program planning and implementation strategies, effectiveness of community preventive measures, community decision-making processes, and the necessary communication, management, and leadership skills.

Research must continue to develop, test, and evaluate new combinations of preventive programs and to evaluate the effectiveness of any new strategies for community dental health education. More must be known about the relationship between plaque and dental caries and about the acquisition of oral health as a value. Community programs must use the approaches most likely to succeed against known barriers to receiving dental care and maintaining good oral health.

If the success of dental health education programs in schools is judged by effectiveness based on knowledge, attitudes, and skill acquisition, evaluators of such programs must be held accountable for conducting evaluation studies in a manner appropriate to these predetermined general objectives.

Dental health education in schools can be more of a priority, however, which involves the efforts of many people. Universities and colleges charged with the responsibility of preparing school personnel must include dental health as a component of the curriculum. School districts also need to explore ways of including dental health education on a permanent basis. Parents must be encouraged to support dental health activities through reinforcement at home and can also join health professionals in demanding that dental health education be a mandatory component of health education in every curriculum. We also need more professional support for proven effective preventive measures such as water fluoridation, appropriate use of fluoride supplements and topical applications, and sealants.

There are several major changes taking place that will affect the dental profession and the oral health of the public: a reduction in tooth decay, an increased awareness of the prevalence of periodontal disease, infection control and dental treatment phobias associated with contraction of HIV disease, population demographics that may affect the prevalence of root caries, periodontal conditions and oral cancer in association with advancing age, an increased demand for services by people with developmental disabilities in accordance with the Americans with Disabilities Act of 1990, issues of domestic violence, and finally an alarming increase in the use of smokeless tobacco among American youth and the increase in oral cancer associated with tobacco use and alcohol consumption. Future planning in community dental health education will include the targeting of preventive measures for specific subgroups with documented unmet needs within the general population. Innovative programs for persons with developmental disabilities residing in the community and in state institutions and programs for the elderly (ambulatory, homebound, and institutionalized) have been developed. Homeless individuals and families, unemployed or underemployed and uninsured people, and children and adults who have HIV disease have a myriad of unaddressed needs, one of which is professional dental care. Creativity and resourcefulness in future program planning are essential in view of our finite resources, especially funding, which is so crucial to program development, implementation, and evaluation.

REFERENCES

1. *Journal of Dental Research* (special issue), vol 75, Feb 1996.
2. American Dental Association: Wake up to prevention for the smile of a lifetime, *J Am Dent Assoc* 116(special issue):3G, 1988.
3. Lang WP, Ronis DL, Farghaly, MM: Preventive behaviors as correlates of periodontal health status, *J Public Health Dent* 55(1):10-17, 1995.
4. Chambers DW: Susceptibility to preventive dental treatment, *J Public Health Dent* 33:82, 1973.
5. Davis MS: Variations in patients' compliance with doctors' orders: analyses of congruence between survey responses and results in empirical investigations, *J Med Educ* 41:1037, 1966.
6. Raynor JF, Cohen LK: A position of school dental health education: behavioral influences on oral hygiene practices, *J Prev Dent* 1:11, 1974.
7. Yacavone JA: Translating research in the social and behavioral sciences for more effective use in community dentistry, *J Public Health Dent* 36:155, 1971.
8. Young MAC: Dental health education: an overview of selected concepts and principles relevant to program planning, *Int J Health Educ* 13:2, 1970.
9. Green LW, Johnson KW: Health education and health promotion. In Mechanic D, editor: *Handbook of health, healthcare and the health professions,* New York, 1983, Wiley.
10. Dworkin SF, Ference TP, Giddon DB: *Behavioral science and dental practice,* St Louis, 1978, Mosby.
11. Frazier PJ, Horowitz AM: Oral health education and promotion in maternal and child health: a position paper, *J Public Health Dent* 50:390, 1990.
12. Frazier PJ et al: Quality of information in mass media: a barrier to the dental health education of the public, *J Public Health Dent* 34:244, 1974.
13. American Dental Association: *Materials you need for your effective practice,* Chicago, 1996-1997, The Association.
14. American Dental Hygienists' Association: *Professional products,* Chicago, 1996-1997, The Association.
15. Bandura A, Cervone D: Self-evaluative and self-efficacy mechanisms governing the motivational effects of goal systems, *J Pers Soc Psychol* 45:1017, 1983.
16. Horowitz AM et al: Effect of supervised daily plaque removal by children: results after third and final year (abstract), *J Dent Res* 1977.
17. Meskins HM, Martens LV, Katz BJ: Effectiveness of community preventive programs on improving oral health, *J Public Health Dent* 38:302, 1978.
18. Winslow CEA: The untilled field of public health, *Mod Med* 2:183, 1920.
19. Green LW: Bridging the gap between community health and school health, *Am J Public Health* 78:1149, 1988.
20. Winnett RA, King AC, Altman DG: *Health psychology and public health: An integrative approach,* Boston, 1994, Allyn & Bacon.
21. Frazier PJ: *The effectiveness and practicality of current dental health education programs from a public health perspective: a conceptual appraisal.* Paper presented at the Dental Health Section Symposium, annual meeting of the American Public Health Association, Miami Beach, Fla, Oct 1976
22. US Public Health Service: *Review of fluoride benefits and risks: report of the ad hoc subcommittee on fluoride of the Committee to Coordinate Environmental and Health Related Programs,* Washington, DC, 1991, US Department of Health and Human Services, Public Health Service.
23. Lockwood SA, Malvitz DM: Public health briefs: trends in state agency oral health and public health expenditures, 1984-1989, *Am J Public Health* 85(9):1266-1268, 1995.
24. *Cancer facts and figures—1993,* Atlanta, 1993, American Cancer Society.
25. Horowitz AM, Nourjah P, Gift HC: US adult knowledge of risk factors and signs of oral cancers: 1990, *J Am Dent Assoc* 126:39-45, 1995.
26. Haber J: Cigarette smoking—a major risk factor for periodontitis, *Dent Hygienist News* 8(3):3-5, 1995.
27. Wagner L: Tobacco use prevention and cessation resource list, *J Dent Hyg* 69(2):56-59, 1995.
28. Wagner L: Upfront—Tobacco control and counseling initiatives taken, *J Dent Hyg* 70(5):185, 1996.

29. Smoking Cessation Clinical Practice Guidelines Panel and Staff: The Agency for Health Care Policy and Research: smoking cessation clinical practice guideline, *JAMA* 275(16):1270-1280, 1996.
30. US Department of Health and Human Services: *Preventing tobacco use among young people: a report of the Surgeon General,* Atlanta, 1994, US Department of Health and Human Services, Public Health Service, Centers for Disease Control and Prevention, National Center for Chronic Disease Prevention and Health Promotion, Office on Smoking and Health.
31. Ripa LW: Nursing caries: a comprehensive review, *Pediatr Dent* 10:268-282, 1988.
32. National Association for Anorexia Nervosa and Associated Disorders: *Surveys on anorexia nervosa and bulimia nervosa,* Highland Park, Ill, 1995, The Association.
33. Brown S, Bonifazi DZ: An overview of anorexia nervosa and bulimia nervosa, and the impact of eating disorders on the oral cavity, *Compendium* 14(12):1594-1608, 1993.
34. Brownridge E: Eating disorders and oral health, *Ontario Dentist* 71(6):15-18, 1994.
35. McGivern T: Oral manifestations and dental treatment of HIV infection, *J Pract Hyg* 3(6):19-26, 1994.
36. Bednarsh HS, Eklund KJ, Klein BH: Courts stike down HIV discrimination in dental offices, *Access Am Dent Hyg Assoc* 10(3):12-16, 1996.
37. Soh G: Racial differences in perception of oral health and oral health behaviors in Singapore, *Int Dent J* 42(4):234-240, 1992.
38. Kiyak HA: Age and culture: influences on oral health behavior, *Int Dent J* 43(1):9-16, 1993.
39. Ronis DL, Lang WP, Passow E: Tooth brushing, flossing, and preventive dental visits by Detroit-area residents in relation to demographic and socioeconomic factors, *J Public Health Dent* 53(3):138-45, 1993.
40. Casamassimo PA: Special patients aren't special anymore, *Dent Teamwork* 8(2):18-22, 1995.
41. Steifel DJ: Preface. In Tesini DA, editor: *Developing dental education programs for persons with special needs: a training and reference guide,* ed 2, Boston, 1988, Massachusetts Department of Public Health, Division of Dental Health.
42. National Oral Health Information Clearinghouse: Oral health clearinghouse for special care patients open, *Dent Hygienist News* 7(1):20, 1994.
43. Chez N: Helping the victim of domestic violence, *Am J Nurs* 94(7):32-37, 1994.
44. *1995 Accreditation manual for hospitals, Standards,* PE. 1.9, 100-101, Oakbrook Terrace, IL, 1994, Joint Commission on Accreditation of Healthcare Organizations.
45. Meskin LH: If not us, then who? *J Am Dent Assoc* 125(1):41-45, 1994.
46. Gibson-Howell JC: Domestic violence identification and referral, *J Dent Hyg* 70(2):77, 1996.
47. Lewin K: *Field theory in social science,* New York, 1951, Harper & Brothers.
48. Bandura A: *Social foundations of thought and action: a social cognitive theory,* Englewood Cliffs, NJ, 1986, Prentice-Hall.
49. Tedesco LA et al: Effect of a social cognitive intervention on oral health status, behavior reports, and cognitions, *J Periodont* 63:467-575, 1992.
50. Tedesco LA et al: Self-efficacy and reasoned action: Predicting oral health status and behaviour at one, three, and six month intervals, *Psychol Health* 8:105-121, 1993.
51. Ajzen I, Fishbein M: *Understanding attitudes and predicting social behavior,* Englewood Cliffs, NJ, 1980, Prentice-Hall.
52. Rosenstock IM: Why people use health services, *Milbank Memorial Fund Q* 44:94, 1966.
53. American Dental Association: Ask higher dental priorities at AMA-Kennedy meeting, *ADA Leadership Bull* 7(16), 1978.
54. Prochaska JO, DiClemente CO: Toward a comprehensive model of change. In Miller DR, Healther N, editors: *Treating addictive behaviors,* New York, 1986, Plenum Press.
55. Farquhar JW et al: The Standford Five City Project: an overview. In Matarazzo JD, Weiss SM, Herd JA, editors: *Behavioral health: a handbook of health enhancement and disease prevention,* New York, 1984, Wiley.
56. Green LW, Anderson CL: *Community health,* St Louis, 1986, Mosby.
57. Perry CL et al: Parent involvement with children's health promotion, the Minnesota home team, *Am J Public Health* 78:1156, 1988.
58. World Health Organization: *New approaches to health education in primary health care,* Geneva, 1983, The Organization.
59. World Health Organization: *Prevention methods and programmes for oral diseases,* Geneva, 1984, The Organization.
60. Silversin J, Kornacki MJ: Acceptance of preventive measures by individuals, institutions, and communities, *Int Dent J* 34:170, 1984.
61. Action for Children's Television: *News release,* Cambridge, Mass, June 3, 1991.
62. Center for Science in the Public Interest: *News release: children's television called a junk food cafeteria,* Washington, DC, June 3, 1991.
63. National PTA statement: *Concern about T.V. advertising of non-nutritious foods to children,* Washington, DC, June 3, 1991.

64. American Academy of Pediatrics: *Policy statement: the commercialization of children's television,* Chicago, 1991, The Academy.

65. American Academy of Pediatrics: *News release: pediatricians suggest eliminating TV food ads aimed at children, criticize children's television,* Chicago, July 23, 1991, The Academy.

66. Center for Science in the Public Interest: *Report: content analysis of children's television advertisements,* Washington, DC, 1991, The Center.

67. Centers for Disease Control and Prevention: Comparison of the cigarette brand preferences of adult and teenage smokers—United States 1989 in 10 U.S. communities, 1988 and 1990, *MMWR Morbid Mortal Wkly Rep* 41:169-181, 1992.

68. Centers for Disease Control and Prevention: Changes in the cigarette brand preferences of adolescent smokers—United States, 1989-1993, *MMWR Morbid Mortal Wkly Rep* 43:577-581, 1994.

69. Dreyfuss R: Tobacco enemy number 1: Joe Camel's tracks, *Mother Jones (20th Anniversary Special Issue): inside the nicotine network* 44, 1996.

70. Pollay RW et al: The last straw? Cigarette advertising and realized market shares among youths and adults, 1979-1993, *J Marketing* 60:1-16, 1996.

71. Ring T: A look at health issues in the presidential election, *Access ADHA* 10(8):54-55, 1996.

72. Rules and regulations, *Fed Reg* 61(168):4616-4617, 1996.

73. Rubinson L: Evaluating school dental health education programs, *J Sch Health* 52:26, 1982.

74. US Department of Health and Human Services, Public Health Service, Centers for Disease Control and Prevention: Current trends: the effectiveness of school Health education, *MMWR Morb Mortal Wkly Rep* 35:593, 1986.

75. Davis RL et al: Comprehensive school health education: a practical definition, *J Sch health* 55:335, 1985.

76. Cohen L, Gift H, editors: *Disease prevention and oral health promotion: Socio-dental sciences in action,* Copenhagen, 1995, Munksgaard.

77. RA Winett, AC King, DG Altman: *Health psychology and public health: an integrative approach,* Boston, 1994, Allyn & Bacon.

78. Potshadley AG, Schweikle ES: The effectiveness of two educational programs in changing the performance of oral hygiene by elementary school children, *J Public Health Dent* 30:17, 1970.

79. Haefuer DP: School dental health programs, *Health Educ Monogr* 2:212, 1974.

80. Potshadley AG, Shannon JH: Oral hygiene performance of elementary school children following dental health education, *J Dent Child* 37:293, 1970.

81. Raynor JF, Cohen LK: School dental health education. In Richards ND, Cohen LK, editors: *Social sciences and dentistry: a critical bibliography,* London, 1971, Dentaire International.

82. Castile AS, Jerrick SJ: *School health in America,* ed 2, Atlanta, 1979, US Department of Health, Education and Welfare, American School Health Association.

83. Taub A: Dental health education: rhetoric or reality? *J Sch Health* 52:10, 1982.

84. Mulholland DN: A comprehensive dental health education program, *J Sch Health* 48:225, 1978.

85. Croucher R et al: The "spread effect" of a school-based dental health education project, *Commun Dent Oral Epidemiol* 13:205, 1985.

86. Kamholtz JD, Wood B: Competing with Ronald McDonald, Cap'n Crunch and the Pepsi Generation, *J Sch Health* 52:17, 1982.

87. Texas Department of Health, Bureau of Dental and Chronic Disease Prevention: *Preventive dentistry program,* Austin, 1992, Texas Department of Health.

88. Texas Department of Health: *Tattletooth program: statewide implementation plan,* Austin, 1986, Texas Department of Health.

89. US Department of Health and Human Services, Public Health Service, Centers for Disease Control and Prevention: Current trends: the effectiveness of school health education, *MMWR Morb Mortal Wkly Rep* 35:593, 1986.

90. Texas Department of Health, Bureau of Dental and Chronic Disease Prevention: *Summative evaluation report for the Texas Department of Health oral health curriculum: Tattletooth II—a new generation,* Austin, 1990, Texas Department of Health.

91. Hide C: *Preschool dental health curriculum evaluation, Texas Department of Health.* Report prepared for Texas Department of Health, Dental Health Services, Austin, Tex, 1993.

92. Bivins EC: *History and development of dental public health in North Carolina.* Report prepared for the North Carolina Department of Human Resources, Division of Health Services, Dental Health Section, Raleigh, NC, 1974.

93. *Program plan,* North Carolina Department of Environment, Health, and Natural Resources, Division of Dental Health, Raleigh, NC, 1991.

94. *A ten-year report,* North Carolina Department of Human Resources, Division of Health Services, Dental Health Section, Raleigh, NC, 1985.

95. *Program report—FY86, program plan—FY87,* North Carolina Department of Human Resources, Division of Health Services, Dental Health Section, Raleigh, NC, 1986.

96. *1986 Conjoint report*, North Carolina Department of Human Resources, Division of Health Services, Dental Health Section, Raleigh, NC, 1986.

97. Fulton J, Hughes JT: *The national history of dental disease*, Chapel Hill, NC, 1965, School of Public Health, University of North Carolina.

98. Hughes JT, Rozier, RG Ramsey DL: *Natural history of dental diseases in NC, 1976-1977*, Durham, NC, 1982, Carolina Academic Press.

99. McMahon EL, Hensey ER: Celebrating 70 years of NC dental public health, *J Public Health Dent* 50, 1990.

100. Rozier RG et al: *Dental health in North Carolina: a chartbook*, Chapel Hill, NC, 1982, Department of Health Policy and Administration, School of Public Health, University of North Carolina.

101. Rozier RG, Dudney GC, Spratt CJ: *The 1986-87 NC school oral health survey* (monograph), Raleigh, NC, 1991, North Carolina Department of Environment, Health and Natural Resources, Division of Dental Health.

102. Special Athletes/Special Smiles: *Mission statement*, adopted 1993.

103. Kaufhold G, Perlman S: Personal communications.

104. *Special Athletes/Special smiles—Statement of objectives, Category C-1: Community service*, Boston, 1995, Boston University School of Dental Medicine and Colgate with Mullen Public Relations.

105. Perlman SP, Friedman C, Kaufhold G: *Special smiles: a guide to good oral health for persons with special needs.* Prepared by Special Athletes/Special Smiles and Boston University; supported by Colgate Oral Pharmaceuticals Boston, 1996.

106. *Special Athletes/Special Smiles—results documentation, Category C-1: Community service*, Boston, 1996, Boston University School of Dental Medicine, Colgate with Mullen Public Relations.

107. Heifetz SB et al: Programs for the mass control of plaque: an appraisal, *J Public Health Dent* 33:91, 1973.

108. Heifetz SB, Suomi JD: The control of dental caries and periodontal disease: a fundamental approach, *J Public Health Dent* 33:2, 1973.

109. Carlos JP, editor: *Prevention and oral health, Fogarty International Center series on preventive medicine*, Methesda, Md, 1973, vol 1, DHEW pub no NIII 74-707, US Department of Health, Education and Welfare, Public health Service, National Institutes of Health.

110. Nash DA: The future of allied dental education: creating a professional TEAM, *J Dent Ed* 57(8):621, 1993.

111. Institute of Medicine: *Dental education at the crossroads: challenges and change*, Washington, DC, 1995, National Academy Press.

112. Wagner L: Upfront—ADHA participates in development of new IOM report, *J Dent Hyg* 69(3):104, 1995.

113. *Healthy people 2000, national health promotion and disease prevention objectives*, Washington, DC, US Department of Health and Human Services, Public Health Service. DHHS pub no (PHS) 91-50213, 1990.

114. Dyke BC: Community water fluoridation from the past toward the year 2000, *Dent Hyg News* 8(2):3-5, 1995.

115. Frankel JM, Allukian M: Sixteen referenda on fluoridation in Massachusetts: an analysis, *J Public Health Dent* 33:96, 1973.

116. Hirakio SS, Foote FM: Statewide fluoridation: how it was done in Connecticut, *J Am Dent Assoc* 75:174, 1967.

117. McNeil DR: Political aspects of fluoridation, *J Am Dent Assoc* 65:659, 1962.

118. Domoto PK, Faine RC, Rovin S: Seattle fluoridation campaign 1973—prescription of a victory, *J Am Dent Assoc* 91:583, 1975.

119. National Health Federation: *This is the National Health Federation* [leaflet].

120. Mecklenberg RE et al: *How to help your patients stop using tobacco* Washington, DC, 1993, US Department of Health and Human Services. NIH pub no 93-3191, pp 9-19.

121. Wagner L: Upfront—Sealant manual available, *J Dent Hyg* 70(5):185, 1996.

122. Gift HC, Corbin SB, Nowjack-Raymer RE: Public knowledge of prevention of dental disease, *Public Health Rep* 109(3):397-404, 1994.

123. Horowitz HS et al: Combined fluoride, school-based program in a fluoride-deficient area: results of an 11-year study, *J Am Dent Assoc* 112:621, 1986.

124. Klein SP et al: The cost and effectiveness of school-based preventive dental care, *Am J Public Health* 75:382, 1985.

125. Review of the national preventive dentistry demonstration program, *Am J Public Health* 76:434, 1986.

126. Niessen LC: New directions: constituencies and responsibilities, *J Public Health Dent* 50:133, 1990.

127. National Institute of Dental Research: *Oral health of United States children: the National Survey of Dental Caries in U.S. School Children 1986-87*, Bethesda, Md, 1989, US Department of Health and Human Services. DHHS pub no (PHS) 89-2247.

128. Wagner L: Upfront—U.S. dental health status revealed, *J Dent Hyg* 70(4):144-145, 1996.

129. Lyons S: Access extra, survey reveals nation's oral health status, *Access* 10(7):27, 1996.

CHAPTER 12

Planning for community dental programs

Madalyn L. Mann

René Dubos[1] has pointed out that most of human history has been a result of accidents and blind choices. When a crisis occurs, our solutions are immediate and involve piece-meal efforts rather than considered and thoughtful planning. The need to develop our ability to predict, plan, and thus prevent the same crisis from recurring should have the highest priority.

Why plan?

As part of our role as health professionals, we are called on to assist health agencies and organizations in developing plans for obtaining dental care. We need to develop our own abilities to take our dental expertise and channel it into the areas of policy development, decision making, and program planning in a system more complex than the one with which we are familiar in the private dental office. This complex system may take the form of a community, an organization, a corporation, or an institution. The system can be better understood if we look on it as a patient, possessing certain needs and characteristics. Because we are dealing with more than one individual,

planning a program for a community or institution requires a deep understanding and analysis of the system as a whole and of the individual members that make up the system.

PLANNING DENTAL CARE FOR THE PATIENT

The steps the dentist takes when seeing a patient for the first time can be compared with the steps a planner takes when viewing a system for the first time. A new patient who walks into the dental office is given a medical and dental history form to complete. This record provides background information on the patient's health, history of diseases, and drug reactions, as well as the patient's history of dental care. In addition, information on the patient's ethnic background, degree of education, and financial status may indicate the patient's attitude about dental care, the type of dental care wanted, and how that care will be financed. A clinical examination with the use of radiographs further reveals the type and quality of dental care received and identifies any existing conditions or disease requiring treatment. For the dentist these steps assess the needs of the patient.

The next step is to identify and diagnose the problem or problems. Perhaps the patient requires full mouth reconstruction to restore the mouth to optimum functioning. The dentist reviews with the patient the ideal plan and acceptable alternatives based on the patient's wants and financial limitations. Once the patient accepts the treatment plan and the method of payment, the plan is ready to be implemented.

The dentist selects the appropriate person to perform the necessary services from a staff of specialists and designs a realistic timetable to coordinate who will do what first, second, and so on until treatment has been completed.

When treatment has been completed, the patient is placed on a 6-month recall and returns to have an evaluation of the care that was rendered. Any modifications or adjustments are done at this time. The patient is then placed on a maintenance plan and returns periodically for a routine examination. This becomes an ongoing process for the patient and the dentist. The difference between the planning steps for an individual patient and the planning steps for a community is that dealing with more than one individual at a time requires more complex steps. Box 12-1 compares the provision of dental care for a private patient with that for a community.

BOX 12-1

A COMPARISON OF THE PROVISION OF DENTAL CARE FOR A PRIVATE PATIENT AND A COMMUNITY

Private Patient
1. The dentist conducts a dental and medical history and a clinical examination of the patient.
2. The dentist diagnoses the oral health of the patient.
3. The dentist develops a treatment plan based on the diagnosis, the priorities, the patient's attitude, and the method of payment for the services.
4. The dentist obtains patient consent for treatment.
5. The dentist selects the appropriate labor to provide the care: dentist, specialist, laboratory technician, dental hygienist, dental assistant.
6. The dentist selects the appropriate dental service for the patient: preventive services, restorative services, endodontic services, and so on.
7. The dentist evaluates the treatment rendered to the patient: clinical examination, radiographs, patient oral hygiene, patient satisfaction.

Community
1. The planner conducts a survey of the community's structure and dental status.

2. The planner analyzes the survey data of the community.
3. The planner develops a program plan based on the analysis of the survey data, the priorities and alternatives, the community's attitudes, and the resources available.
4. The planner obtains community approval of the plan.
5. The planner selects the appropriate labor to implement the program: dentist, dental hygienist, dental assistant, dental technician, nutritionist, health educator, schoolteacher, social worker, health aides, public health nurses.
6. The planner selects the appropriate activities for the community: community water fluoridation, school-based fluoride rinse programs, comprehensive dental services, oral cancer screening and referral programs.
7. The planner evaluates the community program: comparison of baseline survey with subsequent survey, attainment of goals and objective, cost-effectiveness of activities, appropriateness of activities, community satisfaction.

Modified from Young W, Striffler D: *The dentist, his practice, and the community,* Philadelphia, 1969, WB Saunders.

PLANNING DENTAL CARE
FOR THE COMMUNITY

Usually a planner is contacted because a problem has been identified within the community, for example, a high incidence of nursing bottle caries among young children. The planner, like the dentist, begins by conducting a needs assessment of the affected children and their families. Included in the needs assessment are the population's health problems and beliefs, ethnic makeup, diet, education and socioeconomic status, number of children with nursing bottle caries, and the severity of the disease.[2] Again, this information will help the planner in determining an appropriate plan.

Once the information has been gathered and analyzed, the planner, along with the community, sets priorities for dealing with the problem. The planner may decide that the first priority is to treat all existing cases of nursing bottle caries within the community, followed by reeducating the parents of these children and those individuals who recommended sweetening the contents of the children's bottles. The planner then sets a reasonable goal to reduce the incidence of nursing bottle caries within that community within a specified time and proposes methods or objectives to accomplish the goal.

Next, the planner identifies what resources are available to the community. Who will provide the treatment, how will the care be financed, and where will the care be provided? If too many constraints exist (e.g., no transportation available to bring the children to the dental office or a lack of funds necessary to provide the treatment), then the planner needs to consider alternative strategies to accomplish the intended goal. The planner might identify and recruit volunteer dentists or dental students to treat the children at no cost to the community.

Once the decision is made and approved by the community, it is ready for implementation. An implementation timetable is developed to provide a schedule for putting the plan into action.

After the children have been treated, a 6-month follow-up examination is instituted to evaluate the effectiveness of the plan. At that time the planner addresses questions such as the following: How many children identified as having nursing bottle caries were treated? How many dropped out of treatment, and why? How many developed new nursing bottle caries? The answers to these questions will help the planner to modify and adjust the program according to the needs of the community.[3]

The steps taken by a dentist to plan a course of action for the patient are a simplified version of the steps taken by a planner to plan for a community. However, because of time, cost, or labor limitations, the planner may find it necessary to modify the plan by considering various options.

Who are the individuals who do the planning? There are many kinds of planners. Some have been professionally trained or educated, whereas others have received on-the-job experience within their organization. There are two distinct approaches to planning, internal and external: planning by individuals within the system or organization and planning by those brought in from outside.[4] A planner hired from within the system is usually an individual whose work responsibility is to plan for the system on a full-time basis. The advantage of hiring from within is that the planner already has a true understanding of the issues and operation of the system, including the subtleties of that system. This knowledge enables the planner to begin making decisions more quickly regarding appropriate action. The disadvantage, however, is that the planner may already have acquired certain biases about the system that could influence his or her objectivity.

The planner brought in from outside is usually an individual who contracts to work for the company or agency on a consulting basis for a short period. The planner's job is to assist the organization in its planning by formulating a new proposal and/or making recommendations for changing an existing plan. The advantage of this type of planner is that he or she potentially brings to the organization a fresher outlook, less bias, and a greater sense of objectivity. The drawback is that the outside planner requires more time to reach a level of understanding of the system sufficient to plan an appropriate course of action.

One of the most important concerns for any planner should be to take into consideration the human element. Statistics alone do not tell the whole story. For example, a planner who reviews the health labor statistics on a multiethnic community and who sees that, overall, sufficient numbers of practitioners work within the community may think that the community does not need any new practitioners. A closer examination of the practitioner and patient populations may reveal that the practitioners are primarily of a certain ethnic background and do not like treating patients of different ethnic backgrounds, of which there are a great number in the community. Thus there may be large subgroups of the population who do not have access to dental care, even though statistically there are enough dentists available in the community.[5] Although statistics can be most useful in analyzing data, a planner must be aware of their limitations.

Planning: a definition

E.C. Banfield presents a basic definition of the term *planning:* "A plan is a decision about a course of action." In other words a plan is a systematic approach to defining the problem, setting priorities, developing specific goals and objectives, and determining alternative strategies and a method of implementation.

There are many types of health planning. Each varies according to the factors affecting the health system, such as the geography of a region, the sociocultural background of the population, economic considerations, and the political situation.

Some types of health planning, as outlined by Spiegel and associates,[6] include the following:

1. Problem-solving planning involves the identification and resolution of a problem. An example of problem solving was the appearance of dental fluorosis among residents of a community in Colorado. This enamel disorder was identified through a scientific study of possible causative factors.

2. Program planning entails designing a course of action for a circumscribed health problem. School-based fluoride rinse programs are an example of designing a course of action for the problem of dental caries within a community setting.

3. Coordination of efforts and activities planning aims to increase the availability, efficiency, productivity, effectiveness, and other aspects of activities and programs. This stage often involves an adjustment process, such as a merger or a closing of services and facilities. An example is the closing of obstetric and pediatric wards in hospitals located in areas with a declining birth rate.

4. Planning for the allocation of resources involves selecting the best alternative to achieve a desired goal when the amount of resources is limited. Planners are called on to allocate the budget, the labor, and the facilities in a system so that it may meet existing needs and demands. An example is the decision by a state government with limited financial resources for the provision of dental services to cut services to medically indigent adults based on the cost-effectiveness of providing preventive dental care to a younger population.

5. Creation of a plan involves the development of a blueprint or proposal for action containing recommendations and supporting data. It is common for a commission or special task force to be created to prepare the plan. A state health plan that

describes the health status and the distribution of health services for the population in that state is a good example of such planning.

6. Design of standard operating procedures requires planners to come forth with a set of standards of practice or criteria for operation and evaluation. This can be a result of legislation, or it can be created voluntarily by the parties concerned. Guidelines for evaluating the quality of dental care as part of a quality assurance program for an insurance company is one example.

This chapter describes various types of health planning but concentrates specifically on the program-planning process. This process of program planning uses a systematic approach, as seen in Fig. 12-1, and should be used as a guide to solving a particular problem. The process can be compared with the ability of a jazz musician to take the notes of a standard musical scale and use them to create a unique melody. In a similar fashion a planner uses the program-planning steps to create a plan that is unique for the specific situation or system.

The process of planning is dynamic. Within a fluctuating and ever-changing system, the process itself must remain fluid and flexible, responsive to the presentation of new factors and issues.

This chapter discusses the components of program planning and focuses on the various options available to the planner. The initial step in the planning process is conducting a needs assessment.

Conducting a needs assessment

There are several reasons why a planner should conduct a needs assessment. The primary reason is to define the problem and to identify its extent and severity. Second, The assessment is used to obtain a profile of the community to ascertain the causes of the problem.

This information helps in developing the appropriate goals and objectives in the problem solution.

Another important reason to conduct a needs assessment is to evaluate the effectiveness of the program. This is accomplished by obtaining baseline information and, over time, measuring the amount of progress achieved in solving the specific problem.

Suppose the planner designed a program to administer fluoride tablets to all school-aged children in a given community. To determine how effective a fluoride tablet program is in terms of reduction of dental caries, the planner would first take a baseline needs assessment of the caries rate among the school children before implementing the fluoride tablet program. After the initial assessment, the program is implemented. To measure the effectiveness of such a preventive regimen, the planner would then make periodic assessments of the school children at various time intervals and compare these results with the initial assessment.

Conducting a needs assessment for a community can be a very costly endeavor with respect to funds, labor, and time. If the funds are not readily available, the planner has several options.

One option is to coordinate with the research activities of other agencies interested in obtaining similar health information on the given population. For example, a neighborhood health center may be involved in conducting a health survey of all the residents living in a defined geographic area.

Another method is to investigate surveys that have been done in the past by other organizations. Frequently, dental surveys are conducted through research departments of dental schools, through local and state health departments, or by the local health systems agencies (HSAs). If no surveys have ever been done, the planner may either want to solicit the assistance of these agencies and organizations or inform them that a survey will be con-

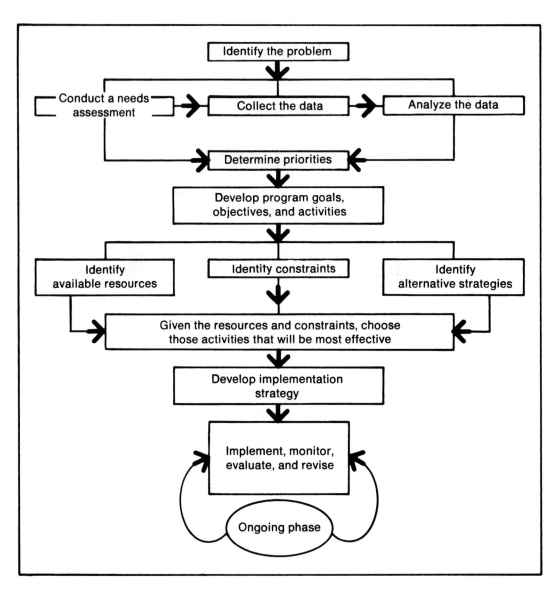

Fig. 12-1. Planning and implementation strategy flowchart.

ducted. This approach prevents overlap or duplication of activities.

Whether the planner conducts his or her own survey, combines efforts with others, or uses information from past surveys, it is important to consider what type of information is needed and how it should be obtained.

Data can be obtained by various techniques such as survey questionnaires or clinical examinations or more informally through personal communications. The technique the planner chooses is based on who is to be examined. Factors the planner should consider are the number of individuals involved, the extent and degree of severity of the problem, and the attitudes of the individuals to be surveyed. The greater the number of individuals to be examined, the more formal the survey. If the problem is clinical, as opposed to attitudinal, a clinical examination might be recommended. If the planner wants to interview a small group of individuals on their attitudes and feelings about a particular issue, a personal communication might be more appropriate.

To gather general information on a population, a population profile should be obtained. Such a profile includes the following:

1. Number of individuals in the population
2. Geographic distribution of the population
3. Rate of growth
4. Population density and degree of urbanization
5. Ethnic backgrounds
6. Diet and nutritional levels
7. Standard of living, including types of housing
8. Amount and type of public services and utilities
9. Public and private school system
10. General health profile
11. Patterns and distribution of dental disease

To gather epidemiologic data on the patterns and distribution of dental disease, the planner can use a clinical examination, review patients' dental records, or consult the National Health Survey for data on a population residing in a similar geographic region with similar characteristics.

In addition to assessing the incidence and the distribution of dental disease, the planner needs to inquire into the history and current status of dental programs in the community. Questions to ask should include the following:

1. What types of programs currently exist?
2. Are these programs oriented toward prevention, treatment, education, research, or a combination?

3. Who or what organization is responsible for the planning, implementation, and/or administration of the program(s)?
4. How successful have those responsible been?
5. What was the community's acceptance of such a program?

The planner must learn the way in which policies are developed and decisions are made within the community to better understand the community as a whole, especially if he or she is new to the community. The following areas need to be explored:

1. Who are the financial leaders (bankers, business people), and who are the political leaders (mayor, city council, other public officials)?
2. Who sets the policies for the community?
3. What is the organizational structure of the community?
4. What are the community leaders' attitudes toward oral health and community dental programs?

After learning how the community operates, the planner needs to examine the types of resources available to the community to implement a program. These include the funds, the facilities, and the labor. The following questions might be asked:

1. Funds
   a. What is the source of funding at the state and local level for dental care?
   b. Is third-party coverage available to the community through the workplace?
   c. Is federal funding available through special eligibility programs?
   d. Are private funds available through foundations or endowments?
2. Facilities
   a. Where is the closest major medical center?
   b. What specialty services does this center provide?
   c. What dental facilities exist, and where are they located (in public schools, health centers, hospitals)?

d. How well are the facilities used by the population?

e. Are the facilities easily accessible to the population served?

f. Are the dental services provided appropriately, adequately, and efficiently?

g. Does the facility meet the required Occupational, Safety, and Health Administration (OSHA) standards for blood-borne pathogens?

h. Is the equipment adequate and running efficiently?

i. How many operatories are available?

j. How many dental laboratories are available?

3. Labor

a. How many active licensed dentists, hygienists, and assistants are available?

b. How many laboratory technicians are available?

c. How many dental and dental auxiliary schools are located nearby?

d. How many active community health aides are available?

e. How many public health nurses are available?

f. How many school nurses are available?

g. How many public health hygienists, voluntary health agencies, and nutritionists are available?

When planning a preventive dental program for a community or institution, it is important for the planner to determine where the population obtains water and the fluoride status of that water. In certain regions of the country, particularly in rural areas, many persons obtain their water from either individual wells or nearby rivers, lakes, or streams. The amount of fluoride in the water sources might indicate to the planner that a fluoride supplement program may not be necessary for that community. If individual wells are being used, the planner needs to obtain a report on the fluoride status of each well because wells may be receiving their water from different sources.

If a community is obtaining water from a central area, the planner needs the following information:

1. What type of drinking water is available to the community?

2. What is the fluoride content of the water?

3. Does the water contain optimum levels of fluoride?

4. What efforts, if any, have been made in the past to provide fluoridation?

5. What are the attitudes of the community, the dental profession, and decision makers toward fluoridation?

6. What are the laws with regard to fluoridation?

7. Is a referendum possible or required?

8. Are the schools' water supplies fluoridated?

To prevent duplication of fluoride administration, the planner also should inquire into the type of fluoride being administered to individuals in private offices, the schools, and the health centers.

1. Do local dentists or physicians prescribe fluoride supplements to their patients?

2. Do schools (preschool, parochial, public) have a fluoride tablet or rinse program?

3. Do the health centers or hospitals administer fluoride to their patients?

4. Do fluoride brush-in programs exist in the schools?

5. If so, how often do children brush with a fluoride toothpaste?

6. How successful have these programs been, and how are they supported?

All the information presented in this section can be obtained easily through the various survey instruments discussed. If, however, a survey cannot be conducted, the necessary information about an institution or a community also can be obtained through other means. This approach requires the planner to investigate all available sources that might have data relevant to the population or the community. Such sources include the local, state, and federal agencies and private organizations.

In a small community one can find a tremendous amount of information on the community's residents by visiting the local health department. The local health department maintains statistics on the population's health status, morbidity and mortality, general health problems, and health service use. A trip to the chamber of commerce and town hall can provide useful information on the community profile, including population distribution, age breakdown, income, educational levels, school systems, and transportation.

In a larger community the state health department can also provide health-related information for all communities, cities, and towns within the state.

The federal government has large volumes of health statistics data from many of its agencies. The most familiar and widely used sources of data are the National Health Surveys and the U.S. Census Bureau. These sources provide longitudinal and comparative data regarding large population groups. Because of the magnitude of the data gathering, these surveys are usually conducted once every 10 years. Consideration of the publication date of such data and its relevancy and applicability to specific populations is important.

Other sources for obtaining such data are research studies and investigative reports. Many of these studies are funded by government agencies and are conducted by local organizations, research companies, or consulting groups. A considerable volume of data is usually generated from their reports. A computer literature search (MEDLINE) may be helpful. The National Library of Medicine provides these computer searches for a nominal fee. Most medical libraries affiliated with universities also provide this service.

Once the data are obtained, the information must be analyzed before it can be put into a plan of action. The data presented in the following case study can be used to consider ways of developing an appropriate program.

Analysis of data: a case study

BACKGROUND

Tide Water is the fifth-largest city in Massachusetts. It is situated in the southeastern section of the state on the shore of Deep Water Bay. Excellent water resources and deep-water shipping potential brought industrial growth to Tide Water, and it became the "spindle city of the world" as the cotton industry flourished. Native granite was used to construct multistorey factories, some of which are still in use. This prosperity ended quickly when the cotton manufacturers moved to the South in the 1930s and 1940s. The problem of vacant mill space, in addition to the Depression, made Tide Water's economic situation one of the worst in the country. Tide Water was able to make a strong recovery with a growing garment industry, which replaced the cotton mills and other manufacturers and provided a more diversified industrial base. The available information about Tide Water is listed in the following sections.

POPULATION

1990 census: 96,988 persons

ETHNIC AND RACIAL CHARACTERISTICS

1. Foreign born: 16%
2. Foreign stock: 48%
3. Race: white, 99%; black, 0.5%; other, 0.5%
4. Density (persons per square mile): 2,946

AGE DISTRIBUTION

	Total male	Total female
Under 5 yr	4,223	4,047
5 - 14 yr	8,120	7,893
15 - 19 yr	3,782	4,028
20 - 64 yr	23,992	27,458
Over 64 yr	4,902	8,453

EDUCATION*

Median number of school years completed: 8.8

*Figures reflect a large immigrant population, principally Portuguese.

EDUCATION—CONT'D

Persons completing high school or more: 25.6%
Persons completing fewer than five grades: 13.3%

PERSONAL INCOME

Salary	Families
Less than $1,000	616
$1,000 - $2,999	2,341
$3,000 - $4,999	2,988
$5,000 - $6,999	3,922
$7,000 - $8,999	4,474
$9,000 - $11,999	5,761
$12,000 - $14,999	2,838
$15,000 - $24,999	2,079
$25,000 - $49,999	407
$50,000 or more	95
TOTAL FAMILIES	25,521
Median income	$8,000

TRANSPORTATION

Bus service: intracity and intercity
Taxi service: three companies, with a total of 65 radio-equipped cabs
Highways and streets: four major highways (2 N-S; 2 E-W); 600 miles of streets, 99% paved

FLUORIDE STATUS

Tide Water has a community water supply that has been fluoridated since 1985.

HEALTH RESOURCES (LABOR)

140 physicians
43 dentists

FACILITIES

Two hospitals (725-bed capacity)
One community health center (diagnosis, primary health dental care, education and prevention; sliding fee)
Mental health centers (many facilities, inpatient and outpatient clinics and residencies; free and sliding-scale fee)
AIDS, venereal disease, and tuberculosis programs (free)
Alcohol and drug programs (free)
15 nursing homes (1,150-bed capacity, representing all levels of care)

GOVERNMENT

City size: 33 square miles
Mayor (two-year term) and council (two-year term; 191 members) form of government
Democrats: 31,311
Republicans: 4,875
Independents: 10,204

EDUCATIONAL FACILITIES

20 day-care centers (50% free and/or sliding fee)

	No.	Enrollment
Public schools		
Elementary	32	10,007
Middle	1	982
Junior high school	2	1,852
Academic high school	1	1,948
Girls' vocational high school	1	214
TOTAL	37	15,003
Catholic parochial schools		
Elementary	15	3,379
High schools	2	992

Other
Regional/technical high school
County agricultural high school
Colleges
Community college: offers wide range of courses, many in health disciplines
Southeastern University: four-year programs in most areas

It is important to first look into the socioeconomic structure of the community and determine the type of employment that exists. Tide Water has a large industrial garment area. This leads to the following questions: Is there a high percentage of industrial workers? If so, are they union employees? If this is the case, are they provided with a comprehensive health benefits package, including the provision of dental care? This information is important because it tells whether this population might be able to afford dental care through their jobs.

The population breakdown shows a large percentage of Portuguese living within the community. This indicates that possible cultural and language issues should be considered. In addition, the age distribution indicates that the highest proportion of people are between 20 and 60 years of age, or in the age bracket for the adult working population. There is a large population of school-aged children between the ages of 5 and 19 years living in the community. The age distribution of a community is important to consider because it tells where the target groups are and thus sets up certain priorities for planning. For example, if the majority of the population were of middle to older age, it would not be effective to design a program that would affect only a young population, such as schoolwide fluoride rinse programs.

The educational status of a community provides two perspectives for planning. First, it tells the educational level, in years of schooling obtained, by the majority of community members. Second, it may indicate what the community's values are toward obtaining an education. Planning a health awareness program centered around an educational institution would be successful only if people are attending schools and value the information they receive there.

Knowing the median income of a community is very important to a health planner because it indicates the population's ability to purchase health services. If a segment of the population's income falls below the poverty level, those individuals would be eligible for federal and state medical assistance programs (provided the individual state participates in such a program), thus making health services financially accessible to these individuals.

Health care must be both geographically and financially accessible if people are going to use it. A look into the community's public transportation system provides the planner with information regarding a population's ability to get to health care services. This is especially true for rural communities where roads are unpaved and public transportation is scarce.

Looking at the health care facilities in the community tells the planner what type of services are being provided, the amount of services, and the cost of receiving those services.

The labor data give information about the number of dentists providing care. (The federal government has developed certain labor-to-population ratios that indicate whether a population is considered to be residing in a medically underserved area.) However, just looking at the number of dentists in the community will not give the planner a true picture of whether the number of dentists within the community is sufficient to provide services to the population residing there.

Although the number of dentists in the community may be adequate, the planner must question whether the dentists are available to provide the care. How long does it take to get appointments? What are the dentists' hours (e.g., do they work after 5 PM and/or on the weekends)? In addition to knowing the number of dentists, it is necessary to consider what types of services are being provided to whom and for what cost.

Another consideration is the type of practice. Do the dentists accept third-party payments or Medicaid payments? Do they provide comprehensive services, including preventive care? Do they provide dental health education to their patients?

Knowing the fluoride status of a community is also essential for dental planning. In the case study community profile of Tide Water, it is stated that water has been fluoridated since 1985. This indicates that those children born in 1985 and after that year will receive maximum benefits from the fluoridated water. However, it is safe to say that those children born before 1985 may need additional attention with other fluoride measures.

In most cases the politics of the community will determine the direction the program takes. A conservative town government attempting to cut costs may be opposed to programs that provide prosthetic services to the medically indigent or elderly. Each local government's policies may vary in its methods of instituting new programs, allocating funds, hiring personnel, or setting priorities. In addition, the politics of the state government will also shape the overall direction taken by the communities within the state.

By looking at the educational system of a community, the planner can determine the number of schools, the enrollment for each, and the distribution of children among the schools within the community. This information can assist the planner who is developing a school-based program for the community. The public and parochial schools are the ideal settings for dental programs. Moreover, as in countries like New Zealand, schools also serve as excellent vehicles for providing routine dental care.

The educational facilities should be designed appropriately to accommodate such programs. Teachers, parents, and school administrators should be in support of the programs, and, most important, the need must exist among the school-aged population to warrant such programs. In this particular community with its high percentage of Portuguese-American children, the schools can be a good meeting place to use to open communication channels with the families and to offer support services when needed.

If the planner is designing a dental treatment program for a specific population that is not receiving any care, there are methods developed by the Indian Health Service to convert the survey data into specific resource requirements for treating the population. The Indian Health Service (IHS) is a federal agency within the Public Health Service. It has been involved with extensive surveys on the oral health status of Native Americans. One method it has developed with the use of specific oral health surveys assesses the dental disease prevalence among the

population and translates the data into time and cost estimates to treat the population. These surveys for disease prevalence include the decayed, missing, and filled (DMF) index, the Periodontal Index, and the Oral Hygiene Index–Simplified (OHI–S). In addition to determining the dental need, IHS assesses treatment needs, which include prosthetic status, periodontal status, orthodontic status, oral pathology status, and restorative status.

With the use of a mathematical model, dental resource requirements can be computed and projected over a period of time. The data are then translated into time, labor, and facility requirements.

The basic measurement is time. Clinical dental services requirements and labor capability both can be expressed in time units. Various time requirement studies have been done by the IHS to determine the amount of chair time that is necessary to complete a clinical service.[7] This unit of time is called a service minute. For example:

Clinical service	Time required (service minutes)
Complete oral examination	10
Prophylaxis	17
Single-surface amalgam	10

LABOR AND FACILITY REQUIREMENTS

The number of dentists and dental auxiliaries, as well as of facilities and operatories necessary to treat the population, is determined by obtaining the total number of service minutes required for a given population. For example, a random sample of a population was examined, and calculations showed that 70,000 service minutes per year would be required to treat approximately 60% of that population. Based on that figure, the amount of staff required to provide approximately 70,000 service minutes would be one dentist and two dental assistants.[7] The number of operatories needed to accommodate this dental staff for maximum efficiency would be three.[7] The ratios (one dentist to two dental assistants to three operatories) have been derived from efficiency studies by the Indian Health Service.

This evaluation is highly statistical. Statistics can set parameters to the problem, but the values and attitudes of persons are equally important. The planner must take into consideration the sociocultural interests or the psychologic readiness of a people to want or use health services. If the community does not agree on which of the array of statistics represents the community's priorities, little will be done to translate the need identified in the data into effective programs.

Determining priorities

"Priority determination is a method of imposing people's values and judgments of what is important onto the raw data."[6] The method can be used for different purposes, such as for setting priorities among problems elicited through a needs assessment. It also can be used for ranking the solutions to the problem.

Given the community profile and analysis of dental survey data, how are priorities established? At this point the community should be involved to assist in the establishment of these priorities. A health advisory committee or task force representing consumers, community leaders, and providers should be established to assist in the development of policies and priorities. Planning with community representation will aid in the program's implementation and acceptance.

Few dental public health programs meet all the dental needs of the population. With limited resources, it becomes necessary to establish priorities to allow the most efficient allocation of resources. If priorities are not determined, the program may not serve those individuals or groups who need the care most.

Certain factors should be considered in determining priorities. For example, a problem that affects a large number of people generally takes priority over a problem that affects a small number of people. However, if the problem is common colds (affecting a large number of people) competing with Lyme disease (affecting few people), then the more serious problem should take priority.

If the health problem is dental disease, generally more than one population group is affected. The following are groups commonly associated with high-risk dental needs:

1. Preschool and school-aged children
2. Mentally and/or physically disabled persons
3. Chronically ill and/or medically compromised persons
4. Elderly persons
5. Expectant mothers
6. Low-income minority groups (urban and rural)

If the community decides to address the problem of dental caries first, specific groups are more susceptible to dental caries, such as preschool and school-aged children and low-income minority groups. The planner then begins to develop plans geared to an identifiable population group.

Once the target group has been identified (based on the dental problem), the type of program should be established. To do this, the planner begins to set program goals and objectives.

Development of program goals and objectives

Program *goals* are broad statements on the overall purpose of a program to meet a defined problem. An example of a program goal for a community that has an identifiable problem of dental caries among school-aged children would be "to improve the oral health of the school-aged children in community X."

Program *objectives* are more specific and describe in a measurable way the desired end result of program activities. The objectives should specify the following:

1. *What:* the nature of the situation or condition to be attained
2. *Extent:* the scope and magnitude of the situation or condition to be attained
3. *Who:* the particular group or portion of the environment in which attainment is desired
4. *Where:* the geographic areas of the program
5. *When:* the time "at" or "by" which the desired situation or condition is intended to exist

An objective might state, "By the year 2005, more than 90% of the population aged 6 to 17 years in community X will not have lost any teeth as a result of caries, and at least 40% will be caries-free." This is known as an outcome objective and provides a means of measuring quantitatively the outcome of the specific objective. This approach helps the evaluator and the community know both where the program is and where it hopes to be with respect to a given health problem. It also aids in establishing a realistic timetable for reducing or preventing principal health problems.

Second, objectives are the specific avenues by which goals are met. Process objectives state a specific process by which a public health problem can be reduced and prevented. For example, by 1995 community X will have a public fluoride program to guarantee access to fluoride exposure via the following:

1. Fluoridation of the public water supply to the optimum level
2. Appropriately monitored fluoridation of school water supplies in areas where community fluoridation is impossible or impractical
3. Initiation of the most cost-effective topical and/or systemic fluoride supplement programs available to all schools if both (1) and (2) are impossible

4. Provision of topical fluoride application for persons with rampant caries and use of pit and fissure sealants where indicated[8]

Once the problem has been identified and program goals and objectives have been established describing a solution to or a reduction of the problem, the next step is to state how to bring about the desired results. This area of program planning is referred to as program activities, and it describes how the objectives will be accomplished.

Activities include three components: (1) what is going to be done, (2) who will be doing it, and (3) when it will be done.

Activity 1. Beginning January 1, 1995, two dental hygienists will be hired to administer a self-applied fluoride rinse program within the public school systems.

Activity 2. On March 1, 8, 15, 22, and 30, 1995, a series of 2-day training workshops for parent volunteers will be conducted by the two hygienists at selected public schools in community X.

In planning these program activities, it is important to carefully consider the type of resources available, as well as the program constraints.

RESOURCE IDENTIFICATION

Selection of resources for an activity, such as personnel, equipment and supplies, facilities, and financial resources, must be determined by consideration of what would be most effective, adequate, efficient, and appropriate for the tasks to be accomplished. Some criteria that are commonly used to determine what resources should be used follow:

1. *Appropriateness:* the most suitable resources to get the job done
2. *Adequacy:* the extent or degree to which the resources would complete the job
3. *Effectiveness:* how capable the resources are at completing the job
4. *Efficiency:* the dollar cost and amount of time expended to complete the job

As discussed previously in the chapter, obtaining the community profile provides the planner with valuable information on available resources. The type of resources needed to develop a dental program and the sources from which they can be obtained are listed in Box 12-2.

IDENTIFYING CONSTRAINTS

When planning any program, there are usually as many reasons not to do something as there are reasons to do it. The former are usually considered to be roadblocks or obstacles to achieving a certain goal or objective.

What should be determined at this point are the most obvious constraints that are associated with meeting program objectives. By identifying these constraints early in the planning stages, one can modify the design of the program and thereby create a more practical and realistic plan.

Box 12-2

RESOURCE IDENTIFICATION WORKSHEET

Resource	Source
Personnel	
Sponsors or supporters	Public health organizations, professional dental organizations, dental and dental hygiene schools, industry, health consumer groups, government, labor, media, business, foundations, public schools
Clinical providers	Dentists, dental hygienists, dental assistants, dental technicians, social workers, health aides, public health nurses, physician's assistants, nutritionists
Nonclinical providers	
Planning	Health planning agencies
Clerical	Volunteers, students, parents, retirees
Educational	Professional organizations, universities, students
Analytical	Universities, consulting firms
Equipment	
Dental units and instruments	Dental supply companies, dental and dental hygiene schools, renovated public health clinics, hospitals, federal government depositories
Computers, calculators, filing cabinets	Business, industry, civic groups, hospitals
Supplies	
Office supplies	Consumer groups, industry, business, government
Dental supplies	Dental supply companies, dental products companies
Dental Health Education Materials	American Dental Association, other professional organizations, public health agencies, dairy councils, local, state, or federal agencies, i.e., National Institute for Dental Research, Centers for Disease Control
Facilities	Hospitals, health centers, nursing homes, public schools, dental schools, public health clinics, industry, health maintenance organizations

Constraints may result from organizational policies, resource limitations, or characteristics of the community. For example, constraints that commonly occur in community dental programs include limitations of the state's dental practice act, attitudes of professional organizations, lack of funding, restrictive governmental policies, inadequate transportation systems, labor shortages, lack of or inadequate facilities, negative community attitudes toward dentistry, and the population's socioeconomic, cultural, and educational characteristics. The community's source of water (type and location), the lack of fluoride in the water, and the community's dental health status are also viewed as constraints to program planning. In addition, the amount of time available to complete a project is considered a constraint if that time is too limited to attain the program goals.

One of the best ways to identify constraints is to bring together a group of concerned citizens who might be involved in or affected by the project. As a group that is familiar with the local politics and community structures, these individuals not only can identify the constraints but also can offer alternative solutions to and strategies for meeting the goals.

Alternative strategies

Being aware of the existing constraints and given the available resources, the planner should then consider alternative courses of action that might be effective in attaining the objectives. It is important to generate a sufficient number of alternatives so that out of that number at least one may be considered acceptable.

The planner must be aware of those alternatives that sound good on the surface but may have certain limitations when closely examined. With limited resources, the planner needs to consider the anticipated costs and the effectiveness of each alternative. A classic example is the use of preventive measures in a community setting. If, for example, the community re-fused to fluoridate the central water supply, or if a community received its water from individual wells, the planner would look at the alternative preventive measures available in relation to dental caries and the cost savings in terms of needed treatment.

If the preventive measure were considered to be cost-effective as well as practical to implement, the planner would then choose that measure as the best of the alternatives.

Implementation, supervision, evaluation, and revision

This chapter has concentrated on the planning process: identifying the problem, determining priorities, defining the goals and objectives, identifying the resources and constraints, and considering the alternatives for implementation. The process of putting the plan into operation is referred to as the implementation phase. This phase is ongoing in situations where close supervision and evaluation of the program will ensure effective operations.

The implementation process, like the planning process, involves individuals, organizations, and the community. Integrating all the external variables, as depicted in Fig. 12-2, to achieve comprehensive planning and implementation requires what Bruhn terms an "ecologic" approach.[9] Only through teamwork between the individual and the environment can the implementation be successful.

DEVELOPING IMPLEMENTATION STRATEGY

An implementation strategy for each activity is complete when the following questions have been answered:

1. *Why:* the effect of the objective to be achieved
2. *What:* the activities required to achieve the objective
3. *Who:* individuals responsible for each activity

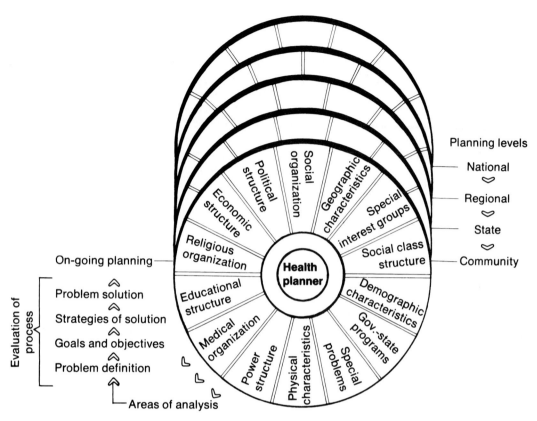

Fig. 12-2. An ecologic approach to comprehensive health planning. *(From Bruhn JG: Planning for social change: dilemmas for health planning,* Am J Public Health *63:604, 1972.)*

4. *When:* chronologic sequence of activities
5. *How:* materials, media, methods, and techniques to be used
6. *How much:* a cost estimate of materials and time

To develop an implementation strategy, planners must know what specific activity they want to do. The most effective method is to work backward to identify the events that must occur before initiating the activity. The National Heart, Lung, and Blood Institute has developed the *Handbook for Improving High Blood Pressure Control in the Community,*[10] which provides examples of implementation strate-gies that can be applied to any type of health program. Box 12-3 lists rules for implementation strategy development. Through a review of these rules the details of operating a program will become clear to those responsible for instituting the program.

MONITORING, EVALUATING, AND REVISING THE PROGRAM

Once it has been implemented, the program requires continuous surveillance of all activities. The program's success is determined by monitoring how well the program is meeting its stated objectives, how well individuals are

---

BOX 12-3

RULES FOR IMPLEMENTATION

1. Specify clearly the activity (who does what for whom).
2. Be sure someone is responsible for the whole activity and coordinates individuals who may carry out the different tasks.
3. Identify all the preparatory steps prior to doing that activity (e.g., prepare training manual, prepare materials, write article, acquire equipment, train volunteers, determine treatment protocol).
4. List steps in the order in which they must occur.
5. Check for missing steps which need to be added.
6. Determine when (date) each step should begin and end.
7. Check your dates to make sure the correct amount of time has been allowed.
8. Consult with organizations affected by the activity; identify potential problems, opportunities, etc.
9. Specify what resources will be needed and their source.
10. Specify what constraints will need to be addressed.
11. Make sure all people involved know what is expected of them and by when.

From National Heart, Lung and Blood Institute: *Handbook for improving high blood pressure control in the community,* Washington, DC, 1977, US Government Printing Office.

---

doing their jobs, how well equipment functions, and how appropriate and adequate facilities are. Before problems arise in any of these areas, adjustments must be made to fine-tune the program.

Evaluation, both informal and formal, is a necessary and important aspect of the program. Evaluation allows us to (1) measure the progress of each activity, (2) measure the effectiveness of each activity, (3) identify problems in carrying out the activities, (4) plan revision and modification, and (5) justify the dollar costs of administering the program and, if necessary, justify seeking additional funds.

Each objective should be examined periodically to determine how well it is meeting the program goals. The objective should be stated in measurable terms so that a comparison can be made of what the objective intended to accomplish and what it actually accomplished.

Evaluation should also address the quality of what is being done. For example, if one of the activities was placing pit and fissure sealants on specific teeth of school-aged children, an evaluator would want to assess how well that sealant was placed, the appropriateness of the tooth chosen, and the time involved in placing the sealant on the tooth.

The attitudes of the recipients of the program should be examined to determine whether the program was acceptable to them. There are many programs that are considered successful by those who run the program; however, the people who have been the recipients of the service may have wanted something very different. Fig. 12-3 illustrates this point and gives us a perspective on planning by showing the concept of the planner, the actual plan, the design, the constraints involved, the alternative strategy, and, finally, what in fact the recipient wanted in the first place.

Summary

Merely hanging up a shingle is no longer all that is necessary for a health care provider to deliver health services to a given community. Consumers of health care are more involved

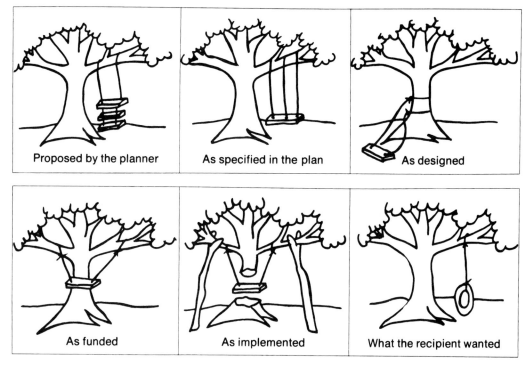

Fig. 12-3. A perspective on planning.

than ever before in learning about the types of health care they should be receiving, and they are actively questioning the choices available to them. We as health professionals need to be responsive to those consumers.

We must be prepared to meet the challenges of the 1990s through the development of good planning skills. These skills can then be used to achieve such goals as the following:

1. The construction of well-planned and accessible health facilities
2. The selection of appropriate, well-qualified, and sensitive health personnel
3. The provision of appropriate and effective health services
4. The time and the funds to provide the needed care
5. The active participation of representatives of those communities, organizations, and individuals who will be the recipients of the health care

Only through fully understanding the needs of the community, the organization, and the individual can we begin to coordinate our planning efforts to develop acceptable, appropriate, and effective health care programs today and for the future.

REFERENCES

1. Dubos R: *So human an animal*, New York, 1968, Charles Scribner's Sons.
2. Striffler D: *Surveying a community and developing a working policy: the administration of local dental programs*, University of Michigan, School of Public Health, Proceedings from Fifth Workshop on Dental Public Health, Ann Arbor, Mich, 1963.

3. Schulbert H and others: *Program evaluation in the health fields,* New York, 1969, Human Sciences.

4. Blum HL: *Note on comprehensive planning for health,* Berkeley, Calif, 1968, Comprehensive Health Planning Unit, School of Public Health, University of California.

5. *Provision of dental care in the community, University of Michigan, School of Public Health, Ann Arbor, 1973,* Proceedings from the Third Annual Course in Dental Public Health, Waldenwoods Conference Center, Hartland, Mich, May 22-26, 1966.

6. Spiegel A and others: *Basic health planning methods,* Germantown, Md, 1978, Aspen Systems.

7. U.S. Department of Health, Education and Welfare, Public Health Service: *Dental program efficiency criteria and standards for the Indian Health Service,* 1974.

8. *Model standards for community preventive health services,* A report to the U.S. Congress for the Secretary of Health, Education and Welfare, August 1979.

9. Bruhn J: Planning for social change, *Am J Public Health* 63:7, 1972.

10. U.S. Department of Health, Education, and Welfare, Public Health Services, National Institutes of Health, National Heart, Lung and Blood Institute: *Handbook for improving high blood pressure control in the community,* DHEW Pub No 78-1086, Washington, DC, 1977, US Government Printing Office.

CHAPTER 13

Program evaluation in health care

David O. Born

Purpose of program evaluation

Program evaluation is concerned with finding out how well programs work by using social and behavioral science research techniques to assess information of importance to program administrators and public policy makers. The fundamental purpose of program evaluation is to provide information for decision making. Ultimately, evaluation is a judgment of merit or worth about a particular person, place, or thing.

Is evaluation research?

The term *research* refers to systematic inquiry that leads one to discover or revise knowledge about a particular subject. Basic research is generally focused on discovering facts, relationships, behaviors, and underlying principles. Applied research often deals with the same phenomena, but the focus is usually less on the discovery of basic knowledge and more on the development of tools or the application of knowledge to develop solutions to actual problems. Evaluation is an example of applied research. Administrators, educators, policy makers, and others face questions (problems) about designing, implementing, continuing, and improving social, educational, health, and other programs. Evaluators assess or evaluate those programs to discover or revise knowledge about them and the problems they were designed to address so that informed judgments can be made, modifications can be implemented, and solutions can be achieved.

As researchers, program evaluators engage in scientific inquiry. They use tests, questionnaires, and other measurement devices. They collect and analyze data systematically by using common statistical procedures. Finally, they typically describe their findings in formal reports.[1]

An important difference between basic research and evaluation research is the generality of the findings. Ideally, the basic scientist is searching for basic knowledge; the more basic or fundamental, the better. Fundamental facts and principles, such as Einstein's theory of relativity, have broad applicability. They generalize across wide areas of knowledge. Most applied scientists—and program evaluators, in particular—are usually dealing with specific problems in specific settings. Their findings or conclusions can seldom be generalized to "similar" problems.

To elaborate on this distinction between the basic science researcher and the evaluator, consider the role each individual might play in the testing of a fluoride rinse. In examining the value of fluoride rinse, the basic science researcher would probably be concerned with the effects of fluoride on teeth, the strength of the solution necessary to produce a reduction in caries, and whether the conclusions could be generalized across the population. The evaluator would be more concerned with determining whether the actual mouthrinse program, initiated to test the researcher's conclusion, was run correctly and followed the objectives that it stated. The evaluator's concern for the fluoride rinse as such is only superficial. Once the evaluator can judge whether the program is an accurate test of the fluoride rinse, the secondary results might then relate to the positive or negative effects of fluoride rinse. In other words the particular program's operation is of prime importance to the evaluator, and the effect of fluoride is important only in terms of its results as applied to a realistic, closely monitored program.

Determining the value of things is another difference between evaluation and basic research. Evaluation eventually comes down to making a decision about what should be done or which course of action is best. Basic researchers strive only to obtain accurate, truthful information. There is no requirement to attach assessments of merit to the discovered knowledge.[1] Theoretically, the basic scientist's task does not involve making value judgments. The evaluator may or may not make decisions based on value judgments, but the evaluation report almost always ends up in the hands of someone who does.

Focus of evaluations

Evaluation studies ultimately focus on the goals, objectives, or intent of the program or activity being studied. At the simplest level we ask: Does this program do what it was designed to do? There are, of course, many other facets to evaluation. One of the most useful frameworks for looking at the evaluation research task has been put forward by Donabedian.[2] He suggests that assessment or evaluation can profitably look at structure, process, and outcome.

Structure refers to the program setting and logistics (i.e., facilities, equipment, financing, human resources). *Process* refers to the actual ways or methods employed in the provision of program services (i.e., delivering health care, educating children). *Outcome* refers to the actual impacts, effects, and changes brought about as a result of the program being evaluated.

Donabedian rightly sees structure, process, and outcomes as inextricably linked: the interrelationships are critical to the program's ability to meet its goals or fulfill its intent. Examining structure, process, and outcomes allows the evaluator to identify more clearly where problems and program liabilities lie and, hence, where corrections can be made if goals are to be met. Looking at goals, structure, process, and outcomes should be the primary focus for the evaluator. A second set of concerns also exists, however. These questions might be classified as "client" questions; that is, for whom and why is the evaluation research being conducted? This is not a trivial question. The researcher must understand, for example, whose decisions will determine the ultimate fate of a program and what their interests and concerns are. The evaluator must also know what kinds of decisions will be made.

To illustrate, a dental school implements a new curriculum for its students. An evaluator who is brought in designs and carries out a carefully planned study to determine if the program has the resources it needs (structure), how well the program is running (process), and how successful the graduates are (outcomes). Such an evaluation is appropriate if the client's interest is to determine if the curriculum is functioning properly and meeting its goals. The design would not be appropriate, however, if the client wanted to know if the graduates of the new curriculum were better trained professionals than those of the old curriculum. The evaluator must understand the client's focus.

Individuals interested in the results of evaluation may include program developers, program staff, program directors, policy makers (state or federal bureaucrats), program directors in other similar agencies, or epidemiologists.[3] Each group seeks different information about the same program. Program developers seek all kinds of information about ways to improve specific parts of the program that affect them directly. The director of the program is usually interested in knowing the overall effectiveness of the basic program, although he or she is generally more concerned with finding out what specific modifications will be needed to improve the organization and operation of the program. Financial issues are usually of concern to policy makers, who question whether a program should be continued as is, given more resources, or canceled. Staff from other programs are interested in whether the program can be generalized for possible adaptation or adoption. Epidemiologists may seek to compare the effect of different program principles and generalize about the factors responsible for success.

Clearly the evaluator faces a number of potentially competing interests. In responding to those interests the researcher must distinguish between different types of evaluation. As we have seen, Donabedian's framework allows us to focus on the critical features or components that make up a program. These factors must be taken into account if evaluation efforts are to be successful and useful. At the same time Scriven[4] draws our attention to the fact that evaluation research may be one of two types. He uses the terms *formative* and *summative* to describe these types.

FORMATIVE EVALUATION

Formative evaluation refers to the internal evaluation of a program. It is an examination of the processes or activities of a program as they are taking place. It is usually carried out to aid in the development of a program in its early phases.

The following situation is one in which a formative evaluation is appropriate: a fluoride rinse program is initiated at a neighborhood health center in which paraprofessionals are trained to administer three types of fluoride rinses under a strict sequence of procedures. After 3 days of operation, the work of the paraprofessionals is observed to determine the extent of adherence to a strict sequence of procedures. The observation and determination of correct or incorrect procedure sequence provide an example of examining the activities of a program as they are occurring (formative evaluation). If the sequence is incorrect, formative evaluation allows the program to make remedial changes at that point and thereby improve performance. Such a strategy is much better than waiting until the program is completed and then announcing that there were procedural errors. Formative evaluation is used primarily by program developers and program staff members concerned with whether various components of a program are workable or whether changes should be made to improve program activities.

SUMMATIVE EVALUATION

Summative evaluation, by contrast, judges the merit or worth of a program after it has been in operation. It is an attempt to determine whether a fully operational program is meeting the goals for which it was developed. Summative evaluation is aimed at program decision makers, who will decide whether to continue or terminate a program, and also at decision makers from other programs who might be considering adoption of the program.

Different evaluation designs are needed to carry out these two types of evaluation. Different types of measures and time schedules also are required. Because most programs are ongoing, with changes often being made "on the fly," a discernible end point or completion date may not exist. In such cases the dichotomy between formative and summative evaluation may not be as precise as described here, and formative evaluation may continue to be important as the program develops and matures.

Most health programs can be divided into four phases of implementation, which should occur in sequence: (1) the pilot phase, the development of which proceeds on a trial-and-error basis; (2) the controlled phase, in which a model of a particular program strategy is run under regulated conditions to judge its effectiveness; (3) the actualization phase, in which a model of the program strategy is subjected to realistic operating conditions; and (4) the operational phase, in which the program is an ongoing part of the structure. Often this ideal progression from phase 1 to phase 4 does not occur, and a program becomes lodged at one state of development. Each phase has different objectives to be met and thus different evaluation designs by which to best assess achievement of program objectives. Formative evaluation plays an important part in both the pilot phase and the controlled phase of program implementation. Summative and formative evaluations are used during the actualization phase, whereas the final operational phase is evaluated with a summative evaluation design.[5]

Specifying health program outcomes and inputs

One generalization that can be made of health program evaluation is that it is primarily concerned with how well a program is meeting its goals, either at some formative stage (so that the information can be fed back into the program) or at the end. The first step in evaluation, then, is to discover what the program goals are and to then restate them as clear, specific objectives written in measurable terms.

This first step is often a formidable task. Many program directors and staff members develop only general goals expressed as vague abstractions. They find it difficult to translate them into concrete specifications of the changes in behavior, attitude, knowledge, or health outcome that they hope to effect. In addition, programs often have multiple goals. Some are more important than others, some are more immediate (as opposed to long-range), some are easier to study, and some may be incompatible with others. Yet each program director and staff member must establish a sense of goal priorities if they, or external evaluators, are to assess the operation of their program. In many instances directors and staff members are unable to sort out goals, objectives, and priorities clearly, and they find it useful to bring in outside evaluators or administrative consultants to assist in this process.

The frequency of ambiguous and unclear goal statements has led some observers to speculate about the underlying reasons for this state of affairs. One view is that it usually requires support from diverse groups and individuals to get a program accepted. Program goals need to be formulated in ways that satisfy the diversity of interests represented. Another speculation is that program planners lack experience with expressing their thoughts in measurable terms and concentrate mainly on the specifics of program operation. In one sense ambiguous goal statements serve a useful function: they hide differences among diverse groups by allowing for a variety of interpretations. However, such differences between groups and staff or within the staff can be disruptive when the program is implemented. Once a program has been initiated, if there is lack of true consensus as to what the program is specifically attempting to achieve, progress is difficult. Each staff member may be pulling in a different direction and trying to implement a different interpretation of the goal. As an outside agent or more objective observer, the evaluation study director can make a substantial contribution to program planning and administration in formulating goals, clarifying priorities, and reconciling divergent viewpoints related to program direction.

Ultimately, of course, evaluation attempts to measure the outcomes of a particular program. If a program's goals cannot be operationalized (stated in a precise, measurable manner), it becomes nearly impossible to determine whether the desired outcomes of a program have been achieved. In other words, without clearly stated goals and objectives, evaluation becomes an imprecise tool of questionable usefulness.

One common difficulty in specifying desired objectives is that objectives are often long range in nature, making it extremely difficult to measure success in meeting those objectives. In the interim, evaluation is conducted by relying on surrogate measures of attitudes, knowledge, skills, or behaviors that presumably are related to the ultimate objectives.

This problem is not unique to evaluation but is also basic to program design. A program may be designed to produce certain intermediate changes on the assumption that they are necessary for the attainment of ultimate goals. In such cases probably the best that evaluation can do, at least under the usual time constraints, is to discover whether intermediate goals are being met. It is up to more intensified research efforts to investigate the relation between these goals and desired final outcomes.

MEASURING OUTCOMES

To evaluate the effectiveness of health programs, specific measurement instruments must be set up for systematic collection of data on the attainment of each program objective and program goal. These procedures follow accepted principles of biostatistical and research design, which are discussed in Chapters 14 and 15.

Establishment of an effective health program evaluation requires specific description and measurement of each objective of a program. Depending on the nature of the program and the evaluation effort, some data will be collected as a part of the day-to-day operations of the program. Examples might include patient visits, staff turnover, program revenue, and supply costs. In most cases data collection instruments addressing specific objectives will also be necessary. Examples of factors to be measured by such instruments might include patient satisfaction, employee morale, sealant wear, and the mastery of skills (such as toothbrushing). Usually, multiple instruments are required. If a program has several objectives, use of a simple summary instrument is likely to be superficial and misleading. If measurement instruments that are truly relevant to program intents are available, they should be used, thus moving the evaluation process several steps ahead. Time is saved, and the program and the evaluation benefit from tested and validated instruments. Use of the same measurement instruments makes it easier to compare the relative effectiveness of one program with many other programs and adds significantly to the overall body of research knowledge. However, if existing instruments are not relevant to the program objectives, new measures constructed for the specific needs of the program must be developed.

INSTRUMENT RELIABILITY AND VALIDITY

Measurement instruments used to assess program objectives and materials must be valid and reliable. A valid measurement instrument is one that provides a score that accurately describes the characteristics it is intended to measure. A reliable instrument consistently or repeatedly produces the same score. Validity and reliability are important because no test or other measurement instrument is perfect. Each time a test is administered, a range of scores results. We know that statistically each score contains a small amount of error because of testing and measurement procedures. If the procedure is repeated 10 times for 10 separate components of a health program, one can see how the amount of error can build, thus reducing the ability of the evaluation to assess program effectiveness accurately. The greater the reliability and validity, the more accurate the information collected during the evaluation process.

A simple example of a test that might be reliable but not valid would be the dental hygiene board examination administered to first-year dental students. Results of that test might prove to be highly reliable and consistent yet not valid. One might guess that if first-year dental students took the dental hygiene board examination several times, their individual scores would not fluctuate much higher or lower than the scores they received the first time. Thus the test would be considered highly reliable. It repeatedly produced the same or nearly the same score. This test would not be considered valid because it measured material totally foreign to the first-year dental student. The test is designed to measure skills of graduate dental hygienists, not first-year dental students. Thus the test is reliable but not valid.

As a second example, assume that a course is offered in which four tests are administered during the course of the semester. No one test was found to be perfectly reliable, thus error as a result of testing would result with each administration. Assume that student A received the following scores:

	Score	Reliability	Testing error	Range
Test 1	80	0.80	5	75-85
Test 2	70	0.63	8	62-78
Test 3	80	0.55	12	68-92
Test 4	90	0.92	2	88-92
AVERAGE	80			73-87

In this example student A obtained an average of 80 and probably would receive a course grade of B− or B. Yet because of normal error associated with the unreliability of the four tests, that student's true performance may be between 73 and 87. These scores indicate that student A's course grade could actually be between C− and B+, a substantial difference for most students. The more reliable the test, the smaller the error. Compare the reliability scores with the test error. The test with high reliability (0.92) has the smallest error (2), whereas the test with low reliability (0.55) has the greatest amount of error (12).

DIFFICULTIES IN OBTAINING NECESSARY INFORMATION

After consideration of what measurement instruments to use and when to measure outcomes, a final concern must be how to measure. In this area two problems are particularly important: bias and sampling. The possibility of bias is great if one evaluates his or her own work. Bias may be avoided by using objective measures (rather than subjective measures) and also by using several people (rather than a single person) to measure outcomes. Sampling is used in evaluating a health program when it is not possible or practical to obtain information from every person involved in an activity or when it is not possible to assess every activity that a program initiates.

Sample size depends on the activity to be studied. The student is advised to consult a standard research design text for a more formal discussion of bias and sampling problems related to evaluation and research.

Constant intrusions into the program for the purpose of collecting data can be a source of friction with program staff. The evaluation is a service to the program, not vice versa; therefore evaluation activities should be limited to those found essential to furthering the effectiveness of the program. One thoughtfully constructed test or questionnaire is often better than three imperfectly conceived ones. When the evaluation is clear about what is needed and why, measures can be constructed and data can be collected with a minimum of disruption.

Programs may intend to bring about changes not only in people but also in agencies, larger social systems, or the public at large. Measures need to be relevant to such changes. Cost-benefit analysis is another measurement technique. This technique is not a suitable substitute for the usual methods of evaluation but a logical extension of them. Evaluation defines the program's benefits; cost-benefit analysis adds consideration of the value of the benefits. Costs of the program are compared with benefits as a way of judging whether the program is a worthwhile investment.

How does one decide which program activities to measure? Difficulties arise when theory and knowledge are inadequate to define the factors that affect success. In most program areas the general rule of thumb is that each stated objective of the program should be measured. A clearly stated objective indicates what achievement is sought, and thus such an objective will aid in the identification of what procedures to use for measuring program outcomes.

Table 13-1 presents six general factors that may serve as starting points for evaluation of health programs. Below each general factor are specific areas in which various program members would find evaluation information of interest. This list is not intended to be all-inclusive. It is designed to provide a few ideas to an individual who is not sure where to begin.

To conclude this discussion of measurement instruments, the following outline identifies three factors to consider in instrument selection: importance, statistical adequacy, and feasibility.[6]

1. Importance
   Is the information that is gained by administering the instrument the measure

that is needed to assess health status or health program effectiveness? Does the program require this information to perform its function?

2. Statistical adequacy
   a. Validity: Does the instrument accurately assess what you are trying to measure?
   b. Reliability: Will repeated application of the computational method for the measure yield similar results? How reliable are the data used to calculate the results?
   c. Sensitivity: Can the instrument adequately distinguish among levels of performance?

3. Feasibility
   a. Clarity of measure: How precise is the measure? Is the wording understandable? Are its limitations explained?
   b. Data availability and cost: Does the program have the information needed to assess the objective? Are the instruments appropriate for their specific use within the program?
   c. Compatibility: Can data collected for this program be compared with similar data on a statewide or national basis? Can they be compared with similar data from different types of programs?
   d. Ease of use and interpretation: Can collection and interpretation of data for implementation of the measure be done without specialized or statistical knowledge?

Study designs appropriate for specific programs

In planning an evaluation study, one is immediately struck by the fact that there are a multitude of possible study designs from which to choose.[7] Choosing the best design is one of the most critical tasks the evaluator faces. In the

Table 13-1. Component factors of health system characteristics

Availability	Accessibility	Cost	Quality	Continuity	Acceptability

Supply of services:
 	
Existing service capacity
 	
Used capacity
 	
Supply of resources:
 	
Personnel
 	
Equipment
 	
Facilities
 	
Financial resources
	Ability to obtain services in terms of these factors:
	
	1. Economic
	
	   Out-of-pocket cost
	
	   Health insurance coverage and benefits
	
	   Opportunity cost to patient/client, family, and others
	
	2. Temporal
	
	   Travel time
	
	   Waiting time
	
	3. Locational
	
	4. Architectural
	
	5. Cultural
	
	6. Organizational
	
	7. Informational
	
	Use of services by specified population subgroups
		Service cost
		
		Costs incurred by providers
		
		Costs incurred by financing mechanisms
		
		Sources of payment for services
			Structure
			
			   Competence and qualifications of resources
			
			   Existence and extent of review and assurance mechanisms
			
			   Minimal volume of specialized services
			
			Process
			
			   Accuracy of services
			
			   Appropriateness of services
			
			   Documentation of treatment
			
			Outcome
			
			   Health status
			
			   Behavior
			
			   Environment
				Coordination of settings among health system components and to/from other nonhealth systems
				
				Regular source of care
				
				Degree of interruptions or delays in service plan given a logical sequence of services
				
				Patient transfer
				
				Medical and health information transfer
				
				Follow-up
					Consumer satisfactions with:
					
					Availability
					
					Accessibility
					
					Cost
					
					Continuity
					
					Courtesy and consideration
					
					Provider satisfaction

Modified from Hadley SA, Gillespie JF Jr: Operational measures: indicators of health system performance, *Am J Health Plan* 3:44, 1978.

broadest sense evaluation research designs are divided into two groups: experimental and nonexperimental. Experimental design has long been considered the ideal for evaluation. The design requires that people, objects, and other factors be randomly assigned either to the program or to a control group. A control group is a set of individuals in an experiment whose selection and experiences are identical in every way possible to the program participants except that they are not part of the program. The control group may receive a pseudoprogram (the social science equivalent of the laboratory placebo), the standard program (the traditional rather than the innovative program), or no program at all. Relevant measurements are taken before and after the program. If the program recipients show greater positive change than the controls, the outcome can clearly be attributed to the program. Experimental design is the study design that most researchers select when given a choice.[8]

Toothbrushing studies are a perfect example of the true experimental design model. For illustration purposes the study shown in Table 13-2 demonstrates the effectiveness of a fluoride toothpaste for the reduction of new carious lesions. The study is of 3 years' duration and of longitudinal design. Both experimental and control groups brush daily under supervision. The study is double-blind; all experimental materials are color coded, and the look and the taste are identical. All participants use the same brand and model of toothbrush, with the type of toothpaste (i.e., fluoride toothpaste and nonfluoride toothpaste) being the one variable examined in the study. Results show a significant reduction in the number of new lesions, thus allowing the researcher to assume that the reduction was a result of the one differing variable (i.e., fluoride versus nonfluoride).

One major problem arises when an attempt is made to implement experimental procedures in health programs. It is nearly impossible to implement the design in the busy day-to-day activities of the program. How can random services be tested on people who come to drop-in, multiservice, or neighborhood health centers. In addition, there is resistance from the program staff and difficulty resulting from the very nature of the recipient groups and from outside events that "contaminate" the controls placed on the study. These contaminations reduce the validity of the evaluation.

Two types of validity affect the ability to implement evaluation research designs according to strict experimental requirements: internal validity and external validity. These kinds of validity are different from the term *validity* used earlier in relation to measurement instruments. A program has internal validity if its outcomes result from the approach or the techniques being tested rather than from other causes that have nothing to do with the program being implemented. Internal validity de-

Table 13-2. Longitudinal results of 3-year fluoride toothpaste study

	Randomly assigned groups	
	Experimental (fluoride toothpaste)	*Control (nonfluoride toothpaste)*
Baseline examination (DMFS) (before beginning testing)	97.4	97.5
After 1 yr	91.5	95.0
After 2 yr	86.3	93.4
After 3 yr	80.0	90.3
Difference	17.4	7.2

DMFS, Decayed, missing, filled surfaces.

termines whether the results can be accepted based on the evaluation design of the program.[2]

A program has external validity if the results obtained can be generalized to similar programs or approaches everywhere. External validity affects one's ability to credit the evaluation results with generality based on the procedures used.[8]

By its nature the process of conducting an experimental evaluation design exercises some degree of control over the program, thus contributing to internal validity, while producing some limitations in external validity. A catch-22 situation is produced. As the circumstances of a program are controlled, the chances that what happens in the program will be exactly what the evaluator hopes to find (internal validity) increase. However, the more conditions are controlled, the less chance there is that the program will continue to work when the controls are removed (external validity).

The constant struggle between external and internal validity is an important one; external validity is of little value without some reasonable degree of internal validity to provide confidence in the conclusions. There is no advantage in being able to generalize results that are based on invalid or inconsistent program activities. The two sets of validity demands must strike a balance. There should be enough internal validity so that an experiment can be conclusive; yet it should be sufficiently realistic to be generalized. In program evaluation internal validity becomes the major concern because most programs involve only a superficial attempt to generalize results beyond their program.

Perhaps the most respected source in the area of research design is Donald T. Campbell. Campbell[9] suggests that experimental design is possible in most health programs with careful planning and administrative backing and that control groups can be used in somewhat turbulent programs.

In reality, it is often impossible to apply rules relating to internal validity fully. To evaluate programs in such situations, the evaluator must choose some approach other than experimental. If circumstances preclude experimental design, quasiexperimental designs developed by Campbell and Stanley[8] are often suitable. Campbell[9] offers three types useful in evaluation: interrupted time series, control series, and regression discontinuity designs. Although the results of these approaches do not provide the certainty and the potential for generalization of experimental designs, they guard against most of the important threats to valid interpretation. For the interested student, a standard research methods text is suggested for more comprehensive discussion of research design. It should also be noted that evaluation is concerned with making decisions about specific programs. Therefore internal validity is often more important than external validity to the evaluator.

Outcomes assessment

Recently in many social and health service sectors attention has been centered on something referred to as *outcomes assessment*. Within the field of dentistry this term is increasingly used in the evaluation of dental educational programs and managed care programs, among others. Although the subject of measuring program outcomes has come up throughout this chapter, the newer term *outcomes assessment* shifts the focus to a somewhat different emphasis than that of standard evaluation research; such differences as do exist tend to derive from the orientation of the evaluators involved in specifying the outcomes to be measured. Additionally, outcomes assessment tends to reflect a broader, more inclusive view of the program and the socioeconomic context within which it operates. In particular, it involves a trend toward identifying outcomes that are ultimately meaningful to the consumers of the programs being evaluated.

In the case of managed care in dentistry, providers, plan purchasers, insurers, and patients all have specific interests in the outcome of the managed care plan. Capilouto,[10] for example, points out that purchasers want lower costs and higher quality, patients want lower out-of-pocket expenses, and providers are struggling to obtain the best "price" for their services. Insurers, like purchasers, are concerned about quality and price but have an additional interest in generating profits. Other authors[11-13] also have addressed the issues of outcome assessment in the highly charged atmosphere being created by the current explosion of managed care programs in dentistry.

Although much of the work being undertaken in the development and assessment of outcome measures in dentistry is essentially evaluation research, much of it is termed *health services research*. This term suggests a broader focus than is usually attached to *evaluation research*. The expanded focus serves to draw our attention to the fact that with the increasing complexity of delivering and financing health care in this nation, programs must be evaluated not only in narrow terms that define their programmatic effectiveness but also in the context of their interaction with elements drawn from much wider reaches of the health arena. New political, financial, administrative, and delivery system networks and alliances are forming as active and reactive forces in the dental care marketplace. At the same time individual patients often find their power in the marketplace diminishing as employers and insurers "wheel and deal" with enormous sums of health care dollars, shaving costs at every turn in the interest of maximizing profits.

Providers, like patients, also find their roles changing dramatically. The dynamics of the entire system have become more wide-ranging, more complex, and more interconnected with nonhealth sectors of the economy. Specific dental care program evaluation (and thus outcomes assessment) must be designed to address the concerns of more and more outside agencies, individuals, and political constituencies. Therefore health services research and outcomes assessment must not only address the issues of quality of care, patient satisfaction, and other variables traditionally specified in evaluation paradigms; they also must be sensitive to and account for the influences of these more fluid, and often very powerful, forces. Given these circumstances, the basic principles of good evaluation are unchanged, but the scope of the studies often must be expanded considerably.[14]

Constraints on using the results of evaluation

Once the evaluation is completed, the logical expectation is that the results will be used to make rational decisions about future programming. All too often, however, the results are ignored. With all the money, time, effort, skill, and irritation that went into the acquisition of information, why do the results generally have so little impact? One reason may be that evaluation results do not match the informational needs of decision makers.

Individuals responsible for conducting evaluations should have a better understanding of decision processes and informational requirements relevant to decision making. A related issue is timing. Evaluation results should be ready in time to be considered, not after the decisions on future programming have been reached. Moreover, the evaluation results may not be relevant to the level of the decision maker who receives them. For example, overall assessments of program merit may be most useful to directors in other agencies who want to know whether a new program strategy works and, if so, under what conditions. Such people may never receive the report, or they may receive it in a nearly unreadable form.

Another constraint on the use of results may be a lack of clear direction for future programming. Results may be ambiguous, and their implications may be unclear. Results need to be translated into terms that make sense for pending decisions and that delineate alternatives indicated. There seems to be a large void between the findings of program evaluation and the planning of future programs. Someone is needed to translate the evaluation results into explicit recommendations for future programs.

In practice, evaluation is sometimes undertaken for dubious reasons. Evaluation may be used by program decision makers to delay a decision, to justify a decision already made, to pass the responsibility of future decisions to others, to vindicate a program in the eyes of its observers, or to satisfy funding conditions of government or foundation agencies.[5] These noninformational reasons for evaluation are not rare, and individuals conducting an evaluation should be forewarned if they learn that one of these is the underlying purpose of evaluation. It is as important to spend enough time investigating who wants to know what and why as it is to carry out the evaluation activities. Evaluations performed for political ends or in situations in which there is no commitment to using the data for decision making might well be eliminated rather than wasting the talents of the individuals involved.[15]

External evaluators (persons called in who are not part of the program) are often reluctant to draw conclusions from their data. However, judgments and recommendations for action need to be made at some point. Unless the evaluator plays a leading role in the process, this important step may not get done.

A further constraint on the use of results is that organizations are comfortable with the status quo. When organizations are presented with negative results, their prestige, ideology, and even resources are threatened. They frequently react by rejecting the results.

Campbell[9] suggests that one way out of this dilemma is for reformers to change their stance. Instead of committing themselves to new programs as though they were proven solutions, they would do better to commit themselves to seeking solutions to the problem. Then they could run a series of experimental programs until genuine solutions were found.

The prevalence of negative findings in a wide range of program fields is not something to bemoan or cover up, even when such results provoke political controversy or organizational resistance. Rather, the evidence that so many programs are having little constructive effect represents a fundamental critique of current approaches to social programming. This is a matter to which society will, in time, need to respond.

Summary

Evaluation involves research into the operation and accomplishments of programs that are usually, but not exclusively, designed to impact on social problems. By their very nature, evaluation efforts are linked, more or less directly, to a set of values that provide the criteria for judging relative success.

In considering programs the evaluator must recognize that program structure, process, and outcomes are all interrelated and that these factors are functionally related to the program's goals and objectives. Performing a good evaluation involves formulating (or clarifying) objectives, specifying the criteria to be used in measuring success, determining and explaining the degree of observed success, and (usually) recommending modifications in program activity to improve performance.[16]

Evaluations are undertaken not simply to reveal success or failure. If that were the case, most evaluations of programs would reveal a lack of total success in attaining goals and objectives. Good evaluation does more than demonstrate the degree of attainment. It also identifies problems and points out how a structural problem, for example, links with and affects process and outcome variables.

Identified problems may also relate to ill-conceived, ill-defined, or simply misdirected goals. Ideally, good evaluations identify opportunities and ways to correct programs and to improve their efficiency. The evaluation of programs assumes that (1) programs have been planned to expend funds to enable materials to be developed and activities to be performed and (2) the activities are intended to cause the achievement of program goals.

A program may not achieve its goals for the following reasons[17]:

1. Resources were not used as planned.
2. The assumptions linking resources to activities were invalid.
3. Activities were not performed as planned.
4. The assumptions linking activities to objectives were invalid.
5. The assumptions linking objectives to the program goals were invalid.

A sixth reason, which is technically included in this list but often overlooked and thus deserving of special mention, is that the behavior of the program staff and/or the client population may consciously or unconsciously undermine program performance. In other words, the best-designed program in the world cannot succeed if the providers and the clients do not like it and are openly or tacitly unwilling to cooperate.

If evaluation can identify the problems, subsequent program planning should proceed more effectively than it would in the absence of evaluation. Thus a successful evaluation in the hands of a thoughtful administrator can improve the planning and management of programs, thereby increasing program effectiveness.

REFERENCES

1. Popham JW: *Educational evaluation*, Englewood Cliffs, NJ, 1975, Prentice Hall.
2. Donabedian A: The quality of care: how can it be assessed? *JAMA* 260:1743, 1988.
3. Weiss CH: *Evaluating action programs: readings in social action and education*, Boston, 1972, Allyn & Bacon.
4. Scriven M: The methodology of evaluation. In Tyler RN, Gagne RM, Scriven M, editors: *Perspectives of curriculum evaluation*, AERA monograph series on curriculum evaluation, No 1, Chicago, 1967, Rand McNally.
5. Suchman EA: Action for what? A critique of evaluation research. In O'Toole R, editor: *The organization, management, and tactics of social research*, Cambridge, Mass, 1970, Schenkman.
6. Schulberg HC, Sheldon A, Baker F: *Program evaluation in the health fields*, New York, 1969, Behavioral Publications.
7. Isaac S, Michael WB: *Handbook in research and evaluation*, San Diego, Calif, 1981, Edits.
8. Campbell DT, Stanley JC: *Experimental and quasi-experimental design for research*, Chicago, 1966, Rand McNally.
9. Campbell DT: *Reform as experiments in evaluating action programs*, Boston, 1972, Allyn & Bacon.
10. Capilouto E: Market forces driving health care reform, *JDE* 59(4):480-483, 1995.
11. Bader J et al: A health plan report card for dentistry, *J Am Coll Dentists*, Fall, 1996, pp. 29-38.
12. Symposium on Self-Reported Assessments of Oral Health Outcomes, *JDE* 60(6):485-519, 1996.
13. Maas W, Garcia AI: Health services research, the agency for health care policy and research, and dental practice, *J Am Coll Dentists* 61(1), 1994.
14. Bader J: Health services research in dental public health, *J Public Health Dent* 52(1):23, 1992.
15. Elinson J: *Effectiveness of social action programs in health and welfare, assessing the effectiveness of child health services*, Report of the Fifty-Sixth Ross Conference on Pediatric Research, Columbus, Ohio, 1967.
16. Glossary of administrative terms in public health, *Am J Public Health* 50:225, 1960.
17. Deniston OL, Rosenstock IM, Getting VA: Evaluation of program effectiveness, *Public Health Rep* 83:323, 1968.

BIBLIOGRAPHY

Anderson SB and others: *Encyclopedia of educational evaluation*, San Francisco, 1976, Jossey Bass.

Baker EL: Formative evaluation. In Popham JW: *Evaluation in education: current applications*, Berkeley, Calif, 1974, McCutchan.

Bloom BS, Hastings ST, Madaus GF: *Handbook on formative and summative evaluation of student learning*, New York, 1971, McGraw-Hill.

Cook TD, Campbell DT: *Quasi-experimental design and analysis issues for field settings*, Boston, 1979, Houghton Mifflin.

Donabedian A: The seven pillars of quality, *Arch Pathol Lab Med* 114:1115, 1990.

FitzGibbon CT, Morris LL: *How to design a program evaluation*, Beverly Hills, Calif, 1978, Sage.

FitzGibbon CT, Morris LL: *How to present an evaluation report*, Beverly Hills, Calif, 1978, Sage.

Guba EG: Development, diffusion and evaluation. In Eidell TE, Kitchell JM, editors: *Knowledge production and utilization in educational administration*, Eugene, Ore, 1968, Center for the Advanced Study of Educational Administration, University of Oregon.

Guba EG: Failure of educational evaluation, *Educ Tech* 9:29, 1969.

Polit DF, Hungler BP: *Nursing research: principles and methods*, ed 2, Philadelphia, 1983, JB Lippincott.

Rosenstock IM: Evaluating health programs, *Public Health Rep* 85:835, 1970.

Rosenstock IM, Welch W, Getting VA: Evaluation of program efficiency, *Public Health Rep* 83:603, 1968.

Rossi PH, Freeman HE: *Evaluation: a systematic approach*, Newbury Park, Calif, 1989, Sage.

Stufflebeam DL and others: *Educational evaluation and decision making*, Itasca, Ill, 1971, FE Peacock.

Suchman EA: *Evaluation research: principles and practice in public service and action programs*, New York, 1967, Russell Sage Foundation.

Tuchman BW: *Conducting educational research*, ed 2, New York, 1978, Harcourt Brace Jovanovich.

Wholey JS and others: *Federal evaluation policy*, Washington, DC, 1970, Urban Institute.

Worthen BR: Toward a taxonomy of evaluation designs, *Educ Tech* 8:3, 1968.

SECTION IV

Research in dental public health

CHAPTER 14

Introduction to biostatistics

Lynda Rose

Familiarity with biostatistics, or the mathematics of collection, organization, and interpretation of numeric data having to do with living organisms, is essential for today's health care professional. Many people, however, are statistics shy. The goal of this chapter is to make clear the basics of biostatistics and to make the reader more comfortable with its usage.*

Dental health professionals have a variety of uses for data: for designing a health care program or facility, for evaluating the effectiveness of an ongoing program, for determining the needs of a specific population, and for evaluating the scientific accuracy of a journal article, to name just a few. These data are helpful only to the extent that they may be ordered and interpreted. Therefore what has been established is a system of managing data by using various techniques. Two statistical techniques are generally accepted: descriptive statistical technique enables an individual to describe and summarize a set of data numerically; inferen-

tial statistical technique provides a basis for making a generalization about the probable results of a large group when only a select portion of the group has been observed. Inferential statistics are used to generalize results to a larger population of interest, whereas descriptive statistics attempt only to generalize the group actually studied.

Before elaborating on terms relating to descriptive and inferential techniques, it is necessary to identify what is meant by the terms *population* and *sample*.

A *population* is any entire group of items (objects, materials, people, and so on) that possess at least one basic defined characteristic in common. Examples of populations might be all dentists, all U.S. citizens, all periodontally involved teeth, all individuals in a given school, or all patients treated at a particular private office. It is often impossible to collect information from an entire population because of the size of the population or because of such limitations as finances, time, or distance between population members. In cases in which it is impossible to collect data on the entire population, complete and reliable information can be collected from a representative portion of the

*A complete treatment of biostatistics is not possible in this text. The interested reader is referred to the standard texts in the bibliography of this chapter, which cover this material in detail.

population called a *sample*. By observing and measuring a sample, it is possible to obtain information and make statements about the total population.

Statistics is a science that describes data for the purpose of making inferences about the population from which the data are obtained. When we collect a specific piece of information—data—from each member of a population, we obtain a characteristic of the population called a *parameter*. Similarly, when we collect a piece of information from each member of a sample, we obtain a characteristic of the sample called a *statistic*. Because most studies are conducted by using samples, statistics are most commonly used. Using statistics (characteristics of a sample), we try to infer what the parameters (characteristics of a population) will be.

Sampling

Samples, by definition, cannot have exactly the same characteristics as a population. However, a sample that is truly representative of the population can be obtained by using probability sampling methods and by taking a sufficiently large sample.

A *random sample* is defined as one in which every element in the population has an equal and independent chance of being selected. The following example illustrates two random sampling procedures: assume a population of 5000 seniors in the predental program at 50 universities. Each senior class has 100 predental students divided into five equal sections of 20 students each. The objective is to determine the grade point average (GPA) of each predental student by selecting a representative sample of 1000 students (i.e., a sampling ratio of one fifth, or 20%). A simple random sample to select the 1000 students would be completed in the following manner: a list of 5000 students needs to be compiled and numbered 1 through 5000. A numbered tag is prepared for each student. From the 5000 well-mixed tags, 1000 are

drawn by a lottery. After each selection the tag is replaced and another tag is drawn. This is the most basic random sample approach.

A similar procedure may be applied for selecting a random sample by using a table of random numbers, which can be found in most statistics textbooks. For this example, it would be necessary to use four columns of digits in the tables so that each student, 1 through 5000, would have an equal probability of being selected. Selection would begin by blindly identifying a number on the table that corresponds to a member of the total population (1 through 5000). The selection process continues by taking numbers horizontally or vertically until the desired sample size is reached. Repeated numbers are omitted when encountered during sample selection in both procedures.

Random sampling is the procedure of choice whenever possible. It prevents the possibility of selection bias on the part of the researcher. What if GPA is related to school? A simple random sample may not ensure representation of the entire population of predental students. It may be necessary to select individuals according to certain strata or subgroups to diminish the chance of sample fluctuation. This method of selection is called *stratified sampling*. It is accomplished by randomly selecting a proportionate number of subjects from each subgroup for the sample. In the preceding example the subgroup would be the university attended. To produce a stratified random sample, one would (1) prepare a list of students at each of the 50 universities and (2) draw at random one fifth of the students at each university. Because the sampling ratio is used in each stratum, there is a proportional allocation by school. This eliminates the possibility of sampling bias, which could result by selecting at random and giving no consideration to school.

Another type of sampling is the *systematic sample*. A systematic sample is not a true random sample because everyone may not have an independent chance of being selected. This type of sample is usually obtained by drawing a number and then selecting every nth individual, for example, having a list of names and deciding to test every even-numbered person on the list. All odd-numbered names are systematically excluded.

Two types of samples that may introduce serious bias in estimating population parameters are (1) the judgment sample and (2) the convenience sample. In a judgment sample someone with knowledge of the population may select a sample in arbitrary ways to represent the population. In a convenience sample a group is chosen because it happens to be convenient and may represent the population; for example, one classroom within a school is selected because the teacher gives permission to work with the pupils, or the patients at a particular private office are used because the dentist allows access to the patient list. Results relating to that particular classroom or that particular dentist's office may be valid, but when generalized to include the larger population of school classrooms or dentists' offices, their reliability is questionable.

Once a sample has been selected, raw data are collected and consideration must then be given to data analysis. Data analysis requires the application of statistical tests to data for the purpose of organizing, describing, and summarizing findings. Among the steps that may be applied in data analysis are the following:

1. Organizing data from lowest to highest
2. Constructing a frequency distribution
3. Grouping and regrouping data, based on relevant information
4. Tabulating scores
5. Constructing tables and graphs for efficient communication of obtained results

Descriptive data display
FREQUENCY DISTRIBUTIONS

To better explain data that has been collected, the data are often grouped according to the variable they measure and ordered into an array. An array is simply a group of scores arranged from lowest to highest score. It can be organized into a frequency distribution by tabulating the frequency with which each score occurs. Three types of frequency distributions may be used: ungrouped, grouped, and cumulative. The following example illustrates the descriptive displays of data.

A group of 33 dental students has taken Part I of the National Boards examinations. Their examination scores have been recorded. The dean of the dental school wishes to summarize these scores at the next school faculty meeting. Here are a few of the ways that the information could be presented.

First, an ungrouped frequency distribution table of the National Board scores is presented in Table 14-1. The variable of interest is the examination score, which is shown in the first column of the table. The exam scores for the group are listed in descending order. The next column of the table contains the frequency with which each score occurs in the data set. Next, the frequency of occurrence is expressed as a relative frequency, that is, as a percent of the total number of scores represented in the table. For example, three students scored 77 on the exam. This represents 9.1% of the group of 33 students.

Second, the data can be displayed as a cumulative frequency distribution. Table 14-1 shows the cumulative frequency and cumulative percent for the National Board scores. These descriptive measures express the frequency of occurrence of scores up to and including any given value in the data set. For example, 25 students (75.8% of the group) scored 80 or below on this exam.

Instead of displaying each individual value in a data set, the frequency distribution for a variable can group values of the variable into consecutive intervals. Then, the number of observations belonging to an interval are counted.

A grouped frequency distribution for the National Board scores is illustrated in Table 14-2. Note that although the data are condensed in a

Table 14-1. Frequency distribution table for national board scores (NB1)

NB1	Frequency	%	Cumulative frequency	Cumulative %
		National Boards 1		
56	1	3.0	1	3.0
57	1	3.0	2	6.1
63	1	3.0	3	9.1
65	2	6.1	5	15.2
66	1	3.0	6	18.2
68	2	6.1	8	24.2
69	2	6.1	10	30.3
70	1	3.0	11	33.3
71	1	3.0	12	36.4
72	2	6.1	14	42.4
74	1	3.0	15	45.5
75	1	3.0	16	48.5
76	2	6.1	18	54.5
77	3	9.1	21	63.6
78	2	6.1	23	69.7
79	1	3.0	24	72.7
80	1	3.0	25	75.8
81	3	9.1	28	84.8
82	1	3.0	29	87.9
83	1	3.0	30	90.9
84	1	3.0	31	93.9
88	1	3.0	32	97.0
89	1	3.0	33	100.0

Table 14-2. Grouped frequency distribution of National Board scores

Scores	No. of students	%
56-61	2	6
62-65	3	9
66-69	5	15
70-73	4	12
74-77	7	21
78-81	7	21
82-85	3	9
86-89	2	6

useful fashion, some information is lost. The frequency of occurrence of an individual data point cannot be obtained from a grouped frequency distribution. For example, seven students scored between 74 and 77, but the number of students who scored 75 is not shown here.

GRAPHING TECHNIQUES

Graphing represents another alternative in displaying descriptive data pictorially and al-lowing rapid assimilation of findings by the reader. A general rule for constructing graphs along the x and y axes is that the vertical y axis usually represents the frequency of scores oc-curring along the scale of measurement, whereas the x axis represents the scale that measures the variable of most interest.

A bar graph is a two-dimensional pictorial display of data that is discrete in nature.

A histogram is a graphic representation formed directly from a frequency distribution. It is a display in which the horizontal (abscissa) and vertical (ordinate) axes of a graph are formed according to the scale values and the frequencies of the distribution, respectively. A histogram consists of a set of rectangles whose base is on the horizontal axis and which ex-tends in height along the vertical axis propor-tional to the frequency. If the points are wide-spread, a double bar (//) or a double curved line ($\approx$) is used to indicate breaks in the graph. Graphically, a histogram is similar to a bar graph except that the rectangles touch one an-other in a histogram (Fig. 14-1).

When the concern is to depict the continu-ous nature of the data, a line graph called a fre-quency polygon is used. To construct it one would place a point at the center of each rec-tangle found in a histogram and connect each point with a straight line. Of all graphing tech-

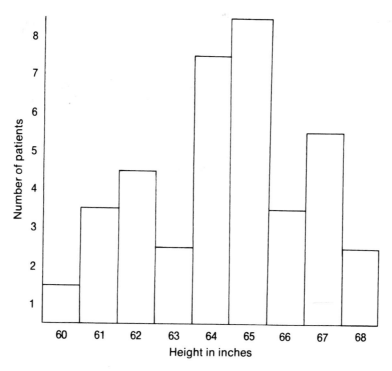

Fig. 14-1. Histogram of patient height.

niques, polygons are used the most frequently. Often polygons are superimposed on a line graph to display pictorially two or more distributions in one figure (Fig. 14-2).

When material is presented in tabular form, the table should be able to stand alone; that is, correctly presented material in tabular form should be understandable even if the written discussion of the data is not read. Following are suggestions for the display of data in graphic or tabular form:

1. The contents of a table as a whole and the items in each separate column should be clearly and fully defined. The unit of measurement must be included.
2. If the table includes rates, the basis upon which they are measured must be clearly stated—death rate percent, per thousand, per million, as the case may be.
3. Whenever possible, the frequency distributions should be given in full. These are basic data from which conclusions are being drawn, and their presentation allows the reader to check the validity of the author's arguments.
4. Rates or proportions should not be given alone without any information as to the numbers of observations upon which they are based. By giving only rates of observations and omitting the actual number of observations or frequency distributions, we are excluding the basic data.
5. Where percentages are used, it must be clearly indicated that these are not absolute numbers. Rather than combine too many types of figures in one table, it is often best to divide the material into two or three small tables.

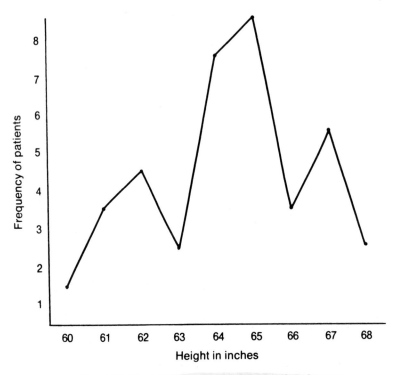

Fig. 14-2. Frequency polygon of patient height.

6. Full particulars of any exclusion of observations from a collected series must be given. The reasons for and the criteria of exclusions must be clearly defined.*

Figures (graphs) are used for a purpose different from that of tables. Figures are the presentation of material in a simplified manner to illustrate a particular set of data clearly. A major concern in the presentation of both figures and tables is readability. Tables and figures must be clearly understood and clearly labeled so that the reader is aided by the information rather than confused. The student is again directed to standard biostatistic texts for a formal discussion on summarizing data in graphic and tabular form. Also, standard writing style

*From Hill AB: *Principles of medical statistics*, ed 7, London, 1961, Lancet.

manuals generally contain discussions on the formal display of tables and graphs.

MEASURES OF CENTRAL TENDENCY

The display of data in graphic or tabular form may be tedious, time-consuming, and unwieldy when every piece of data is not necessary. Sometimes a summary that can describe the total collection of data with just one number is preferable. Three measures in common use describe the central tendency of a distribution of scores: the mode, the mean, and the median.

The *mode* is that value that occurs with the greatest frequency. When two or more values have equally large frequencies, it is possible for a distribution to have more than one mode. For example, the distribution of scores in Table 14-1 has two modes, 77 and 81. Both occur with the equally high frequency of three. The primary value of the mode lies in its ease of computation and in its convenience as a quick indicator of the central value in a distribution. Beyond this, its statistical uses are extremely limited.

The measure of central tendency called the *mean* is the same as the arithmetic average that one learns to calculate in the elementary grades. It is computed by adding a list of scores and then dividing by the number of scores. The symbol for mean is a capital letter X with a bar above it $(\overline{X})$. The mean is by far the most common measure of central tendency used to describe a set of data because it fluctuates least from sample to sample and is sensitive to any change in any score in the distribution. The presence of a few extremely high or extremely low scores can change the value of the mean considerably.

The *median* is that point that divides the distribution of scores into two equal parts, that is, the point at which 50% of the scores lie above it and 50% lie below it. For example, given the scores 1, 3, 5, 6, 8, 9, and 10, the median is 6, because two equal-sized parts (1, 3, 5 and 8, 9, 10) are above and below 6. The median is not affected by extreme scores in a given direction and is more stable than the mode.

An area in which the median is most often used and one that clearly illustrates its advantage over the mean or the mode is salary or dollar values. Suppose that seven dental hygienists and two dentists work in a productive private office. Their salaries are as follows:

$88,500	$36,500	$28,300
$80,000	$34,000	$28,300
$41,000	$32,000	$28,300

The owner of the office declares that the average member's salary is $44,100—the mean. In a later report the business manager declares that the average salary is $28,300—the mode. Neither person has intentionally reported false results. Both have used a measure of central tendency. However, the statistical tool reported

was the one best suited to the reporter's objective rather than the one that best described the data, in this case the median. In this example the median is $34,000. This value gives a much clearer picture of where the salaries lie for the individual in the middle of the salary range. The mode in this example was extremely low compared with the majority of salaries, and the mean was inflated by the two very high salaries of $80,000 and $88,500.

VARIABILITY

Measures of central tendency indicate the typical performance for a group. However, this is not enough information to describe a distribution of scores. How widely scores are dispersed around that central point must also be known. Suppose Dr. A has a class of dental hygienists whose mean intelligence quotient (IQ) is 110. Some students in this class have IQs of 80 to 90, and others have IQs of 130 to 140. Dr. B's class of hygienists also has a mean IQ of 110, but the lowest is 100 and the highest is 124. The two hygiene classes have the same mean; however, we can see that the abilities of one class are definitely different from those of the other class because we know something about the spread of scores around the average.

Three terms are commonly associated with variability: range, variance, and standard deviation. The *range* is the difference between the high score and the low score in a distribution. In Table 14-1 the range is 33 (89 to 56). Often, ranges are stated as lowest and highest score, that is, the range is 56 to 89. The range has the advantage of being easy to calculate. However, it is unstable and is affected by one extremely high score or one extremely low score. Also, only two scores are considered, and these happen to be the extreme scores of the distribution. Standard deviation and variance have much more utility than the range.

The *variance* is a measure of the average deviation or spread of scores around the mean. The variance, as is the standard deviation, is based on each score in the distribution. It is possible to have zero variance. However, it is impossible to have negative variance. Zero variance would occur when all scores in a distribution are equal, for instance, when everyone gets 100% as a test score or when everyone in a group has the same weight or height. The following steps show how the variance is calculated:

1. Obtain the mean of the distribution.
2. Subtract the mean from each score (deviation scores).
3. Square each deviation score.
4. Add these squared deviation scores.
5. Divide the sum by the number of cases added.

The *standard deviation* of a set of scores is simply the positive square root of the variance. Table 14-3 illustrates the calculation of variance and standard deviation for the IQ scores of 10 students.

The variance and the standard deviation (s) are relatively easy to interpret. The greater the dispersion of scores from the mean of the distribution, the greater the standard deviation and the variance. A large standard deviation indicates a wide dispersion around the mean. Consider the following statistics:

$$A. \ \bar{X} = 60 \quad s = 4$$
$$B. \ \bar{X} = 60 \quad s = 9$$
$$C. \ \bar{X} = 60 \quad s = 21$$

Group A is the most homogeneous group with a small standard deviation and therefore a small dispersion around the mean. Group C is the most heterogeneous group, with $s = 21$, indicating a major spread of scores around the mean.

NORMAL CURVE

The normal curve is one of the most used frequency distributions in biostatistics. It is a bell-shaped curve that is symmetrical around the mean of the distribution. The normal curve may vary from narrow distributions that are pointy in the center to wide distributions

Table 14-3. Calculation of variance and standard deviation for sample of 10 students

IQ scores χ	Deviation from mean ($\chi - \bar{\chi}$)	(Deviation)^2 ($\chi - \bar{\chi}$)^2
109	-2	4
99	-12	144
123	12	144
116	5	25
131	20	400
98	-13	169
116	5	25
89	-22	484
128	17	289
101	-10	100
1,110 = Sum of IQs	0	1,784 = Sum of deviation squared
111 = Mean IQ		

Variance (s^2) = 1784 ÷ 10 = 178.4
Standard deviation (s) = 13.36

whose center is flat. The mean of the distribution is the focal point from which all assumptions and statements may be made. The mean is used for two reasons: (1) most distributions do not have a zero point to be used as a starting point (what is zero intelligence?), and (2) the normal curve theoretically does not touch the baseline at any point because of the remote possibility of an extreme score in the distribution. Curves that meet the criteria for normality can be separated into areas under the curve. Fig. 14-3 shows an example of this separation.

The total area bounded by the curve is 1, or 100%. A curve that meets the criteria of normality has the mean equal to the median, which is equal to the mode. The total area is broken into segments of single units (1 standard deviation). As indicated in Fig. 14-3, the portion of the area under the curve between the mean and 1 standard deviation is 34.13% of the total area. The same area is found one unit below the mean. Similarly, two units above and below the mean cut off an additional

13.59% of the area under the curve, and so on for 3 standard deviations. The area under the curve can best be understood by imagining a test that is administered to a large group of students. When the tests are scored, the distribution will probably take the form of a normal curve. In that case 34.13% of the students who took the test would score between the mean and 1 standard deviation above the mean; another 13.59% would score between the first and second standard deviations above the mean; and 2.21% would score between the second and third standard deviations above the mean. Thinking of the area under the curve in terms of percent of persons makes it easier to interpret the distribution of the normal curve.

Significance related to inferential statistics

With large populations, it is often impossible to study each member in the group because of time, cost, and so on. Instead, we select a sam-

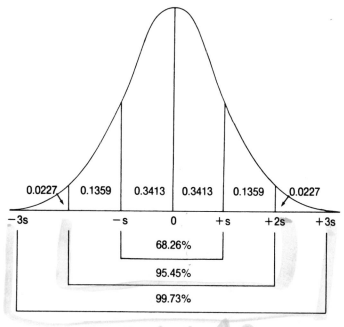

Fig. 14-3. Normal frequency curve.

ple from the population and from that sample attempt to generalize to the population as a whole. In using inferential statistical procedures (trying to infer about a group larger than our sample), we must deal with statistical probability—the mathematical assumption that a certain situation will occur according to chance a specific portion of the time. For example, if a coin is flipped an infinite number of times, by chance the coin will come up heads 50% of the time and tails 50% of the time.

The main thing to remember in inferential statistical procedures is that we are trying to generalize about a group larger than the one for which we actually have data. If we have a good sample, our generalization will be accurate; if our sample is poor, we will be hampered in our ability to generalize to the population. For example, suppose we are interested in determining the general status of a patient's oral health. We could examine each tooth of an individual and then make our judgment. However, if we had 1000 persons to examine in a limited time, we might look for an alternative method. Perhaps we would select four teeth, one from each quadrant, and then base our decision regarding the oral cavity on the results of examining those four teeth. In this case we have taken a sample of four teeth from the population of 32 teeth. Our assessment of the oral cavity will be accurate if the teeth we have chosen are the best representatives of teeth in each quadrant. Needless to say, we should be certain to examine the same four teeth of each individual when making our assessment.

A more detailed example may serve to clarify the use of inferential statistical procedures: a graduate student in public health wishes to implement a community-based education program for a group of urban mothers. He finds through the literature that an education program has been offered to a similar group of mothers using an entirely different approach. The student is interested in testing how much the participants in his program learn as compared with the other program. Assume that both groups started with the same knowledge level. The student tests the mothers and compares the mean result of his program with that obtained in the other program. He finds that his group tests higher, but he is not sure if it is such a difference that he can clearly say that his program is better. There is a procedure available called *Student's t-test* that allows the graduate student to compare the mean results from his program with the mean results of the other program. The purpose of using Student's t-test is to determine the probability that the difference between the two means is real and is not a result produced by a chance difference. What this public health student wishes to find is a statistically significant difference between the first mean and the second mean, that is, the mean produced by his program and the mean produced by the other program.

The distinction between statistically significant and practically significant results is important. For example, in the case just discussed, two programs are offered in health education and one is found to produce greater test scores among participants than the other—say 5 points greater. Based on test results, the program of choice is the one producing the greater score. Suppose this program, which produces a 5-point gain, also costs $100 more per participant to produce. In all likelihood a group of decision makers might decide that $100 per participant is too high a price to pay for the "moderate" gain; although the greater test scores were statistically significant and statistically better, the difference between program results was not practically significant. Pragmatic decisions play a much greater role in research than many scientists are willing to admit.

Correlation and inferential statistics

The science of statistics has given us a large number of tests that can be applied to public health data. Only a few of these are discussed in this section. Discussions here center on the chi-square test, the calculation of the coefficient of correlation, and the Student's *t*-test. Each method is best adapted to data of a certain type. An understanding of the tests will guide an individual toward the efficient collection of data that will meet the assumptions of the statistical procedures particularly well.

CHI-SQUARE TEST

The chi-square test is based on the comparison of the observed measurement of a given characteristic and the expected measurement if the sample differs in no way from what is expected by chance. The chi-square statistic (X^2) measures the discrepancy between observed and expected frequencies by adding together all values:

$$\frac{(\text{Observed number} - \text{expected number})^2}{\text{Expected number}}$$

The X^2 test is set up in such a way that the original number of cases entering into each sample becomes part of the calculation and affects interpretation of the answer. Therefore all observations play an equally important role, whether negative or positive. A zero observation is as important as a large positive or large negative value.

Chi-square will equal zero if all comparisons between observed and expected values are zero. The accurate interpretation of X^2 depends on the computation of a figure called the *degrees of freedom (df)*. This figure indicates the number of cells in a two-dimensional grid that can be filled independently without the totals for the problem being incorrect. It is calculated by subtracting 1 from the number of rows (*r*) and 1 from the number of columns (*c*) in the grid and then multiplying these figures together:

$$(r - 1) \times (c - 1) = df$$

After the X^2 value and the degrees of freedom have been calculated, the next step is to use a master table and find the numbers closest

to the value computed for X^2 in the line of the table that represents the figure for degrees of freedom. Having located the number, one then goes to the head of the column and reads the probability of chance occurrence of such a value of X^2.

The following problem illustrates the procedure for calculating the X^2 value. Suppose that we are interested in whether vaccination, apart from whether it has only prophylactic effect, reduces the severity of any actual attack of smallpox. Chi-square could be used to determine whether vaccination has an effect.

First we must discuss several areas illustrated in Table 14-4. To perform X^2 analysis, it must be possible to place each piece of information into only one cell. For instance, an individual who was never vaccinated cannot be placed in both the abundant and the sparse categories. This would cause one person to be counted twice and invalidate the results. Next, expected frequencies must be determined before it is possible to make comparisons with the observed frequencies. The formula for calculating expected frequency follows:

$$eij = \frac{(\text{Tr} \times \text{Tc})}{N}$$

where *e* is the expected frequency of cell *ij*, *Tr* is the total for row *r*, *Tc* is the total for column *c*, and *N* is the total frequency. Table 14-5 provides an example showing the expected frequencies used in Table 14-4 and how they were calculated.

The master table value for X^2 with 2 degrees of freedom is 5.99 at the 5% confidence level. Because our calculated value was 230.17, we have determined that there is a statistically significant difference between what was expected by chance and what actually occurred. Therefore vaccination in this example had a significant effect.

With X^2, we deal with one variable but test its occurrence in a number of different situations. This comparison of categorical-type information is the type of problem for which X^2 is best

Table 14-4. Calculation of chi-square

	Hemorrhagic or confluent	Abundant	Sparse	Row totals
Observed frequencies				
Vaccinated within 10 years of attack	10	150	240	400
Never vaccinated	60	30	10	100
TOTAL	70	180	250	500
Expected frequencies				
Vaccinated within 10 years of attack	56	144	200	400
Never vaccinated	14	36	50	100
TOTAL	70	180	250	500

$$\chi^2 = \frac{(10 - 56)^2}{56} + \frac{(150 - 144)^2}{144} + \frac{(240 - 200)^2}{200} + \frac{(60 - 14)^2}{14} + \frac{(30 - 36)^2}{36} + \frac{(10 - 50)^2}{50}$$

$\chi^2 = 230.17$

$df = (r - 1)(c - 1)$

$df = (2 - 1)(3 - 1)$

$ds = 2$

Table 14-5. Expected frequencies calculated for Table 14-4

	Confluent	Abundant	Sparse	Total
Vaccinated within 10 years of attack	$\frac{(400 \times 70)}{500} = 56$	$\frac{(400 \times 180)}{500} = 144$	$\frac{(400 \times 250)}{500} = 200$	400
Never vaccinated	$\frac{(100 \times 70)}{70} = 14$	$\frac{(100 \times 180)}{180} = 36$	$\frac{(100 \times 250)}{250} = 50$	100
TOTAL	70	180	250 = 500	

suited. Therefore in a sense we are really dealing with two variables, although values for the second variable need not be related to the other in any recognizable pattern.

CORRELATION

Correlation analysis allows us to deal with another common type of problem in which there are two variables, each measuring some different characteristic. Each unit in the data being tested consists of a pair of measurements, and our objective is to determine the strength of the relationship. One measurement in the unit is for the first variable, and one is for the second variable. Correlation is best applied when the number of pairs is very large; the larger the number, the more reliable the re-

sults. The relationship between pairs is easiest to grasp by using what is called a *scatter diagram* (Figs. 14-4 and 14-5).

In Fig. 14-4 there appears to be no relationship between the two variables and no way to predict the value of Y from a value of X. In Fig. 14-5, however, a relation becomes apparent, not perfect but recognizable: as one variable changes, the second variable changes in the same direction.

The measure of the direction and strength of the relationship between two variables is summarized by the correlation coefficient. Fig. 14-4 has a correlation coefficient of 0; Fig. 14-5 has a correlation coefficient of +0.87. A correlation of +1 would mean that all the points in Fig. 14-5 were located exactly on the ascending diago-

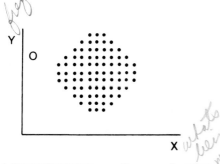

Fig. 14-4. Hypothetical scatter diagram showing correlation coefficients of 0.

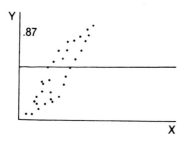

Fig. 14-5. Hypothetical scatter diagram showing correlation coefficients of +0.87.

nal line. Values for X would thus increase as values for Y increased (although the ratio need not be 1:1), and for every possible value of X it would be possible to predict exactly the corresponding value for Y. Inverse or negative correlation would imply a descending line, with values for X decreasing as values for Y increased. If the correlation coefficient were -1, then all points would be located exactly on this descending straight line. The plus or minus sign indicates the direction of the relationship, same or inverse, respectively, whereas the absolute value indicates the strength of the relationship. The closer the coefficient is to 1, the stronger the relationship. Confidence can seldom be given to a correlation coefficient built on less than a dozen pairs of observations unless the correlation is almost perfect, that is, where r approximates either $+1$ or -1. Often 30 cases are used as the recognized minimum

number of pairs, and most researchers believe that using 100 pairs produces stability and confidence in the correlation coefficient.

STUDENT'S *T* TEST

The t statistic is used to compare two means to determine the probability that the difference between means is greater than that expected by chance. Note that if more than two means are to be compared, then another statistical procedure, such as analysis of variance (ANOVA), is indicated, not the t-test. The student is cautioned against performing analyses or accepting results that have more than two means and proceeding to calculate a large series of t-tests with different combinations of means, two at a time. This is blatantly incorrect statistical application, although it may be found in many published articles.

The theoretic distribution for testing statistical significance is Student's t distribution. The t distribution varies. Graphs for t distributions with different degrees of freedom are pictured in Fig. 14-6 in three examples. As the degrees of freedom approach 30, the curve begins to closely approximate the normal curve.

A calculated t value can be positive or negative. The following example helps to clarify the use of the t-test.

	Group 1	Group 2
Number of individuals	10	10
Mean	14.8	8.8
Variance	22.84	25.96
Standard deviation	4.78	5.09

Based on this information, the t-test is the statistic of choice. Assume that the level of significance is 0.05 because no level is specified and after calculation, $t = 2.101$ is produced. One more step remains before the determination can be made about the degree of difference between means: calculation of the degrees of freedom. The number of degrees of freedom is equal to the number of independent scores that

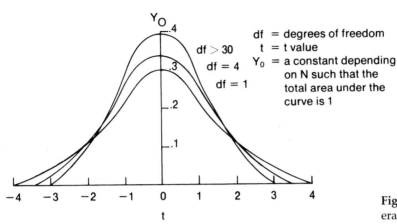

Fig. 14-6. Distribution of *t* for several different degrees of freedom.

are used to estimate a parameter. For the *t*-test the parameter estimated is the standard error. For each sample a standard error is estimated. Thus for most examples with two samples:

$$df = n_1 + n_2 - 2 = 18$$

The previous discussion has dealt primarily (with the exception of the X²) with statistical tests called *parametric tests*. The user of these tests must accept the following two assumptions:

1. Normal distribution. Scores are equally distributed (systematically) around the mean. There are equal numbers of low and high scores, and most scores are found within 3 standard deviations of the group mean.
2. Continuous equal interval measures. A score must be a whole number or a fractional part, that is, 1, 2, 3, 6.9, or 7.1. This is not a situation in which the only possible scores are whole numbers.

One final type of statistical test is nonparametric. Such a test is used in situations where the data clearly does not fit the two assumptions just indicated. These tests have minimal assumptions specific to each test, but generally these assumptions are less rigorous than those for parametric tests.

BIBLIOGRAPHY

Boyer EM: *Basic statistical concepts and techniques applied in dental health*, Des Moines, 1975, University of Iowa.

Darby ML, Bowen DM: *Research methods for oral health professionals: an introduction*, St Louis, 1980, Mosby.

Dunning JM: *Principles of dental public health*, ed 2, Cambridge, Mass, 1975, Harvard University Press.

Emory CW: *Business research methods*, ed 3, Homewood, Ill, 1985, Richard D Irwin.

Hill AB: *Principles of medical statistics*, ed 7, New York, 1961, Oxford University Press.

Richards LE, LaCava JLJ: *Business statistics: why and when*, New York, 1983, McGraw-Hill.

Snedecor GW, Cochran WG: *Statistical methods*, ed 6, Ames, 1971, Iowa State University Press.

CHAPTER 15

Analysis of the dental literature: more accessibility through informatics

Eugene Hittelman

The importance of staying informed

Society has entered the "information age." For the health professional, keeping current is a requirement.[1] The rapid changes in health policy and delivery, the evolving economic pressures and health regulations controlling the practicing provider, and the accumulating standards regarding health care delivery and maintenance, disease prevention, and treatment all require constant vigilance and continual reeducation. The practicing dentist is not only responsible for staying current with the latest techniques and materials but must also evaluate and respond to a constant stream of product advertisements, changes in reimbursement strategies and insurance policies, and modifications in public and professional practice regulations.

Becoming a sophisticated consumer of "information" is not easy; the practitioner must go beyond using "common sense" and assessing the validity and importance of assertions and product statements made in dental journals and at professional meetings, by dental product salespersons, dental researchers, and other practitioners on a "makes sense to me" basis. This challenge requires a critical yet open-minded approach to new information, changing theories, and new ways of thinking. The task is further complicated because science does not yield facts and truths but merely "the best guess we have for the moment." The dentist must be able to search out, gather, and filter relevant information; evaluate the importance and validity of reported findings; and incorporate this new information into existing practice.

On a daily basis, the practitioner is expected to respond, with confidence and knowledge, to questions about the efficacy and dangers of a vast number of medications, dental products, and dental procedures. Patients want to know the success rate of implants ("Will it work for me?" "Are implants safe?"), the dangers of amalgam fillings ("Should I have my fillings removed?" "You know, I saw this program on

TV and . . ."), and the use of antibiotics in the treatment of periodontal disease ("Do I really need surgery? I heard that you can stop the infection with antibiotics and treatments with peroxide and baking soda."). Community leaders want to consult with the local dentist regarding the appropriate use of fluoride in their water supply and the value of fluoride rinses in their school classrooms. They want to know that their constituents will not contract diseases when they visit the dentist for care. The courts and the profession expect the practicing dentist to be current in the requirements of "standards of care" such as when to premedicate a patient, how much radiation is safe, and appropriate infection control. In addition, the dentist must be able to evaluate and perhaps join or recommend managed-care organizations, direct reimbursement programs, and related insurance strategies.

Keeping current is a requirement of modern professional practice. Public health dentistry is dedicated to improving the level of health in the population through appropriate prevention and treatment at the lowest cost to society. The dentist is part of the societal health delivery system and must function both as a participant and a leader.

New information is available in professional newsletters and journals, books, published empirical reports, advertisements, newspapers and popular magazines, and on the Internet.

Everywhere the dentist is confronted with the challenge of accessing, selecting, evaluating, incorporating, and retaining valuable information and of discarding the excess. And this must be done while still providing care and not exhausting the most valuable resource of all: time.

The primary focus of this chapter is on strategies for critically reading and evaluating empiric reports and on the "new" approach to acquiring and productively incorporating professional information called "informatics."

Reading public health research studies
THE GOAL OF RESEARCH

Science is a search for regularities in the universe. It involves a quest for discovering meaningful explanations for events that are encountered daily: disease, health, growth, behaviors, etc. Public health research is one branch of that scientific process in which we attempt to identify relevant causal factors related to dental disease prevalence and to develop strategies for improving the health of the society.[2] The objective of public health research is to recognize, describe and document, and explain variations in health and disease and to develop better strategies for delivering health care to individuals and to society.

Research is a complex activity involving the accurate gathering of data, the appropriate organization of observations, the "correct" interpretation of those findings, and the honest and accurate reporting of those findings to the profession.[3] Research, both applied and basic, involves a systematic process of collecting and organizing observations with the intent of developing accurate descriptions and explanations of interactions between "hosts," their environments, and "pathogens and pathogenic processes" that assail the host, with a goal of understanding health and disease.

Basically, the primary purpose of research is to capture the variance. By this is meant the separation of that portion of variation that is due to chance, measurement error, and outside factors from the systematic variations that can be explained by the variables identified for study.

In public health research two types of research studies are typically found,[4] as shown in Box 15-1. The first type involves documentation. Epidemiologic research serves to identify the rates of disease and health in the population. It is intended to describe the demographic characteristics of the population and

---

Box 15-1

TYPES OF PUBLIC HEALTH RESEARCH

I. Documentation—descriptive research
  A. Epidemiologic research
  B. Descriptive epidemiology
    1. Documenting a population
    2. Census
  C. Risk assessment: correlational studies to identify risk factors for disease
  D. Identifying trends in the population
  E. Product testing: reports on product quality and use
  F. Financial and manpower documentation
II. Hypothesis testing and empiric research
  A. Randomized controlled trials
  B. Field experiments (e.g., original fluoride study)
  C. Laboratory studies (Food and Drug Administration studies)
  D. Program evaluations

Box 15-2

CRITERIA FOR EMPIRIC RESEARCH STUDY

1. It is based on prior research and the existing empirical and theoretical literature:
  It is relevant to current scientific knowledge.
  It is relevant to current clinical and health policy questions.
  It extends previous findings and questions.
2. It is replicable:
  Experimental method is well described.
  Measures used are operationally defined.
  It is manageable in scope.
3. It is based on theory or, at least, on established understandings of phenomenon:
  Data will fit into explanatory schema.
  Measures are derived from clearly defined question.
  It tests or assesses the usefulness of current formulations of the phenomenon studied.
4. It is heuristic:
  Findings lead reader and researcher to ask new and more incisive questions.
  Findings lead to new knowledge or test existing paradigms.
5. It is generalizable:
  Results can be applied to other populations.
  Reader can apply results to his or her own situation.

---

to identify areas of unmet needs and changes in disease prevalence. This documentation may also involve the characterization of properties of dental materials and therapeutics and the availability of dental manpower and may predict future needs of the society. The second type of research involves the testing of theories and hypotheses, the evaluation of the effects of program interventions, and the practical comparison of various strategies and methods of dental treatment and of new medications and dental materials.

REQUIREMENTS OF A RESEARCH STUDY

Beyond asking interesting questions, research should satisfy the five criteria listed in Box 15-2[5]:

1. *It is based on the work of others.* Scientific progress is incremental, each new insight or regularity discovered opens up new questions or takes on meaning within the context of earlier beliefs, findings, and theories. Most research either extends and further clarifies a current scientific paradigm or challenges the current paradigm by opening new approaches for understanding known phenomena.[6] The discovery that caries are transmitted as an infectious disease from the care provider to the child can change strategies of caries prevention with young children. New research studies have the potential of filling in a piece of the puzzle in our search for understanding. However, work that occurs out of context tends, no matter how brilliant, to wither without producing fruit or to lie dormant until the scientific establishment catches up. Before the work on osseointegration

and the use of biocompatible materials such as titanium was performed, dental implant proposals tended to be disregarded and, at times, severely criticized. It is crucial that the research study be set and conceptualized within the growing body of understanding that lead to the proposed study and its findings.

2. *It is replicable.* A well-designed study will describe its methods and variables measured in such a manner that future researchers can repeat or modify the study to observe whether the findings are reproducible. Current trends in clinical research include the use of meta-analysis[7] to aggregate clinical trials and multisite studies; use of reliable and well-defined measurement and experimental design is essential to the building of a body of usable and valid findings.

3. *It is based on theory, or at least on established concerns.* A good theory will guide observations and provide a structure in which to organize and explain the data collected. A theory is an organized explanation of phenomena (data) observed and predictions (hypotheses) of data to be collected. The questions that are asked will determine the answers obtained. Research is not value free; the assumptions of the researcher to a large extent determine what data is gathered and what is discovered. The researcher, in the introduction to the study, should make the assumptions and beliefs clear and accessible to the reader. A theory helps provide the specific questions and determines the variables selected for study.

4. *It is heuristic.* A well-designed and conceptualized study will open the door to future studies. No one study answers all questions; many valuable studies yield more questions than answers. At the conclusion of any research project, the researcher and the readers should be able to ask new and better questions with greater precision and clarity. A study that provides a finding that does not stimulate new exploration and interest is probably not valuable other than to provide specific information

such as the hardness of one material as opposed to another or the setting time of five different cements or the percentage of patients in the target population who require bridgework. Product information is helpful to the practitioner in daily work but does not tend to lead to new knowledge.

5. *It is generalizable.* One test of a good study is whether the findings and the knowledge obtained can be exported into other situations. Generalizability implies that readers can extrapolate findings from the study into predictions for the population. A study of the local high school may not yield much information concerning the health of the children in the city; a case study from one dental office may not provide much information regarding treatment in another. The reader must determine whether what was found will be applicable in the office or community.

READING A RESEARCH STUDY

One form of crucial information is the research study publication. Reports are issued by university scientists, drug companies, governmental agencies (e.g., Food and Drug Administration), and professional organizations. The dentist cannot possibly research or even test all the possible medications, dental techniques, and dental theories that appear but must rely on the professional community. However, studies vary in quality, accuracy, and validity.

The format of a research study

With very little variation, most published research studies adhere to the organization shown in Box 15-3.

Title. The title of the report briefly indicates the topic and focus of the study. The text of the title should contain an indication of the central question posed by the study because many electronic searches scan the title for "key words" indicating the focus of the study.

Abstract. At the beginning of the paper, an abstract of the study is usually provided. By

> **BOX 15-3**
>
> **FORMAT OF A RESEARCH STUDY**
>
>   I. Title of study: topic and focus of study
> II. Abstract
>   A. Research focus
>   B. Method
>   C. Summary of results
>   D. Concluding statement
>   E. Key words
> III. Introduction and literature review
>   A. Importance
>   B. Literature review
>   C. Statement of intent, theory, and hypothesis
> IV. Methods
>   A. Subjects and recruitment strategy
>   B. Measurement strategies and instruments
>   C. Research design
>   D. Method for statistical analysis
>   V. Results
> VI. Discussion
>   A. Review and summary of results
>   B. Discussion of results and comparison to theoretic presentation or hypotheses
> VII. Summary and conclusion
> VIII. Bibliography and references

Introduction and literature review. In the introduction the researcher attempts to provide a background to the problem or question. Past controversies will be summarized, key studies will be mentioned, and the questions considered in the study clarified. The goal of this introduction is to prepare the reader to read the study. It is the obligation of the researcher to review for the reader the key questions and primary importance of the problem, to make the reader aware of relevant past research, to define key issues and terms, and to create a context for the current study so that the reader can intelligently follow the argument.

The introduction will also frequently develop a theoretic framework for the current study, present the hypothesis (developed from the theory) in terms of expected outcomes, and state the importance of the study for current practice or research.

Methods section. The methods section is the heart of any research paper. For this reason I will return later to a more detailed discussion of the key elements involved.

In the methods section the reader is provided with specific and operational information about how the study was conducted. From the descriptions offered in this section, the reader should be able to replicate the study. Often the reader may be tempted to skip this section (and possibly the results section) and go on to the discussion section and the conclusion. However, it is in this section and the one that follows that the reader is able to develop a clear understanding of the actual outcomes (in terms of what really was measured and observed) and the meaning of the results and to verify the legitimacy of the conclusions. Although the researcher may be tempted to extend the assertions beyond those of the actual findings, the reader can reintroduce reality by carefully examining the study method.

The methods section should include four subsections. The *sampling strategy*[8] is a description of the population being sampled, the sam-

scanning this abstract, busy dentists can quickly determine whether the study is relevant to their interests. This abstract will include a brief summary of the research focus and importance of the topic, identification of the population sampled or objects of study, and a brief statement of the experimental strategy. This will be followed by a summary of the findings and a concluding statement. The abstract may also list key words that allow the study to be entered into the database of the discipline involved. Often the abstract is also published in one or more databases so that individuals can screen studies for those they wish to read.

pling method, and the method of assigning subjects to conditions. Readers will want to assess whether the population (or sampling frame) is appropriate for their concerns (external validity). In experimental studies readers will want to know whether the study is being conducted in vivo (in human or animals) or in vitro (in a simulated environment, on extracted teeth, or in a test tube). Readers will want to assess whether the sampling strategy or the experimental assignment introduces bias into the study and clouds the results. The reader also should be informed of the sample size, the selection criteria (rules for accepting, rejecting, and discarding subjects or samples), and the experimental setting.

The *measurement strategies and measurement scales* should be described.[9] Although the question and variables involved will have been described in the introduction and discussed in the results and discussions sections, each variable is operationally defined by its measurement. It is important for the reader to carefully examine the measurement strategies and actual measurements involved. For example, it is quite different if the level of periodontal disease is quantified by assessing actual loss of attachment and bone loss or by an indicator such as an assessment of the level of inflammation and gingival bleeding. Compliance can mean regular taking of medications, sitting still in the dental chair, keeping an appointment, or any of a myriad of other indicators. A careful reader will recognize that the measurement itself serves as the only actual definition; all other assertions are conjecture and must be validated. Validity of a measure is the degree to which the measure can be demonstrated to actually assess the (theoretic) variable in question.

Second, the reader will want to be assured that the measurement scale used supports (contains enough information) the descriptive and inferential statistical procedures used. Reporting, for example, ordinal data with means

and standard deviations adds a precision to the findings that did not exist in the measurement.

Finally, the experimenter should report strategies for ensuring the reliability of the measures taken. If observers or judges are used, the calibration method should be described. If normed instruments or standardized instruments are used, they should be documented and prior use of them in the literature noted. If the study is using uniquely or newly developed measures, these measures should be validated and standardized.

A description of the experimental study design should be provided. The experimenter should describe operationally the experimental study design in a step-by-step sequence. The description must be detailed enough so that the reader could replicate the study. As will be discussed later, readers, before reviewing the results, should try to predict the outcome using their own expectations and experiences.

The experimental conditions of the experiment, the experimental or assigned groupings of the subjects, and the strategies for controlling for alternative explanations (controls) should all be carefully explained. It is helpful if the experimenter can use conditions or measures that are consistent with those reported in prior studies so that results can be compared and combined. This is especially important when the research project is a randomized clinical trial that, for practical reasons, cannot include a large number of subjects.

Finally, *the proposed statistical analysis strategy should be presented.* The researcher should describe the proposed strategy for evaluating, quantifying, and analyzing results. In this discussion the researcher should state the effect size being considered, the level of statistical significance that will be acceptable, and the strategy for statistically evaluating the data.

Results section. In the results section the experimenter will present a descriptive and inferential statistical review of the outcomes from the study. At this point the findings should not be interpreted but instead presented as clearly and descriptively as possible. The experimenter will summarize the findings in tables, charts, or graphs where appropriate and will provide a narrative that reviews the descriptive and inferential statistical analysis. All descriptive statistics should include the number of subjects and observations made as well as summary statistics (measures of central tendency, range, frequency, and correlation).

The experimenter will usually begin with demographic data and descriptive statistics that directly relate to the questions presented in the introduction and to the actual measurements of the dependent variables. Then the experimenter will present a statistical analysis of the data, including a statement regarding the statistical significance of the findings. After the presentation of this basic information, the experimenter may continue with additional observations and findings that were not originally anticipated but were discovered in the data. This "post hoc" analysis may often be as important to future research as the initial findings of the study. A mark of a skilled and intuitive researcher and reader is the ability to be "surprised" by unexpected findings.

Discussion and interpretation of the results. Having clearly presented the outcome of the research in objective terms, the experimenter will then attempt to interpret and explain these results. In this section the researcher has more latitude to play with the data and to make sense of the findings. The reader can, by reviewing the measurement strategies and the experimental design, decide whether this interpretation and extension of the actual findings is justified.

The first step in this discussion is usually to return to the hypothesis, or, in the case of descriptive epidemiologic studies or product documentation, the assumptions and questions that elicited the study, and evaluate the results in terms of the expected outcomes. Although statistical analysis of observations is a consid-

eration, questions of the effects of the methods involved in gathering data and interpreting observations are far more critical. Statistical significance, which has currently taken on an importance of almost religious significance, is actually less important than developing an understanding of what has been observed. Because research never actually proves the correctness or falseness of a theory or hypothesis, the researcher will instead discuss the level of statistical support for the theory and compare the findings with those discussed in the introduction. If the study is a demographic or epidemiologic study, the report will estimate the health status and characteristics of the populations studied. If the study is experimental, the discussion will focus on the ability of the experimental formulation to efficiently answer the questions asked in the introduction.

The second step of the discussion involves explaining unexpected negative or positive findings. The researcher will describe additional observations from the study that will help the reader understand the study outcome (the reader might be reminded of the "lab notebook" for recording incidental observations and data that was required in college science classes). Perhaps the subjects did not comply with the experimental conditions (noncompliance with medication regimens or the missing of appointments). Perhaps the study was contaminated by outside events. The discussion section provides the researcher an opportunity to have a dialog with the reader and propose alternative ways of conceptualizing the results and for developing strategies for continuing or redesigning the study.

Summary and conclusions. In this section the researcher asserts the importance and the interpretations of the study results. Often the researcher will feel it necessary to editorialize or go beyond the data by using the analysis presented in the discussion as a basis. It is tempting, when trying to read a large number of studies to get a handle on a topic or to decide whether to use a product or to determine whether to support a proposal, to read only the introduction and the conclusion. However, without the methods and the results section, it is very easy to be misled and to accept findings that are speculative at best. The reader may draw very different conclusions from the data. However, it is the conclusions that appear in the product brochures, the popular press, and the summary reports. It is the professional's obligation to independently critically evaluate the conclusion and to be prepared to educate patients and fellow professionals and to engage in a dialog with the scientist.

Bibliography and references. The researcher should provide accurate primary references for the introduction and assertions. These references can be valuable for the reader who wishes to pursue the problems further

and to learn more. Also, the references allow the reader to go back and review the actual studies in cases where the reader feels that the researcher may have misinterpreted or misread prior studies.

A strategy for reading a research study critically
SELECTING THE STUDY[10]

The issue of selecting what to read among the massive amounts of information available is often quite challenging (Box 15-4). The reader must first decide on the level of information desired. Sources containing information regarding recent research and related topics can be classified into three levels.

General sources often provide the first indication to the private practitioner that some new

---

Box 15-4

ISSUES TO CONSIDER WHEN SELECTING A STUDY

I. Type of resource source
  A. General sources
    1. Material intended for the general public
    2. Newspaper articles (including topical articles: science or health section)
    3. Popular magazines
    4. Television or radio reports
    5. Popular science book (popularized report)
  B. Secondary sources
    1. Scientific reviews and educational texts
    2. Textbooks intended for specialist or generalists
    3. Review articles in professional and scientific journals
    4. Dedicated journal issues, monographs, and audiovisual reports
  C. Primary sources
    1. Scientific reports of specific experiments
    2. Journals from commercial publishers (e.g., throwaways, free journals for advertising, publications from pharmaceutical houses)
    3. Journals published by scientific publishers
    4. Journals sponsored and published by professional organizations
    5. Journals sponsored and published by learned societies (e.g., International Association for Dental Research
II. Editorial policy and editorial board
  A. Solicited articles reviewed by an editor but not peer reviewed
  B. Refereed or peer-reviewed articles
  C. Reputation of publication: *Ullrich's Index of Periodicals*
    1. Citation reputation
    2. Quality of editorial board
    3. Timeliness of publications (time to publication from submission)

information is available. These sources include newspaper articles (a good example might be the Tuesday *Science* section of the *New York Times*), magazine articles, television special programs, popular books, and news reports. Often these reports signal an important issue or new procedure. The practitioner will want to follow up with more scientific sources to separate the journalistic interpretation from the facts. Often a new cure or innovation is still a promise or speculation, and the practitioner will want to be able to clarify the issue for patients.

Secondary sources include textbooks, review articles in which the topic is summarized and a large number of studies reviewed, and topical issues (for example, *Dental Clinics of North America* publishes review articles in a dedicated issue of the journal). The major problem with secondary sources is that they tend to be several years behind the scientific findings and trends. As will be seen below, the turnaround time from research to professional publication in a primary source (after the research is completed and written up) is seldom less than 9 months. The preparation and publication of the secondary sources is usually another year. Secondary sources provide background and a reasoned discussion of topics, but they are unable to catch the "breaking wave" of new findings. A second problem with the secondary source is that it tends to be selective and interpretative. The reader is separated from the actual study as it was conducted and must rely on the author for interpretation, selection of important issues, and guidance. The major value of the secondary source is its ability to organize the information and guide the reader to the primary sources of information.

Primary sources consist of journal articles, conference reports, and published abstracts (including reports that appear on the Internet and in websites). In this media the researcher directly reports studies, the methods used, and the results. There are several levels of scientific rigor and objectivity in primary sources. Jour-

nals are published by four groups. Scientific societies such as the International Association for Dental Research, the American Association for Public Health, and the American Association of Dental Schools publish scientific research in their interest areas. These studies tend to represent current issues and concerns of the society. Professional organizations such as the American Association of Public Health Dentistry, the American Dental Association, and the American Medical Association also publish primary research journals. Scientific publishers such as Mosby–Year Book publish journals for the profession. These journals typically focus on speciality areas and provide publishing outlets for study groups and specialty groups in the profession. Commercial publishers and groups such as pharmaceutical houses and dental material groups publish articles for the profession. Many of these journals, which include the "throwaway" journals that contain targeted advertising, provide opinion pieces and case studies of product usage.

Most well-regarded and trusted journals use peer review[11] to ensure the scientific merit and objectivity of their publications. For these journals, the editor, after screening the articles submitted for relevance and importance, sends those articles with the identifying information (author's name and institution) removed to several referees who have been selected for their expertise in the subject area. These referees are asked to determine if (1) the paper is relevant and interesting, (2) the paper adheres to appropriate and ethical scientific methods, and (3) the paper meets the standards of the journal. They are also asked to give the article a priority score. The editor then decides whether to (1) accept the article outright, (2) accept the article with suggested revisions, (3) reject the article but suggest revisions that the author can make and then resubmit the paper, or (4) reject the article outright. This process may take up to a year to complete. Rejection rates for the better journals may reach 75% of the articles submitted.

In selecting the article, the reader will want to determine if the article is peer reviewed. The reader can consult *Ullrich's Index of Periodicals* to determine the reputation of the journal and its peer review policies. The reader should also consult the journal in question (typically the journal lists its reviewers and editorial board members on the title page) to determine its editorial board and their qualifications. Finally, most journals provide a statement regarding the sponsorship of their journal and their policies regarding acceptance and screening of new articles.

A STRATEGY FOR READING A RESEARCH ARTICLE

Box 15-5 lists the suggested steps for critically reviewing a study.

Read the methodology section first. After selecting a study to read, the reader will probably gain the most from a research study by turning to the methods section before reading the introduction and literature review. The credibility of any study resides in the method for gathering data and the actual study design.

The reader should begin by assessing the *validity* of the study (Box 15-6). By reviewing the

---

Box 15-5

Suggested Steps for Critically Reviewing a Study

1. Select a study for review by reading abstract.
2. Carefully read the methods section first.
   a. Assess the external validity of the study.
      - Is the subject or sample selection appropriate?
      - Are the experimental conditions relevant to your concern?
   b. Is the measurement strategy appropriate?
      - Are the measures valid, reliable, sensitive, and specific?
      - Are the variables actually measured related to your concerns?
   c. Is the research strategy appropriate?
      - Is the "right question" being asked?
      - Are there adequate controls for alternate explanations?
      - Is the study ethical and appropriate?
   d. Is the statistical approach appropriate for the measures used and for analyzing the data?
3. Read the results section next.
   a. Before reading the results predict what you expect should happen given the method.
   b. Review the results.
      - Are any questions or measures from the method neglected?
      - Are the results reflective of the study method?
      - Are the statistical analyses appropriate and reflective of the methods?
      - Are the tables and graphs accurate?
   c. Compare your predictions with the actual results.
4. Read the discussion section next.
   a. Before reading the discussion, try to explain the results from your own knowledge.
   b. Compare your explanations with those of the experimenter.
   c. Assess whether the discussion follows from the results.
5. Read the introduction and literature review.
   a. Is the theory, hypothesis, or focus satisfied by the study?
   b. Compare your theory with that of the experimenter.
   c. Identify those areas in which you were surprised.
6. Read the summary and conclusion.
   a. Are the conclusions appropriate?
   b. What questions are left unanswered?
7. Review the bibliography for sources that you can follow up to learn more.

method the reader can determine what is actually being studied instead of being told what is supposed to be the target of investigation.

Validity refers to whether the questions asked by the study are answered by the method. There are two kinds of validity: external validity and internal validity. External validity refers to the generalizability of the study findings to the real world. When an experi-

---

Box 15-6

Validity and Reliability

I. External validity
   A. Sampling
      1. Is the sample representative of the population?
      2. Is the sample large enough to reduce sampling error?
      3. Does the sample capture all the subgroups in the population?
   B. Methodology
      1. Are the experimental conditions representative of the real world?
      2. Can the results be generalized to the target population?
      3. Are the results applicable to other populations?
II. Internal validity
   A. Methodology
      1. Does the method control for alternative explanations of the results?
      2. Does the method allow for alternative outcomes?
   B. Measurement
      1. Are the variables, as defined by the measurement strategy, appropriate for the question?
      2. Are the measurement scales used appropriate for the measure?
III. Reliability of measurement
      1. Are the measures described objectively so they can be replicated?
      2. Are examiners' techniques calibrated?
      3. Are measurement instruments standardized?

---

mental sample—either subjects or materials—is selected, is the sample representative of the target population or materials under consideration? Are the experimental conditions similar enough to actual conditions to make the study a test of regularities in the world of interest to the dentist? To determine the external validity, the reader will want to examine the subject recruitment strategy. If individuals are the target, did the research use a random sample, a stratified random sample, a convenience sample, or a targeted sample? If the experimental samples are materials, tissue samples, or devices, were they selected in such a way that they would be similar to those the dentist must confront? And are the experimental conditions representative of actual conditions that exist in treatment or the community?

Internal validity relates to whether the study is designed to answer the questions asked. Is the study designed so that it captures relevant variance and excludes important alternative explanations or distinguishes itself from explanations from other possible formulations of the problem?

A number of issues are raised by considerations of internal validity. The first issue is that of appropriate controls for alternative conditions. Most clinical research and field research studies will apply the principles of quasi-experimental design to control for built in-bias. The basic principle of study design is the building in of controls to either randomize (statistically control) or eliminate contaminating or confounding sources of variance. For example, typically both subjects and experimenters are, when possible, kept blind to condition so as to eliminate subject bias (or placebo effects) and experimenter bias. Because subjects assigned to conditions are not all the same, it is customary to randomize subjects to condition so as to eliminate subject differences and minimize preexperimental group differences. Where it is difficult to distinguish the process or effects of doing the experiment (for example, the giving of an injection may confound the effects of what is in the injection), a control group that is given a sham intervention is also included.

A second issue relates to the validity of the variables used. A variable is any target observation or condition that can take on more than one value (be measured systematically). In most studies a set of independent variables and a set of dependent variables are selected for study. An independent variable consists of a set of conditions or characteristics that are controlled (either by assignment or statistically) by the researcher. Thus the researcher may divide up the sample into "tall" and "short" individuals. The study may consider two different strategies of restoring a tooth. The dependent variables are those the researcher will measure as outcomes of the independent variable. Thus bone density in "tall" and "short" individuals or "recurrent decay" after two different strategies of restoring a tooth might be assessed. The researcher might include one or more intervening variables. An intervening variable is similar to an independent variable in that it is controlled and creates subconditions of the independent variable. Thus the "tall" and "short" individuals might be selected from groups of "over 40" individuals and "20- to 25-year-old individuals." Because the measurement defines the actual variable, the reader will want to determine whether the measured variable really is a valid estimate of the desired phenomena.

There are several ways to establish validity.[12] Box 15-7 lists five types of validity. Face validity implies that the measure is, by its very measurement characteristics (on its face value) valid. For example, if the experimenter wants to see how fast a subject can run 100 yards and times the subject running 100 yards, it would be hard to question the validity of the measure. Concurrent validity involves demonstrating that the measurement provides the same values as some measure that has already been established as valid (comparison to a standardized

---

BOX 15-7

TYPES OF VALIDITY

Face Validity
Measure is obviously valid because its definition is its measurement

Concurrent Validity
Results of measurement are consistent with those of established measures

Predictive Validity
Predictions of measure are consistent with actual outcomes

Content Validity
Measurement contains aspects of the variable (information) that is being measured

Construct Validity
Measurement is derived from theory related to the measure

---

test). For example, if a diagnosis using three signs and symptoms is able to provide the same result as an established diagnostic protocol, the new diagnostic strategy would be accepted as having concurrent validity. A third type of validity is predictive validity. If a measure (e.g., a stress test) has been shown to predict accurately the probability of a cardiac episode, it would be considered a valid measure of cardiac susceptibility. Content validity is based on the appropriateness or representativeness of the measures selected to the actual phenomenon. For example, an examination must include the topics studied. Finally, construct validity implies that the measure is consistent with the theoretic formulation it is testing. An aptitude test based on the expected tasks the subject is to perform would be an example. The reader, before accepting the researcher's approach, must evaluate the validity of the measurements used to collect the data.

A third issue, although not directly a validity issue, is the sensitivity and specificity of the measurement strategy. Sensitivity is defined as the number of true positives divided by the total number of potential positive findings (true positives and false negatives) in the sample. In other words, the reader will want to know how capable the measure is of detecting the target variable or changes in the target variable (e.g., tooth decay). Specificity is defined by the number of true negative results divided by the total number of false positive plus true negative results in the sample. In other words, the reader will want to know how capable the measure is of discriminating between true and false positive results in the sample. If the measure is too sensitive (and lacks specificity), the experimenter will tend to overestimate prevalence or the presence of the dependent target variable (effects) in the sample. If the measure is too specific (and lacks sensitivity), the experimenter will tend to underestimate prevalence or presence (effects) of the dependent target variable.

Validity and reliability are not the only issues to be considered when the methods section is reviewed. A second issue relates to the amount of variance being captured by the study. The effort of the study will be to explain the source of the variations in the dependent variable. The sources of variation in the dependent variable will include error of measurement, individual differences in the subjects, random variations caused by subject selection, other outside factors, and the influence of the independent (and possibly the intervening) variables.

The captured variance—that percentage or portion of the total variation (variance) in the dependent variable explained by the experimental conditions (differences in the independent variable)—is called the *effect size*. When reading the study the reader will want to know the amount of variance being explained or the effect size, for several reasons. If the effect size is very small, the differences or effects discovered may have no meaning in the world of the practicing dentist.

Sample size is also critical. If the sample size is too small to provide enough *power* (the ability of the study to detect a difference if one exists) to test the hypothesis, the dentist may miss an important finding.[13] For example, a dentist reviews a randomized control trial that has compared a generic medication with a brand-name licensed and accepted medication. If the study is too powerful and detects a clinically insignificant but statistically significant difference, the dentist may be unwilling to prescribe the generic drug (leading to higher costs to the patient unnecessarily); if the study lacks sufficient power, an important difference between the generic and the brand-name drug might be missed.

Power is determined by (1) the desired effect size, (2) the sample size, and (3) the level of statistical significance selected. Effect size can be increased by increasing the precision of measurement (reducing error of measurement) or by increasing the influence of the independent variable. The larger the sample size, the greater the power (the lower the probability of a false-negative finding). Finally, reducing the criteria for statistical significance (increasing the level of chance tolerated) decreases the probability of accepting the null hypothesis when it is, in fact, incorrect (lowering type II error).

A third issue involves the research design itself.[14] Often the study design forces the outcome by eliminating alternative possibilities or it asks the wrong question in assessing the usefulness of a theoretic construct. It is also possible the results obtained are due to phenomena independent of those included in the theory (individuals may brush more often because they were asked how often they brushed and not because they were given oral health instruction). A related issue is the possibility that the findings are trivial in that they do not reveal new information or unexpected results.

Read the results section second. One way the reader can test the informativeness or usefulness of the study is by predicting the results before going to the results section. If the reader, especially one who does not use the theoretic structure and hypotheses from the introductory section but merely applies personal experience, can predict the results with some accuracy, the existing knowledge and experience may make this study unnecessary or irrelevant.

Readers might then go back to the introduction and compare the experimental predictions with the findings of the study and their predictions made from reading the methods section.

Critically review the discussion section. After predicting the results and comparing their predictions with the actual study findings, readers can further assess the study by developing an explanation for the results obtained and comparing that explanation with that offered by the researcher. Readers might wish to develop an alternative hypothesis or theory that accounts for the results and compare that with the theory suggested in the introduction. If the explanations differ, perhaps a new study should be developed to test the two formulations.

Read the introduction, the literature review, and the conclusions. At this point, readers are able to assess the value, validity, and contribution of the study. They can decide whether to purchase or recommend the medication, use the method, or purchase the equipment. They may decide to explore further, using the bibliography as a source to develop a new study which can clarify, extend, or contradict what went before.

Accessing and exploring informational sources

Immediate and comprehensive access to scientific and professional literature is an unfulfilled dream of most professionals. In fact, the task of finding and digesting the information needed for intelligent practice is becoming increasingly difficult. The amount of professional communication is massive and beyond the scope of the individual.[15]

The professional must monitor six types of information:

1. *Scientific information:* Current findings regarding the etiology of disease, methods of preventing or curing disease, and strategies for maintaining individual and public health.

2. *Product and treatment modality effectiveness:* The latest findings on materials, therapeutic devices, and medications. The dentist will want to know what is available, what is acceptable, and what has been found to be ineffective.

3. *Laws, regulations, and standards:* The dentist will want to be current in infection control, waste management, and standards of care.

4. *Economic issues:* Currently, managed care and insurance strategies are changing rapidly. The American Dental Association is actively involved in developing strategies to maintain the individual dentist's economic viability, to protect patients' interests, and to respond to the need to control the cost of care.

5. *Political and social issues:* Society is constantly involved in a political process related to public health issues. Currently, the dentist must be up to date on issues related to fluoridation, mercury, and infection control. Tomorrow's issue is waiting.

6. *Local and national epidemiologic findings and current trends in dental care.* The trends in the health of the public are directly related to the cost of care, public health planning, and the distribution of providers. Ten years ago society was worried that there would not be enough dentists to provide care to a growing population; today, the elderly population is growing and the types of care needed are changing.

DENTAL INFORMATICS
How can the dentist stay current with this onslaught?

Originally, the practicing dentist relied on a combination of continuing education, reading journals, communications from supply houses and sales personal, belonging to a variety of professional societies (meetings, conferences, and newsletters), personal communications, and the popular press. Many practitioners continue to rely on these sources. However, the information explosion and the speed of change quickly makes current information outdated. A new possibility has developed over the past 10 years, and increasingly private dentists, dental educators, and public health officials have begun to access the electronic media. The rapid proliferation of an international network for the rapid access and interchange of information in electronic format will change the way care is provided. Computer-based dental records that are coupled with knowledge bases developed in cooperation by academics, educators, researchers, and practitioners can provide the source for decision-based dental diagnosis and treatment. Dentists will be able to move to evidence-based practice based on professional consensus.

The Internet[16] is a worldwide network of computer sites that maintain communications based on the TCP/IP (transmission control protocol/Internet protocol). This system supports E-mail (electronic communications), file transfers (FTP [file transfer protocol], a system for transmitting documents electronically), and interactive connections. This network is a collection of local, regional, national, and international networks that can be accessed by the individual dentist working in the office or home, by means of a "gateway." This gateway allows the practitioner to communicate, collaborate, share resources, and access information.

Many practitioners now use electronic claims submissions[17] to file insurance claims. Electronic Data Interchange (EDI) protocol uses a standardized, structured data format that allows direct compatibility between users. It is used for submitting claims information, claims payment requests, and insurance communications. This movement toward electronic claims submission with a standard format allows the rapid assimilation of usable and accurate data for local, state, and national health planning. Computer-based dental records coupled with knowledge bases developed cooperatively by dental organizations, academics, and dental educators can provide an improved source for diagnosis and treatment planning at the provider level and support the growth of accurate and fair quality assurance. With electronic exchange dentists can participant in informational links with other dentists, insurers, dental associations, academics, biomedical libraries, and public health planners.

The inclusion of E-mail and Telnet connections allows the provider the opportunity to consult and work with speciality centers and dental researchers. It has become possible to share information regarding patient characteristics, disease patterns, new clinical findings, and economic changes throughout the professional community.

Informational search

Schools and organizations maintain national networks that connect directly to the Internet. Some important web sites are listed in Box 15-8. An increasing number of continuing education programs are available to the practitioner through these connections. Currently the American Dental Association, through its web page, offers on-line continuing education programs. Many dental schools now have web pages with hyperlink capability that allow practitioners to access documents, new studies, and audiovisual, on-line courses.

With a variety of "browsers" (software systems that can search throughout the Internet system) and "hypertext" (the ability to "click" on a word or phrase and be connected to other documents at other sites that the word or phrase "pointed to") connections between websites, the individual can explore and capture (download) a worldwide range of relevant documents.

Original organized collections of scientific materials indexed for ready access are called libraries. Searchable, online versions of these libraries, called digital libraries, now exist.

Box 15-8

IMPORTANT WEBSITES

http://www.ada.org	American Dental Association:
	News
	Practice and profession: includes important legislation
	Continuing education multimedia units
	Products and services
	Consumer information
http://www.sciencemag.org	Science magazine
http://www.iadr.com	International Association for Dental Research
http://www.aads.jhu.edu	American Association of Dental Schools
http://indy.radiology.uiowa.edu	Academy of General Dentistry
http://www.sci.lib.uci.edu/HSG/Dental.html	Martindale's Health Service Guide: web page that through hyperlinks leads to variety of dental journals, dental newsletters, and dental resources; includes "Virtual Dental Center"
http://www.cdc.gov/cdc.html	Centers for Disease Control and Prevention: variety of reports on demographic patterns of disease prevalence plus number of studies
http://www.nature.com	Nature Magazine: table of contents and brief reviews
http://thomas.loc.gov	Up-to-date bulletins on current national legislation before Congress
http://www.elibrary.com	Electric Library: a good source for medical informatics; search engine for finding topical information

---

They allow the searching of electronic collections distributed across many physical sites. With the Internet, literature search is directly accessible by all. The first stage of this process involved the collection of literature indexed as a bibliographic source (title, author, journal, and key words). This database was made available electronically. The first major medical index made available over the networks was MEDLINE (National Library of Medicine). The individual lists, much as one might use a card catalog, the desired terms and the computer compiles a list of available articles, journals, and books. With a Boolean algebra of logical "AND," "OR," and "NOT" statements, the dentist is able to develop a topic search that identifies articles appropriate to his or her interest. However, this process, with the advent of faster hardware and better software, has been expanded to include multimedia documents and distributed browsing (multiple collections stored in physically distributed localities are experienced as a single logically connected coherent collection). Documents are linked through hyperlink so that "search engines" can explore a universe of knowledge in a very short time. It is now possible to access and review a tremendous range of current information without becoming overwhelmed.

The dentist can also join "chat groups" (electronically connected like-minded individuals who can "discuss" topics of mutual interest) and be listed through a "LISTSERV" (a subscription list for E-mail distributed electronically) for immediate notification of important bulletins. The Internet, through the World Wide Web, allows the dentist to visit web pages (informational page bulletin boards with hyperlink) developed by professional organizations to further serve their members. (A list of important web page addresses can be found in Box 15-8.) For example, the American Dental Association online web page (http://www.ada.org) provides current news bulletins, lists of products and services with the American Dental Association seal of acceptance, consumer information, and practice and professional education and career information. This information can include not only textual information but also brief video tapes and multimedia materials that can be accessed in the office on the office computer monitor.

Even journals have moved to electronic editions. Journals such as *Nature* and *Science* have electronic editions that supply tables of contents, abstracts, and indexes of recent editions. A number of commercial publishers now have online abstract and index services.

A final note

With the advent of informatics, the Internet, and the move to decision-based treatment, the practicing dentist can no longer afford to hide in the dental office and hope to survive as a professional. As the government moves to guarantee health care of all citizens at a reasonable price, as the middleman participation of third-party insurers grows, and as quality assurance becomes part of all health delivery, the dentist becomes a member of the public health team. The dentist must stay current to survive. The resources are available but can be overwhelming. Just as is required in all good research, it is important to begin with an informed question and to search for answers within the context of current knowledge. Using electronic data exchange protocols and the current resources for computer-based record keeping, the individual provider becomes a contributor and consumer of a modern public health care delivery system that can be based on an economically sound footing and be professionally and ethically acceptable to any professional practitioner.

REFERENCES

1. Preston J: The practice of dentistry, year 2005: a vision, *J Dent Educ* 60(1):68-78, 1996.
2. Grembowski D: The role of health services research in the renaissance of the dental profession, *J Dent Educ* 61(1):10-15, 1997.
3. Emling R: Understanding laboratory and clinical research: an overview, *J Clin Dent* 6(3):157-160, 1995.
4. Ahlbom A, Norell S: *Introduction to modern epidemiology,* Chestnut Hill, Mass, 1990, Epidemiology Resources.
5. Hulley S, Cummings S: *Designing clinical research,* Baltimore, 1988, Williams & Wilkins.
6. Kuhn T: *The structure of scientific revolutions,* ed 2, *Foundations of the unity of science,* vol 2, no 2 Chicago, 1970, University of Chicago.
7. Oxman A, Guyatt G: The science of reviewing research, *Ann N Y Acad Sci* 703:125-134, 1993.
8. Atchison K: Understanding and utilizing qualitative research, *J Dent Educ* 60(8):716-720, 1996.
9. Haynes RB: Some problems in applying evidence in clinical practice, *Ann N Y Acad Sci* 703:210-224, 1993.
10. Kassirer J: Dissemination of medical information: a journal's role. *Ann N Y Acad Sci* 703:173-179, 1993.
11. Brunette DM: *Critical thinking: understanding and evaluating dental research,* Chicago, 1996 Quintessence.
12. Salkind N: Exploring research, New York, 1991, Macmillan.
13. Sackett D, Cook D: Can we learn anything from small trials? *Ann N Y Acad Sci* 703:25-31, 1993.
14. Brook R: Using scientific information to improve the quality of health care, *Ann N Y Acad Sci* 703:74-84, 1993.
15. Altman L: Bringing the news to the public: the role of the media, *Ann N Y Acad Sci* 703:200-208, 1993.
16. Zimmerman J: The electronic window to the world, *J Dent Educ* 60(1):33-40, 1996.
17. Narcisi J: The American Dental Association's committment to electronic data interchange, *J Dent Educ* 60(1):28-32, 1996.

SECTION V

Ethics and the law in community dental health

CHAPTER 16

Ethical issues in community dental health

Muriel J. Bebeau
Jeffrey P. Kahn

What does it mean to become a professional?

Have you been chosen by members of the dental or dental hygiene profession to become a dental professional? If so, those in the profession are telling you that they want to give you the opportunity to become their colleague. Have you thought about what it means to become a member of the dental profession? Are you aware of what distinguishes a dentist or dental hygienist from persons in other occupations or professions? Do you know what is expected of you as a student of the profession and as a future professional?

This chapter will begin by describing the attributes of a profession and the implications for persons who wish to become a member of the dental profession. We will describe the general moral obligations of the dental professional and then turn our attention to ethical issues that arise in community dental health. We will provide a brief discussion of the principles of biomedical ethics that apply to cases that arise in community dental health before presenting some cases to think about. We suggest that you read and discuss the cases with others before

you read our analyses of them. Our hope is that this chapter will help you think more clearly about some of the problems you are likely to encounter in your professional life. In particular, we hope this chapter will help you to think more clearly about responsibilities that extend beyond those you have to the individuals you will serve—responsibilities to the larger society. We hasten to add that we do not envision a set of professional responsibilities that are limitless. Rather, we hope to engage you in examining the nature of responsibility to others, to engage you in thinking about the limits of obligation, and to help you consider strategies that will effectively meet the profession's responsibilities to prevent disease and promote the nation's oral health.

CHARACTERISTICS OF A PROFESSION

What distinguishes a profession from some other occupation? Are there characteristics that distinguish among occupations in ways which suggest that some really are held to a higher ethical standard than others? Sociologists[1] list as many as six attributes that emerge as an occupation becomes professionalized. Briefly, an occupation is given *authority* (i.e., to make judgments on behalf of clients or patients, to determine the standard of practice, to set standards for admission to professional school and standards for accreditation of professional schools, to self-govern, etc.) in proportion to the amount and stability of the *knowledge* it takes to gain access to the profession and in direct proportion to the amount of harm potentially caused by incompetent practice. *Power and privilege* are awarded in exchange for the profession's *promise* to place the rights of the client over self-interest and the rights of the society over the rights of the profession. To guide members of the profession in application of the promise, *codes of ethics* are developed. The canons of a code provide guidance to appropriate behavior in various circumstances and enable the profession to monitor itself. Codes are expanded as new issues emerge or as views of professional morality change. Professions value the powers and privileges granted by society and, through *social organization,* strive to maintain them.

Professions emerge over time, usually as a result of scientific advancement. Dentistry, for example, emerged and became more formalized in direct response to social conditions and scientific advances. In the mid-1800s some dentists made overstated claims about the benefits of treatment. The efforts to organize dentistry were based on a desire to protect the public from unscrupulous practitioners whose practices were not based on the latest scientific knowledge. The prohibitions against advertising—traced to codes of ethics developed by barristers in medieval England—were a direct effort on the part of the profession to control outrageous advertising practices and thereby make the profession more trustworthy. There are positive and negative outcomes of the professionalization process. Let's consider what might be referred to as the paradox of professionalism in contemporary society. On the one hand, professionalization and organization en-

able standard setting that protects the public—a positive outcome. On the other hand, professionalization creates a kind of monopoly that tends to increase costs and reduce access to care—a negative outcome. The challenge for any profession is to maintain a balance between these positive and negative outcomes. Failure to do so undermines public trust in the profession's commitment—to place the interests of society above self-interest—and reduces society's interest in helping the profession maintain the powers and privileges granted.

IMPLICATIONS FOR THE PROFESSIONAL

By considering the attributes that distinguish each occupation or profession, we notice that dentistry possesses each of the essential attributes. Society has conferred powers and privileges on dentistry commensurate with the level of power and privilege reserved for the most highly professionalized occupations (e.g., law and medicine), thereby implying that society views the provision of dental care as essential for its health and welfare.

The possession of essential attributes implies that persons who wish to become members of the profession have these responsibilities: (1) to *acquire the knowledge* of the profession to the standards set by the profession, (2) to *keep abreast of changing knowledge* through continuing education, (3) to make a *commitment to the basic ethic* of the profession—that is, to place the oral health interests of the patient above the interests of the professional and to place the rights of society above the rights of the profession, (4) to *abide by the profession's code of ethics* or work to change it if it is inconsistent with the underlying ethic of the profession, (5) to *serve society* (i.e., the public as a whole), and (6) to *participate in the monitoring and self-regulation* of the profession.

Power and privileges are granted to the profession on the basis of the assumption that each professional will take these responsibilities or obligations seriously. The profession has a right to expect that each individual who is chosen and then decides to become a dental professional will commit to these responsibilities.

Fulfilling these responsibilities is easier said than done. Professionals often find themselves in situations where personal and professional values conflict or where their professional obligations conflict. Many of the common conflicts are addressed in the American Dental Association's *Principles of Ethics and Code of Professional Conduct*. The field of dental ethics attempts to prepare professionals to recognize, reason about, and effectively resolve the common dilemmas of the profession. In particular, dental professionals need to develop skills in ethical reflection that enable them to make good decisions about new problems that are likely to emerge during the course of professional life. Although membership in professional organizations is not legally required, no person can participate in monitoring and regulating the profession or influence the direction the profession takes by standing on the sidelines.

Because this book is devoted to issues of community dental health, this chapter will focus specifically on the obligations of the profession and the professional to serve society. Individual dentists meet that responsibility through service to the individual patient, to the patient's family, to the community, and to the profession. The profession collectively meets that responsibility through a variety of efforts aimed at preventing disease and promoting the nation's oral health.* We will not only advocate for obligations that go beyond the obligation to the individual patient but will also point out the limits of professional obligation. We are not advocating that dental professionals engage in the kind of selfless commitment to others that

characterizes individuals such as Mother Teresa, but neither are we advocating that it is acceptable to exhibit the all-engrossing commitment to self exhibited by some of the more notorious examples of our time: inside-trader Ivan Boesky (his famous quote "greed is good"). We are advocating that the dental professional has obligations to others that are somewhere on a continuum that has Mother Teresa on one end and Ivan Boesky on the other.

Principles of bioethics

One way to think about the ethical obligations of dental professionals is through a popular approach focusing on three basic principles. In this approach, moral action guides are identified on the basis of duties or responsibilities to (1) show respect for persons, (2) avoid causing harm, prevent harm, remove harm, or provide benefit, and (3) act justly. These three bases for the duties are often referred to as the three principles of bioethics and sometimes called the principle-based approach, or principlism. The principles of beneficence (including nonmaleficence) and justice were first enunciated by Frankena[2] and popularized through their application to health care by Beauchamp and Childress.[3]

The distinctions among the duties to avoid harm, prevent harm, remove harm, and provide benefit are very important, even though the duties may all be seen to arise out of the principle of beneficence. Frankena[2] holds that duties to avoid and prevent harm are stronger or more basic than duties to remove harm or provide benefit. These are crucial distinctions for dental health professionals, suggesting that the first duty is to avoid injuring someone through malice or incompetence. After that, the duty to prevent dental disease would be stronger than the duty to help someone who has the disease, and the duty to remove the disease would be stronger than the duty to re-

*For a more extensive discussion of the public duties of the professions, see Jennings B, Callahan D, Wolf SM: The public duties of the professions, *Hastings Center Rep* Special supplement: February, 2-20, 1995.

store oral health. In fact, some do not consider restoring oral health as a duty but rather the discretionary act of a virtuous professional.

The principle of respect for persons is based on the contention that individuals ought to be free to determine what will happen to their bodies. In the health care setting this principle is the basis for the practice of informed consent, by which patients are given sufficient information to make an informed decision about whether to accept a proposed treatment—and the decision itself must be well-considered and voluntary. Dentists are likely to consider this principle often as they consider patient requests for particular treatments and offer patients advice and options. The principle of justice questions what kinds of treatment to provide and for which patients treatment should be provided when resources (time, effort, budgets) are limited. The principle of justice directs us to allocate or distribute resources in ways that are fair.

These principles should not be viewed as absolute but rather as important principles to respect and follow in making decisions about ethical issues. For example, how should a dental professional respond to a patient who requests that all his or her teeth be extracted because it would save having to brush them every day? The dental professional ought to consider the request in light of the duty to respect the decision of the patient, drawn from the principle of respect for persons, while at the same time honoring the commitment to avoid causing harm and doing what is in the best interest (doing good) for the patient. This example illustrates the potential and frequent conflict between important principles. How are we to resolve these conflicts, which are what make the consideration of ethical issues both interesting and difficult? One way to resolve a conflict between principles is to ask whether any particular principle is stronger than the others at issue. In the example above we might ask whether the principle directing us to re-

spect a patient's request is more important (or stronger) than the principle directing us not to cause harm. A long history of protecting the right of individuals to make decisions for themselves may lead us to conclude that respect for persons takes precedent over all other ethical principles, but let's look a bit further at the example. Before respecting the decision of a patient, we must be sure that the decision is one the patient fully understands, including that the patient really means to make the decision. Another way of saying this is that the dental professional must be sure that a patient has the mental capacity to make health care decisions.* Once the dental professional makes sure that the patient is making a real, or autonomous decision, a true conflict between principles exists in the above case. It is important to assess ethical situations in this way so that the ethical issues surrounding a case are being addressed and not disagreement about the facts or other aspects of the case.

The dental professional seems to have two choices in the example we've been discussing: respect the patient's decision and extract the teeth as requested or argue that even if the patient's request is autonomous that the harm that would be caused to the patient by the request is too great, so the principle to avoid causing harm ought to win out. These kinds of conflicts are the source of debates about the so-called paternalistic model of the health care provider, where the professional effectively overrides the autonomous decision of patients on the basis of a claim to superior knowledge of what is best for patients, regardless of whether the patient agrees. Such paternalism has been roundly attacked and is almost universally discredited. But even so it would be a paternalistic decision that many would sup-

---

*For a discussion of strategies for assessing cognitive capacity and achieving consent for treatment, see Shuman SK and Bebeau MJ: Ethical and legal issues in special patient care, *Dent Clin North Am* 38(3):553-575, 1994.

port if the dental professional decided to override the autonomous decision of the patient to have all the teeth extracted. A way out may be to inform the patient that you respect his or her right of choice but cannot violate your professional obligation to avoid actions that are harmful.

The third principle mentioned above—the principle of justice—comes into play most frequently in considerations of allocating scarce resources, such as choosing which patients to treat when there is a shortage of dental services or dental care providers. Fair treatment is often the stated goal when such choices must be made, and reference to the principle of justice helps us decide what is fair. Fairness is another term for justice, and it can mean anything from equal treatment (the same for all) to equitable treatment (unequal but fair distribution). The principle of justice helps us to determine what method of distribution is most equitable. Methods can include distribution that is equal or based on need, merit, ability to pay, or a host of other factors. Justice requires that the method of distribution be justified and applied consistently. With these three principles, outlined here in general terms, ethical issues in dental care can be more effectively understood and examined, and we hope resolved. The case study analyses that follow attempt to apply these principles to real-life dental practice and the ethical issues that may arise in them.

Cases and case analyses

Case 1: The Jeremy Lee Case

Jeremy Lee is a 33-year-old black male. He suffers from a heart valve disease and had an aortic valve inserted 7 years ago. Since surgery he has been receiving antibiotic therapy intermittently for infections. Also, he has been taking the anticoagulant warfarin to prevent clotting of the blood. This medication is necessary to prevent clots from forming and traveling through the blood stream to distant organs. As a result of clots that lodged in small vessels of the brain, Jeremy has had several strokes. However, to date, the strokes have not caused any substantial deficit in his neurologic abilities. In part, his difficulties are related to his failure to consistently take his medications. He has been a Medicaid recipient from time to time, is currently unemployed, and is again on Medicaid.

Jeremy has 5 or 6 badly broken and neglected teeth remaining in the maxilla and about 12 teeth in the mandible. At least 7 anterior teeth in the mandible are in good condition in that they have no caries and no mobility. The gingiva is inflamed, but there is no pocketing more than 3 mm. There is some calculus, but a routine prophylaxis could improve the tissue. Jeremy has been given oral hygiene instruction but, according to the record, has shown no interest in improving his hygiene.

Because of his medical problems, Jeremy needs to be hospitalized to have his teeth removed. His health care team has to stop the warfarin, switch to heparin (which can only be given intravenously), and perform surgery under general anesthesia. After surgery intravenous antibiotics must be continued for 48 hours and the warfarin resumed and monitored until appropriate levels are reached. The procedure requires 5 days of hospitalization, services of an oral surgeon (who will extract the teeth, contour the ridges, and prepare the tissues for a denture), and an anesthesiologist for 1.5 hours, recovery time, etc., all at a cost of approximately $4800.

Restoration of the teeth is out of the question because it would be costly and is not covered by Medicaid. As the oral surgeon, you need to decide whether to challenge the referring dentist's decision to remove all the teeth in the mandible. Perhaps you should advocate leaving the seven sound teeth. Normally, this would be preferable because wearing a full lower denture is difficult. In a person as young as Jeremy, after long years of wearing a denture resorption would occur, making it increasingly more difficult to achieve a good fit. However, if Jeremy doesn't change his oral hygiene habits, a partial denture could even accelerate the loss of the remaining teeth. Also, any infection could further complicate his health problems, and the teeth might need to be extracted at a later date, requiring hospitalization and further expense. If Jeremy is still on Medicaid, the added expense will be borne by society. On the other hand, the experience of wearing an upper denture might influence him to change his ways to avoid having a lower denture as well.

Should you remove all the teeth? Why? What reasons would you give to support your position?

ANALYSIS
Professional-patient issues

This dilemma raises questions about rights of patients who are unable to pay for their own care and must rely on public assistance. Should such patients have the same rights—to be informed of alternatives, to choose the preferred treatment, or to refuse treatment—as patients who are able to pay for the treatment? Should the fact that Jeremy Lee seems to have difficulty complying with the directives of his health care providers be considered by the oral surgeon in deciding what to do? In this case no information is provided about the patient's involvement in the treatment decision. Should we presume that the referring dentist achieved consent for the proposed treatment? The oral surgeon has a referral for extraction of all the teeth. Should the oral surgeon follow the directive of the referring dentist or overrule that decision and make a judgment as to the best interest of the patient? Although we might argue that the referring dentist should be consulted to determine whether the patient participated in the decision, it is interesting to explore whether to remove all the teeth, given the circumstances in this case.

One factor to consider is the limitations placed on Jeremy's autonomy by his lack of financial resources. As a medical assistance recipient in most states, Jeremy is provided with relief from pain, swelling, and infection, but restorative services are usually very limited. For example, he may be entitled to new dentures every 5 years. Or, if the dentist decides to leave the seven sound teeth, Jeremy would be

eligible for a partial denture, but more functional and esthetic restorations (e.g., crowns and bridges) typically are not covered.

Although we might argue that many people would be likely to change their health care habits after receiving an upper denture, Jeremy has a history of noncompliance, at least as it relates to his general health. Failure to take his medications has life-threatening consequences. He has experienced these consequences without improving his compliance. Although there may be important questions as to whether Jeremy understands the consequences of his actions and is making an informed decision when he fails to comply, the surgeon cannot ignore his past noncompliant behavior because it is the single best predictor of his future actions. It is important to consider the range of possible reasons for lack of compliance: (1) A patient simply lacks understanding of the consequences, in which case he may be educable. (2) A patient lacks understanding of the consequences and has cognitive deficiencies or beliefs that make education difficult, in which case he may need a guardian or supervision if the provider cannot achieve comprehension. (3) A patient may be consciously or unconsciously engaging in self-destructive behaviors because of depression, mental illness, or chemical dependency. In such cases, mental health interventions are needed.

People usually do not make major changes in health habits and behaviors. The oral surgeon needs to consider prior behavior in assessment of this case, especially in view of the patient's serious medical problems.

Profession-society/community issues

Conflict of duties. One thing that makes this dilemma so difficult is that dentistry has become much more focused on preservation of tooth structure and on restoration of function rather than on extraction of teeth. The incredible decreases in dental disease we have witnessed in the last 20 to 30 years is responsible for this change of focus. But this has turned the focus from the prevention or removal of harm to the provision of benefit as the preeminent value of the profession. The idea that removing seven sound teeth in this case might be in the patient's best interest, given his health habits and the significant health risks associated with a second surgery, seems to fly in the face of the profession's emphasis on restoration of function and the idea that removing healthy teeth is in and of itself harmful.

In this case it seems the surgeon would actually be "doing harm" to "prevent harm" that may come about if the teeth and surrounding tissue were left to fall victim to disease that is likely to result from the patient's continued habits.

A second conflict of duties arises between the surgeon's obligation to serve as an advocate of Jeremy's interests and his obligation to the rest of society (e.g., not to spend a disproportionate amount of public money on this patient). Many situations involving public funds are predetermined. This is one situation where the dentist may be able to argue that the patient's seven sound teeth have resisted decay and disease in the face of Jeremy's health habits and are therefore less likely to become diseased in the future.

Rights of Jeremy versus the rights of society. Some practitioners will take the view that health care is a privilege rather than a basic right. They may feel that Jeremy should not be given any care that he cannot pay for. Other practitioners may take the view that there should be no discrimination on the basis of ability to pay, that the same packages of benefits should be available to all irrespective of ability to pay. Such differences in views are often grounded in deeply held convictions. Rather than to argue which is the "right" view, it may be helpful to explore the beliefs that are at the root of these conflicting ideas. Many of

us have been socialized to believe that anyone could take care of himself or herself if only he or she would put forth the effort to do so. Even though we may recognize that such a view is only partially true, such ideas are rooted in concepts of individualism and the puritan ethic, values that underlie much of American history and culture.* Irrespective of personal perspective, American society currently provides basic care for those who are poor and disadvantaged, but the benefits provided do not represent optimal oral health.

Rights to oral health care versus rights to medical care. Indeed, Medicaid programs often do not cover any adult dental care or are restricted to emergency services. Sometimes episodic procedures for relief of pain and infection are provided, but generally dental care is viewed as elective rather than as an integral part of an individual's overall primary health care. For example, before the recent implementation of the Oregon Health Plan, a patient could have a benign mole removed from the neck but could not have decayed teeth restored.[4] When the Oregon Health Plan created a state-approved list of medical and dental health services by an open public process, many dental services previously excluded from the Medicaid list of benefits were suddenly included. "Oregon now has one of the most generous dental Medicaid benefit packages in the country, including coverage for services such as endodontic treatment, scaling and root planing, along with basic preventive, restorative and prosthodontic services. Cast crowns and bridges are included with limitation. Further, over 100,000 individuals not previously covered by Medicaid were brought into the plan and provided dental coverage."[4]

---

*For a discussion of the origin of societal views about the right to health care, see Burt BA, Eklund SA: Ethics and responsibility in dental care, In: *Dentistry, dental practice, and the community,* Philadelphia, 1995, WB Saunders, pp. 23-28.

From the perspective of increasing access to dental care, the profession may want to reconsider the wisdom of advocating for the separation of medical and dental benefits.

Rights of Jeremy versus other Medicaid patients. Although we may be tempted to raise larger questions about the overall prioritization of medical and dental health benefits, when society sets aside limited funding for care to the poor and disadvantaged, questions arise about the distribution of those scarce resources. For example, is it fair to use a disproportionate amount of public money on one person, if so doing diminishes the resources available to others? Other cases to follow will discuss this issue in greater detail.

Case 2: The Dr. Lester Case

Dr. Jim Lester has a suburban practice that suits him fine. He lives in a midwestern community consisting of a city of 60,000 with surrounding suburbs of about 40,000. He works 5 days a week for 40 hours and has time for his family and his current passion, creating a bird sanctuary outside town. His hobby is environmental protection and he belongs to the local Sierra Club. Further, his wife is also a member and this is something they do together.

Dr. Lester's community has been hit hard by the economy. Two years ago two manufacturing plants laid off large numbers of workers. Efforts have been made to attract new businesses, and many workers have stayed in the community hoping some new opportunities will develop. Many are still drawing unemployment, but medical and dental benefits expired some time ago. Several dentists have started a program through the local dental society to contribute time—mostly nights and weekends—at a downtown clinic to provide emergency and preventive care. They ask Dr. Lester to join. He refuses. He points out that he is already contributing to the community through the Sierra Club, that he feels personally fulfilled through his current practice, and that his personal goal has never been to become that involved in organized dentistry. He does a good job with suburban kids and that is his interest. He has always felt that he is the kind of person who does better with a wider range of commitments.

"But Jim," his friend Dr. Al Felding argues, "your lack of professional involvement means the rest of us have to contribute more, and lack of cooperation for this project makes us look bad at the state meetings. You're the third suburban dentist to turn me down this week."

"Look Al," Jim counters, "you chose to do this. I'm not proselytizing you to become a member of the Sierra Club. To each his own. You're fulfilling your mission in life, I'm just choosing a different track for my extracurricular activities. Come off it, will you?"

Should Dr. Lester volunteer to help? Why or why not? What reasons would you give to support your position? As you reflect on the reasons, consider self-interested reasons for participating (or not) and reasons derived from the moral principles that might apply in this case.

ANALYSIS

This dilemma raises questions about the limits of professional obligation. Dr. Lester is already serving his community by performing dental services in his private practice 40 hours a week. He is also contributing to society through activities he enjoys—work with the Sierra Club. He does have obligations not to work so much that he is too "burned out" to give adequate time and attention to himself, his dental staff, his patients, and his family. Further, he has a responsibility to maintain a viable practice, because if he doesn't, he can't serve anyone. Dr. Lester has a right to make a living, perhaps even a very good living, as long as he does not compromise his patients' right to competent care in the process. Balancing responsibilities to patients, staff, self, and one's family are challenging enough. But does Dr. Lester, as a health professional, also have dental responsibilities to the larger community and to the profession regardless of his activities and commitments to the environment?

Professional-patient issues

What if a patient tells Dr. Lester that he can't keep his and his family's regular dental appointments because he is out of work? Does Dr. Lester have any different obligations to this family of patients when they face economic hardship than he has to the community and the dental profession? We can argue that he does indeed, on the basis of the relationship he has with his patients, his obligation to provide dental care, and the relative importance of those obligations to current patients compared with the community at large. Dr. Lester might argue that he had no extra time to provide free care to community members in urgent need of care because he was trying to meet demands of patients in his practice for elective or non-emergency care. We ought then argue that Dr. Lester had an obligation to postpone some of his patients' elective work to assist his colleagues in meeting the more urgent needs of the community.

Profession-society/community issues

Apparently, the local dental society is responding to an obvious need—to provide emergency and preventive dental services to members of the community whose access to care is limited by economic misfortune. Note that the dentists are providing the kind of services that meets basic needs, care that, according to one of the principles described above, might be classified as "preventing evil or harm" or "removing evil [disease] or harm" rather than care that would "do or promote good." In this case the local dental society and the dentists cooperating with Dr. Felding have decided to provide the kinds of care gratis that the families would be entitled to if they were eligible for medical assistance. Is the local dental society obligated to take on this responsibility, and is Dr. Lester obligated to help?

Let's take the obligation of the local dental society first. It could be argued that the obligation for emergency and preventive care rests with the community's citizens and taxpayers rather than with the local dental society and that dentists are responsible only to the extent that they have responsibilities as taxpayers and citizens. On the other hand, dentists are not ordinary citizens. Although all citizens are entitled to a basic education, only those with special ability are granted access to professional education. Dentists have special status in a society based on special knowledge gained through education that is subsidized, in some instances heavily subsidized, by tax dollars.* On the basis of its specialized knowledge and the power given to the profession, it would seem the profession has specific responsibilities (e.g., to advise about the efficacy of public health programs, to participate in the development of public assistance dental programs, and to engage in other activities that promote the oral health of the public). Beyond that, does the profession have a moral duty to provide free dental services to those who have no access to care? Nonetheless, the dental society decided to take on this project.

It could be argued that Dr. Lester, as part of the professional society, has a responsibility to his peers to support the group's decision in some way. Certainly the burden for those that have volunteered would be less and the number of affected families would be more if each dentist in the community and surrounding areas participated in the group's access program. But if we can't argue that it is obligatory of Dr. Lester to help his colleagues, are there other compelling reasons to do so?

Is it in Dr. Lester's interest to help out in his community? When there is a downturn in the economy, dentists are likely to be among the first to notice. People tend to view dental care

*The percentage of the true cost of dental education subsidized by the state varies from state to state, but even in private schools tuition and clinic income covers no more than 65% of the total cost of education. Meskin LH: Do we need another dental school? *J Am Dent Assoc* 127(8):1146-48, 1996.

as expendable or as a need that can be postponed. The economic downturn seems not to have affected Dr. Lester's suburban practice—at least not yet—but the interdependence of business and service in most communities suggests that unless the community works together to attract other sources of employment for laid-off workers, there may be far-reaching consequences. Suburban residents may not feel the economic pinch as quickly as those who have lost their jobs, but in time the effects may reach Dr. Lester's dental practice.

Aside from the potential, and possibly eventual, negative consequences to the economic health of Dr. Lester's dental practice, he might also think about the positive consequences of helping his community and his colleagues in time of need. The most important asset any dentist has is his personal and professional reputation. Volunteering to help people in the downtown area in a time of need is likely to enhance his reputation in the community; conversely, failure to participate could have negative consequences. Further, if compromising time with his family is a significant issue for Dr. Lester, he might consider ways to involve his family in the volunteer activity, thereby teaching his children important lessons about community and social responsibilities. Perhaps his wife and children could accompany him to the clinic on the night he works. Family members may be able to assist him, even if it is something as simple as visiting with people who are waiting to receive care or caring for children while their parents receive care.

Case 3: The Managed-Care Medicaid Proposal

As the dental director* for the health department in your state, you have been working for some time to improve access to dental care for your medical assistance population. Few dentists have

*Typically a dental director has a master's degree in public health in addition to a degree in dentistry or dental hygiene.

signed up to participate in the program because of the low rate of reimbursement for dental benefits. Thus many Medicaid-eligible individuals have been unable to gain access to care. Further, as a result of the general economic problems the state faces, the legislature has been unwilling to raise the rate of reimbursement. In fact, because of a recent budgetary shortfall, your state's Medicaid program dropped all dental coverage for adults, including emergency care, to maintain coverage for children through age 18. When you complain to the state commissioner of health, she points out that if you save money in the dental program for children, you may at least be able to restore emergency care for Medicaid-eligible adults. She suggests that you contact Medicaid Dent-Tell, a benefit company that has been providing a managed-care plan for a state on the East Coast.

You learn the following: Medicaid Dent-Tell (a fictitious for-profit dental benefit company) contracted with an eastern state to provide school-based dental benefits to Medicaid-eligible children. The state reimbursed at a capitation rate of $4.50 per child per month. Medicaid Dent-Tell enrolled all Medicaid-eligible students in the public schools and hired dentists to go into the schools and do screening examinations and prophylaxis. Fluoride treatments were not routinely provided because dentists stated that the portable equipment provided was inferior because it did not have adequate suction equipment to prevent excessive swallowing and nausea. On the basis of the screening, notices were sent home to the parents of children who needed care and followed up with a second notice if parents failed to respond. The notices gave the name and address of the participating dentist closest to the family's residence and included information about the child's needs and indicated which of the needed services would be covered under the plan. Medicaid Dent-Tell claims the program is highly successful, that Dent-Tell has had little difficulty recruiting dentists to participate, and has effectively solved the access problems for the state.

The representative of Medicaid Dent-Tell indicates that the company is interested in expanding to other states. You realize that under such a plan you could provide care for the Medicaid-eligible children and still have money for adult services. *Would you support this plan? Why or why not?*

ANALYSIS

This case points out the conflicts that may arise when dental care resources are limited, as they often are, and choices must be made between providing less-than-optimal care versus no care at all. The Medicaid-eligible population is by definition needy, so cost for dental (and medical) treatment is covered by the state. A continuing issue for those charged with managing Medicaid services is the justice-based question of how to divide a pie of limited size between competing services and among those eligible for coverage. As your state's dental director, you are charged with balancing the provision of all needed dental services to all eligible for coverage, against the limited resources you have at your disposal.

Should you provide all needed dental care for children and use whatever remains for the elderly, do the opposite, or provide limited services to both populations? What level of limited service is acceptable? Also, what questions should you ask about the plan? For instance, you know how many individuals you need to cover. What percentage of the eastern state's children received care? If a fairly large number of dentists signed up, how many of the plan's patients were seen and what treatments were provided? At the end of the year, how much did the state pay the plan? How much did the plan pay the dentists? How many patients received treatment? In reality, the director probably won't get answers to these questions but should ask them.

The professional-patient relationship

Professionals have duties both to prevent or remove harm and to provide benefit to their patients. By choosing the Medicaid Dent-Tell option, you have the opportunity of identifying children in need of dental care and informing their parents about the need to seek care and how to do so. This is the first part of fulfilling the obligations to remove harm and provide benefit, but it does not go far enough from an ethical standpoint. To identify needed ser-

vices without either providing them or offering a means to do so falls short of the obligation to remove harm (treat disease), let alone of providing the full benefit at your disposal to your patient(s). But failing to opt for this partway approach will mean no services at all for the eligible elderly in your state, which would be a failure to live up to your ethical obligations to them.

More important is the obligation to design a plan that enables the population to get the needed care. This plan fails to take into account, or perhaps even exploits, the shortcomings of the population it is intended to serve. Parents of economically and socially disadvantaged populations are highly unlikely to take advantage of a plan that requires (1) that they receive and understand the letter sent to them and (2) that they have the means and perseverance to make the necessary appointment, travel to the office, and perhaps pay some portion of the services not covered by the plan. Although the plan is "successful" in using resources and recruiting dentists, it is unlikely that patients will actually access needed services. Given that no care is provided, not even fluoride treatments, the dental director must ask whether this is an acceptable and responsible use of resources, even if it covers all eligible children.

The professional-society relationship

As the state's dental director, your role-related obligations extend to the community (or society) in addition to whatever obligations you might have toward individual patients. Your title and job duties place you in a position that requires that you consider the good of the community, possibly even before the good of individual patients. Public policy decisions about the allocation of scarce resources generally rely on utilitarian calculations about what will yield the greatest proportion of benefit over harm for a particular community. In this case, the communities to be considered, in the order of their priority, are (1) the population eligible for state-supported dental services and (2) the state's population as a whole. The question you must answer as the state dental services director is whether it is better to provide some level of dental services to all eligible or to provide needed services to one subset of the eligible population at the exclusion of the rest of those eligible? If you cannot provide all needed services to everybody eligible, as is the case here and in most other states, what level of service would be minimally acceptable as a matter of ethical dental practice?

The profession-society relationship

As is the case with any profession, dentistry has moral duties to the society in which its members practice. Those duties include meeting acceptable standards for the provision of dental services, not discriminating against particular groups of patients, and acting in ways that advance the oral health of the public. When faced with the problem of limited resources demonstrated by this case, what does the relationship between the dental profession and society tell us the state dental director ought to do? If you choose the Dent-Tell option, you need to enlist the services of sufficient numbers of dentists to provide the services involved. You may argue that your colleagues have some obligation to participate in programs that benefit those in need. But simple participation of dentists is not sufficient to satisfy the profession's obligations to society. Dentists must also live up to the standards of practice set by them as a profession. In this particular case, you must weigh whether the provision of limited treatments required by the state as part of the Dent-Tell program meets the standards of dental practice required by the profession of its members. In particular, you must weigh whether dental examination without further treatment and prophylaxis but no fluoride treatments are acceptable as a matter of dental practice. If the choice is between offering this reduced level of dental services versus none at all, what is the ethically acceptable choice? Greater services for children could only be provided at the cost of denying all dental services to eligible adults. Which population ought to win out, or is the most humanely acceptable action to provide some, albeit less than optimal, care for all? How would you best serve justice while respecting your obligations to prevent and remove harm and do good? Is it appropriate for you to try to recruit your dental colleagues to participate in plans that fail to meet professional standards of care?

Case 4: The Triage Proposal

As the dental director* for the health department in your state, you have been working for some time to improve access to dental care for your public assistance population. Few dentists have signed up to participate in the program because of the low rate of reimbursement for dental treatment. Thus many Medicaid-eligible individuals have been unable to gain access to care. Further, as a result of the general economic problems the state faces, the legislature has been unwilling to raise the rate of reimbursement.

In fact, because of a recent budgetary shortfall, your state's Medicaid programs dropped all dental coverage for adults, including emergency care, to maintain coverage for children through age 18. When you complain to the state commissioner of health, she points out that if you save money in the dental program for children, you may at least be able to restore emergency care for Medicaid eligible adults. She suggests you consider some school-based dental health programs that would reduce the overall cost of care and suggests you talk to Dr. Harry Reagan, who has been running a kind of triage program in the inner-city schools of your state capital.

Dr. Reagan describes the program. He says there is no way we can address all the dental needs of Medicaid-eligible children in this city. We have decided to go into the schools with a triage approach.

---

*Dental directors typically have a master's degree in public health in addition to a degree in dentistry or dental hygiene.

The dentist does a very quick screening to identify children who need more extensive treatment. These are identified for later treatment by a mobile unit that comes to the school within a week or two. Meanwhile, a team of hygienists does fluoride treatments (without prophylaxis) and then seals the teeth of all program-eligible children. The mobile unit is supported by private contributions and staffed by volunteer dentists and one public health dentist. The unit provides emergency care, diagnostic and some additional preventive services (i.e., prophylaxis and space maintainers, because of the high rate of extraction), and routine restorative care (mostly amalgams).

Dr. Reagan says the program is effective because it is prevention oriented and treats those with the greatest need. He points out that initially the program offered the fluoride treatments and sealants to all school children for a fee. Medicaid paid the fee for those who were Medicaid eligible. Parents, especially single parents and families with both parents working, liked the program because their children could get preventive care without having to take the children out of school and without their taking time off from work. Although the program was successful, it was so heavily criticized by the dental community that organizers decided to limit the program to children on Medicaid. Despite this adjustment, the dental community still claims that the program does not meet standards of dental care. Dentists object to applying sealants without a complete diagnostic assessment (including radiographs); they think prophylaxis should precede fluoride treatments, and so on.

Dr. Reagan thinks they have not pushed the issue because it applies to a rather limited population and because Medicaid reimbursements are so low that local dentists are just as happy to avoid treating this population.

On the other hand, Dr. Reagan doubts that the program could be expanded on a statewide basis without encountering formidable opposition from the dental community.

Should you advocate a similar program? Why or why not? How should you address the dental community and its complaints?

ANALYSIS

Like case 3, this case points out the ethical issues presented when resources are limited. But unlike case 3, in which it is proposed that the same minimum level of services be provided to all, this case suggests a different approach to justice. As in other aspects of health care, limited resources force decisions about how to fairly allocate what is available.

The professional-patient relationship

As the state's dental director, you have an obligation to serve the best dental interests of your patients, who include all those who may receive state-supported dental care. Because there is not enough money to pay for the necessary dental care for all eligible citizens who need it, you must decide how best to accommodate your duties of justice while also respecting your duties to prevent and remove harm and provide benefit toward patients. So, while you know that the program can't provide optimal care to all eligible patients, you must decide whether you can purchase sufficiently acceptable care to all so as to at least meet the obligation to avoid or remove harm. The provision of examinations followed by emergency dental services to those who need them seeks to remove and prevent harm. The provision of only prophylaxis, fluoride treatment, and sealants to everyone else should be seen as only marginally serving their best interests. In a climate of severely constrained resources, however, this may be the best you can hope to achieve.

The professional-society relationship

Triage, or the process of treating those in greatest need first, is a common way of allocating scarce resources. Emergency cases receive priority, and others are treated in the order of urgency until treatment resources run out. In dealing with community needs the dental professional has a duty to provide the best care possible. Under circumstances of limited resources, this may mean allocating care after assessing patient needs and then providing treatment so that all patients are eventually brought to a maintenance level. In this case that means treating emergency cases first and then providing the level of services possible to the remaining patients consistent with the remaining level of resources. Although this approach may not yield the optimal results from the perspective of each individual patient, the dentist must take the community's good into account.

The profession-society relationship

Your colleagues in the profession rightly question whether a triage program adequately meets the needs of Medicaid patients. The profession has a duty to ensure that the dental care provided by its members meets the needs of patients (doing what is safe and effective, what prevents or removes harm and provides benefit) and lives up to the standard set by the profession. This is especially true for state-supported and endorsed programs meant to serve the public health. A quick examination followed by fluoride treatment and sealant without prophylaxis does not meet these standards in many dentists' minds. Although most dentists would not give a fluoride treatment without a prophylaxis, it does not mean that the treatment will be ineffectual.[5]

The question that you and your dental colleagues must ask yourselves is whether such cursory care that covers all eligible patients is worse than providing more adequate care for some at the expense of failing to provide any care to some proportion of this population. A more general question is why such limited resources are available for dental services. Should you and the dental society lobby the state for a larger budget for such services? Why should you be content with the current division of the budgetary pie?

Case 5: The Margo Stinson Case

Margo has worked as a dental hygienist for a periodontist for the last 18 years. She likes her work because she is able to arrange her schedule to accommodate her growing family. Margo and her husband Tom live next door to Stanley Freedman, who is the personnel manager for a manufacturing plant that employs about 700 semiskilled workers. In addition to his responsibilities for personnel management, he also purchases the medical and dental health benefits for his company. Seven months ago the company signed a 3-year contract for dental benefits that provided company employees with a list of dentists who agreed to participate in the plan. The plan cost the company $18.00 a month per employee and provided diagnostic and preventive services (with a limit of two prophylaxes per year) free of charge and required a 50% copayment for restorative services and a one-time $500 reimbursement for orthodontic care. The company had published brochures informing employees of the benefits and listing all participating plan dentists.

Lately Stan had been getting complaints from supervisors about the plan. Employees were requesting to take a half day off work to go to the dentist, and others were complaining about the long delays to get appointments with plan dentists or the long drive to gain accessibility to plan dentists. During an evening visit with Margo and Tom, Stan mentioned his frustration with dentists in the community. He said he thought his company was paying plenty for the dental benefit package. He mentioned that when he asked the benefit company why they had not signed up dentists who were more accessible the company blamed the dentists for engaging in a conspiracy to blackball their plan and control the costs of dental services. Margo was stunned by the direct attack on the dental profession. She wondered what her role and responsibility was with respect to the issues Stan raised.

Does Margo have a responsibility to Stan? To the patients covered by the plan? To the profession? Why or why not? What could Margo do?

ANALYSIS

Margo is in a tough spot. If she responds defensively to an attack on the profession, she may miss an important opportunity to help Stan to help the company employees secure dental care that better meets their needs. How prepared is Margo to address the various questions raised by the situation Stan finds himself in? Is it Margo's responsibility, as a dental hygienist, to know enough about the financing of dental benefit plans or the ways plans are marketed to benefit managers such as Stan to be able to counsel Sam? Actually, unless Margo knows some basics about the distinctions between medical and dental health needs of the population and some basics about the various methods for reimbursement of dental services, she cannot meet basic responsibilities she has to patients, to the public, and to the profession.

What basic information does Margo need? First, she needs to be clear about the following characteristics of dental disease, some of which are markedly different from medical illness and disease[6]:

- Dental disease does not heal without therapeutic intervention, so early treatment is the most efficient and least costly intervention.
- The need for dental care is universal and continuing, rather than episodic.
- The need for dental care is highly predictable and does not have the characteristics of an insurable risk.
- Patient cooperation and posttreatment maintenance is critical to the success of dental treatment and the prevention of subsequent disease.

Understanding third-party reimbursement

Next, to help Stan evaluate why his plan is not working, Margo needs to be aware of the five basic strategies[7] for reimbursing employees for dental care and the advantages and disadvantages of each.

1. *Capitation programs* pay contracted dentists a fixed amount (usually on a monthly basis) per enrolled family or patient. In return, the dentists agree to provide specific types of treatment to the patients at no charge (for some treatments there may be a patient copayment). The capitation premium that is paid by the employer may differ greatly from the amount the plan administrator provides for the patient's actual dental care. The disadvantage of capitation plans for the dentist is that it totally shifts the financial risk to the dentist. If the plan is not adequately funded, the dentist is placed in the position of rationing care or delaying needed treatment to keep from losing money.

2. *Preferred provider organization (PPO) programs* are plans under which contracting dentists agree to discount their fees as a financial incentive for patients to select their practices. If the patient's dentist of choice does not participate in the plan, the patient will have a reduction in benefits if the plan has a point-of-service option or a complete loss of benefits if the plan does not allow the employee to seek out-of-network care. Also, switching providers may actually increase the overall cost of care to the patient. For example, the new dentist will need to conduct a diagnostic assessment even if records are transferred, travel time may be increased, rapport will need to be developed, and so on. Further, if fees are heavily discounted, the dentist is often encouraged by the plan to give scheduling priority to fee-for-service patients and use the PPO patients to fill down time.

3. *Usual, customary, and reasonable (UCR) programs* usually allow patients to go to the dentists of their choice. The plan administrator calculates a "customary" fee limit (reimbursement level) that is based on collected usual and reasonable fee data from dentist's offices in specific geographic areas (e.g., zip codes). There is wide fluctuation and lack of government regulation on how a plan determines the "customary" fee level.

4. *Table or schedule of allowance programs* determine a list of covered services with an assigned dollar amount. That dollar amount represents just how much the plan will pay for those services that are covered. It does not represent the dentist's full charge for those services and the patient pays the difference. It is possible to manipulate the use of certain benefits by setting the reimbursement level so low that persons at the lower end of the socioeconomic scale cannot afford to use the benefit.

5. *Direct reimbursement programs* reimburse patients a percentage of the dollar amount spent on dental care, regardless of treatment category. This method typically does not exclude coverage that is based on the type of treatment needed and allows the patients to go to the dentist of choice.

Then, much as Margo would empower a patient to reflect on his or her choices with respect to the use of a dental benefit package, she will need to empower Stan to ask better questions and make better choices when purchasing dental benefits on behalf of the company's employees.

Employer issues

Benefit purchasers like Stan are probably sincere when they say they want to purchase dental and medical plans that benefit the employee not only in the short term but also in the long term. The challenge Stan faces in selecting among competing plans is the challenge we all face. How do we buy the best plan for the least money? How do we sort through the options? How do we figure out which is the best plan and the best deal?

First, Stan needs a clear view of what employees need. Because, as outlined above, dental needs are predictable and depend on personal health habits, timely care-seeking behavior, and occupational safety, employees need a plan that encourages prevention and early intervention. Employees really may only need to be "insured" against accidental dental

injury or catastrophic illness, which is typically covered under workers' compensation and medical plans.

If Stan purchases a plan that reimburses dentists for diagnosis, prevention, restorations, crowns, and other procedures at cut rates, he can save the company (and patients) money in the short run, but he may be promoting a disease model rather than a health model of dentistry, which is unlikely to promote oral health and will likely be much more expensive in the long run. Costs that accrue to Stan's company include (1) time lost from work by employees whose dental problems grow more serious and more costly and may result in compromised general health if neglected, (2) increased dissatisfaction with the company when increased needs for care are not covered by insurance, and (3) decreased quality of life, which often influences job performance. Thus it is in the interest of the employer to design a plan that promotes access to care and avoids rationing by inconvenience, as the current plan seems to be going. A plan that reimburses at rates that are near or below the actual cost of providing services interferes with access and quality because dentists are prompted (by the low reimbursement rates) to think of these patients as filler for their schedule. A plan that pays a capitated rate for dental services encourages undertreatment, whereas a plan that pays for services at the *dentist's* usual fee for services or requires very minimal copayments encourages overutilization. The designer of a plan needs to consider a plan design that emphasizes preventive care and regular check-ups, that allows patients freedom to choose their dentists, and that is flexible enough for smart treatment planning between patient and dentist.

The benefits of dental coverage

But why provide any kind of dental benefit? Why not simply let employees take care of their own dental needs out of pocket? Why incur any expense in administering dental benefit programs? Dental benefit plans have been effective because they tend to reduce patients' inhibition to seeking care and encourage employees to take advantage of preventive care. Plans that encourage preventive care and early intervention are particularly important for employees at the lower end of the socioeconomic scale. In general, the dental benefits industry has been an asset for employees and the dental profession because of its influence on utilization.

Another thing Margo must realize is that Stan may not be completely free to select a plan or plans (some states require that employees have choices) that he thinks is best. Employees, through their union leaders, may direct the benefit purchaser to ratchet down costs, and employees may think their employer is willing to switch providers to secure lower costs. Capilouto notes, "Individuals are willing to switch medical plans in the face of relatively small increases in premium price. Dental insured, if faced with similar price differential, should act similarly."[8] As we pointed out earlier, frequent changes in providers or delivery systems disrupts the continuity of care and leads to a duplication of services. If a company is faced with an economic downturn, cutting costs by interrupting continuity of care could be costly in the long run. Stan's company may be better off switching to a direct reimbursement plan to have more control not only of the cost of care but of the proportion of premium dollar that is returned to the employee in terms of direct benefit.

Employee issues

Once a benefit plan has been selected, Stan has an obligation to educate employees about their benefit plan. For most employees the task of comparing plans is tedious and very often the plan documents are written in language that obscures the plan's limitations and restrictions. Stan needs to educate patients about the plan(s) in simple language that anyone can understand. He needs to be held accountable for the ratio of premiums paid to payments made.

After all, the benefit he is purchasing is something the employee has earned—it is part of the employee's compensation package. Stan has a moral and a fiduciary responsibility to see that the benefit is a real benefit and not an opportunity for third-party payers to realize higher profits. It is easy to manipulate plan descriptions to make a lesser plan appear better. It is easy to influence employee choice on the basis of relatively small cost savings. It is also easy to claim that you cannot provide desirable benefit packages with convenient providers because of the greediness of some dentists and the generally "unreasonable" cost of dental services. But, if Stan buys into strategies that befuddle the employee or shift blame for problems with care to the dentists, he may not only undermine the employees' trust in himself and his employer, but he may put the employer at risk for liability if an employee is harmed by the plan.

How can Margo empower Stan to become a more responsible steward of the employees' compensation? Employees trust Stan to use his power to bargain on their behalf for benefits. When thinking of cost containment, Stan needs to understand the ratio of premiums paid to payments made. For example, in 1986, $6.1 billion were paid in dental insurance premiums and $5.3 billion were paid to patients (13.4% went to administrative costs, etc.). By 1988, 19% went to administrative and other costs.[9] Today, some estimate that administrative and other costs are around 27% with some egregious instances where payout is less than 50%.[10] And, employers can't rely on regulation of the benefit industry because most states don't regulate on the loss ratio. Most employees would not choose to contribute a substantial proportion of their hard-earned dental benefits to a third-party payers' profits and administrative costs, especially if the choice of provider is restricted.

What could Margo do?

First, she needs to avoid responding defensively. Active listening, to learn as much as she can about the plan, would be most effective. She may want to express some empathy for the challenging job Stan has. If Stan feels understood, rather than challenged or criticized, he may be willing to rethink his problem and learn new information.

Although Stan's comments may suggest a misconception about (1) the distinction between medical and dental health benefits, (2) the reasons dentists haven't signed up for the benefit program his company has purchased, (3) the real cost of the plan he has purchased and the benefit to employees, (4) other alternatives to putting more benefit in the employee's pocket, etc., Margo may wish to phrase these apparent misunderstandings as questions. For example, it is better to ask, "What is your understanding of the differences between purchasing dental and medical health benefits?" or "Has your carrier been *willing* to tell you the ratio of premiums paid to payments made?" or "What is the real cost of that dental benefit plan if employees need to take extra time to travel to plan dentists?" or "Have you asked any of the local dentists why they didn't sign up for your plan?"

Rather than try to answer all these questions herself, Margo may want to refer Stan to the American Dental Association's Council on Dental Benefit Programs. Recognizing the important role dental benefits have played in improving access to dental care for millions of Americans, the council has prepared brochures and other services to help employers of all sizes to design cost-effective, high-quality dental benefit plans for their employees.

Finally, the local or state dental association undoubtedly has persons available who could help Stan and other employers, union leaders, and concerned citizen groups to evaluate competing plans and to recommend plans that would be in the best interest of the employee and the company. Does Margo have an obligation to have some familiarity with alternative plans and the resources available to help the members of the public make informed choices?

Case 6: The Dr. Ellis Case

Dr. Ellis has always been a leader. She was very active in community dentistry programs during dental school and served as class president her last 2 years. After dental school she completed a general practice residency and earned a master's degree in dental public health in another state while her husband completed specialty training in ophthalmology. After returning to her home state, she opened a general dentistry practice. On the basis of her public health background, she took a real interest in treating Medicaid recipients, although she realized she needed to limit the number of medical assistance patients if she were to maintain a viable practice. As did many dentists in the community, she recognized that the level of reimbursement for services barely covered overhead. Further, this population of patients often had trouble complying with the regimens thought necessary to maintain a successful practice. Cancellations and tardiness were just a few of the problems. More important, the time and effort required to complete the paper work associated with reimbursement, together with denial of treatment Dr. Ellis thought essential, made working with this patient pool frustrating at best.

After exploring the problems associated with trying to lobby the legislature for increases in the reimbursement rate for dental benefits, Dr. Ellis decided that she would set aside one afternoon a week in which she would treat—free-of-charge—any Medicaid eligible patients. By providing services free she avoided the frustration associated with completing paper work, and by taking patients on a first come, first served basis (emergency cases excepted) she found she enjoyed the work more and served her patients better. Nonetheless, she realized she could not advocate this for everyone, and, even if she could, she wasn't sure it was a fair solution to the problems Medicaid-eligible people faced as they attempted to gain access to care. Over the years she had served on a number of committees and boards that addressed access to care and dental disease prevention and oral health promotion. She was well versed in the issues and thought that access to care was impeded by the low rate of reimbursement for dental service. Although she didn't agree with her colleagues, many of whom took the position that if society wouldn't adequately reimburse they would not treat, she recognized that the profession had a responsibility to advocate for the disadvantaged. The profession had tried to influence the legislature. The legislature tended to view the profession's efforts as self-serving. Some viewed the profession as self-serving and unwilling to sacrifice anything for the welfare of others. Dr. Ellis was also aware that some states had successfully argued that inadequate reimbursement rates paid to dentists who participated in Medicaid programs severely hindered the ability of recipients to obtain necessary dental services and violated federal law.

Dr. Lisa Ellis has just been elected president of the state dental association. One of her primary goals is to improve access to care for the disadvantaged.

What strategies should she use?

ANALYSIS
Profession-community/society issues

We have argued that the profession has a responsibility to put the oral health interests of society above the interests of the profession. But are there no limits to that responsibility? Does that mean that the profession must care for the underserved with little or no help from society at large? It does not. The provision of dental and medical care for the economically disadvantaged is a responsibility of the larger society. And society cannot shift a disproportionate share of that responsibility to the profession. Thus a state that designs a Medicaid dental plan that reimburses at rates that are near or below the actual cost of providing services may be in violation of federal law because the plan has the effect of denying equal access to care. In a 1992 California case,[11] the court found that the reimbursement rates set by the State of California's Denti-Cal program were in violation of recipients' rights to equal access to dental care, statewide availability of care, timely receipt of care, and comparability of services in the Medi-Cal program (the state's Medicaid plan). The

trial judge ordered the state to increase fees from approximately 30% to 80% of the average amount billed. It took a class action suit, filed on behalf of Medicaid recipients of California to bring about such a change in reimbursements, but such lawsuits have been successful in other states as well. Although the profession did not initiate these lawsuits, their success shows how society can be prompted to assume its share of the responsibility for promoting the oral health of the nation.

Dr. Ellis might develop a strategic plan to, first, educate the public about the cause and prevention of dental disease and about the cost/benefit ratio of early intervention in dental disease. Consider how a good public education program might motivate the 40% of the population that does not regularly seek care or even how such a program might motivate the substantial number of people (35% to 40%) who have dental coverage, but do not use their benefit. Second, focus the profession on the underserved and on unmet need. One of the constants that ran through the recent health care reform debate was that it was intolerable to have 35 to 50 million (14% to 20% of the population) medically uninsured.* But by comparison, only 40% of the population has dental benefits. There is an enormous unmet need. In estimating the need, it should not be assumed that people who do not have coverage do not get dental care. Indeed, many people do not see a dental benefit plan as much of a benefit and prefer to pay out of pocket. Nonetheless, it is reasonable to assume that an increase in dental benefit plans, especially of the type that keep administrative costs low, would enhance utilization of dental services. Also, patient expenditures tend to be greater (as much as 15% greater according to one study[12]) for those who

---

*We do not know, however, the proportion of the uninsured who are financially able to purchase care but choose not to. There is no mandate to have health insurance as there is to have auto insurance.

have dental coverage. Third, challenge the state legislature to consider medical and dental benefits simultaneously when considering a package of primary health care benefits. Then challenge the state to provide adequate reimbursement for dental benefits—through class action suits, if efforts to persuade are ineffectual. Fourth, collaborate with the state and national professional associations to design alternative models for the delivery of dental care to the underserved as well as to the employed. Consider how direct reimbursement plans enable employers to manage costs while preserving consumer sovereignty and eliminating interference in the care-giving partnership. Fifth, remind the profession of its public responsibilities. Like most of us, professions and professionals have a tendency to focus on self-interest rather than the interests of society. Being a dental professional in the modern world means equally treating patients one-to-one and paying attention to epidemiologic, economic, and social elements of practice. Practicing dentistry means working in operatories, on committees, and in communities. The profession needs a cadre of professionals who are well trained to proactively engage legislatures, union leaders, employers, purchasers, and patients to buy benefits that are in the employee's interest.

REFERENCES

1. Hall RH: The professions. In *Occupations and the social structure*, ed 2, Englewood Cliffs, NJ, 1975, Prentice-Hall.
2. Frankena W: *Ethics*, ed 2, Englewood Cliffs, NJ, 1975, Prentice-Hall.
3. Beauchamp TL, Childress JF: *Principles of biomedical ethics*, ed 4, New York, 1995, Oxford University Press.
4. Block LE, Freed JR: A new paradigm for increasing access to dental care: the Oregon Health Plan, *J Am Coll Dent*, 63(1):30-36, 1996.
5. Johnston DW, Lewis DW: Three-year randomized trial of professionally applied topical fluoride gel comparing annual and biannual applications with/without prior prophylaxis, *Caries Res* 29:331-336, 1995.
6. Council on Dental Benefit Programs: *Policies on dental benefit programs*, Chicago, 1994, American Dental Association.
7. Council on Dental Benefit Programs: *Managed care: making choices—a guide for patients*, Chicago, 1995, American Dental Association.
8. Capilouto E: Market forces driving health care reform, *J Dent Educ* 59(4):480-483, 1995.
9. Health Insurance Association of America: *Source book of health insurance*, Washington, DC, 1990, The Association.
10. Bramson JB, Feldman ME: A review of dental HMO expenses: where do the premium dollars really go? *J Am Dent Assoc* 127(1):118-122, 1996.
11. *Clark v Coye*, 1992 WL 370801 (E.D. Cal. Oct. 14, 1992).
12. Martens LV, Bird DL, Davidson GB, Burton KL: Business trends in private general practice (abstract), *J Dent Res* 67:182, 1988.

CHAPTER 17

The impact of transmissible disease on the practice of dentistry

Helene Bednarsh
Bennett Klein

Acquired immunodeficiency syndrome

No single factor has affected the practice of dentistry since the early 1980s more than acquired immunodeficiency syndrome (AIDS). "Once upon a time, no one in the world had ever heard of the acquired immunodeficiency syndrome (AIDS). Neither was the human immunodeficiency virus (HIV) known. That state of innocence has ended forever."[1]

Dealing with the HIV epidemic and its consequences may prove to be the greatest challenge ever faced by the dental profession. The manner in which dentistry responds to this challenge may, to a large degree, shape dentistry's future. This ribonucleic acid (RNA) virus has forced dentistry to reassess its ethics, legal obligations, and ability to protect dentists, staff, and patients from transmissible disease. It has exposed innermost fears and prejudices

NOTE: The material in this chapter necessarily simplifies complex legal issues and is not intended as legal advice. Dental health care workers with specific questions about legal rights and obligations should consult an attorney.

and clouded the ability to distinguish fact from fiction.

HIV is an epidemic that must be understood within its historic perspective. In June 1981 the Centers for Disease Control and Prevention (CDC) reported through their *Morbidity and Mortality Weekly Reports (MMWR,* the disease status and policy reports of the CDC) that five young homosexual men had required treatment for *Pneumocystis carinii* pneumonia, an opportunistic infection previously seen almost exclusively in immunodeficient patients such as transplant recipients and those under treatment for cancer. Its occurrence in five previously healthy individuals without a clinically apparent underlying immunodeficiency was unprecedented. These men also had cytomegalovirus (CMV) infection and oral candidiasis, further indications that they had a "cellular-immune dysfunction relative to a common exposure that predisposes individuals to opportunistic infections."[2] One month later the CDC reported the occurrence over a 30-month period of an uncommon malignancy, Kaposi's sarcoma, "among (26) previously

307

healthy homosexual men."[3] The CDC noted that the clinical characteristics of these cases differed from those usually seen with Kaposi's sarcoma, which had generally been regarded as a disease of elderly men. Again, the situation suggested a common underlying factor— immune suppression.[4]

In 1984 evidence implicated a retrovirus as the etiologic agent of AIDS and two prototypes were isolated, LAV (lymphadenopathy-associated virus) in France and HTLV-III (human T-lymphotrophic virus type III) in the United States, which were later shown to represent the same virus. In 1985 serologic tests became available to detect the presence of antibody to HTLV-III/LAV.[5] The availability of this test had many and varied consequences. First, it permitted investigation of the prevalence of the virus, and these studies demonstrated that infection with the virus itself was more common than the clinical illness (AIDS) in populations with an increased incidence of AIDS. Second, serologic testing gave an opportunity to study the progression of the disease within populations. Third, with the ability to detect antibodies, it became possible to screen blood and plasma donations for the virus. Surveillance of health care workers exposed to the virus also became possible.

Thus in June 1982 there was a hypothesis that a sexually transmitted infectious agent was causing disease in homosexually active men.[6] Now, in 1997, the landscape has changed considerably. Now there is an identified agent, a case definition, and a realization that groups other than homosexual men are being affected. Because of this realization, the focus of prevention has changed from risk groups such as homosexual males and intravenous (IV) drug users to risk behaviors such as homosexual sex, IV drug use, and multiple sex partners. There are clinically well-defined signs and symptoms, some of which are oral. Now, there are markers available for the disease, there is treatment, and there are tests to measure viral load.

Unfortunately, there is still no cure and no vaccination is available.

In 1993 the CDC proposed a change in the case definition of AIDS to more realistically measure the extent of disease. The new case definition was defined by a T cell count of 200 or less and the presence of specific AIDS defining conditions. These were expanded from the original definition to include, for example, cervical cancer and other conditions that would capture groups without previously recognized symptoms. This was important from a surveillance standpoint in terms of tracking disease but was also important to individuals in terms of their eligibility for medical benefits that required an AIDS diagnosis. Therefore the increase in AIDS cases in that year was more a product of a change in reporting than to an overall increase in HIV incidence.[7]

The HIV antibody test was licensed in 1985.[8] This test detects the presence of antibodies to HIV, not the virus itself. The test thus indicates only that infection with HIV has occurred, with no implications as to health status. A person who has antibodies to HIV is referred to as *seropositive*, and one without detectable antibodies is termed *seronegative*. Seroconversion is said to have occurred when an individual's test becomes positive after some time previous to which test results had been negative. It is important to note that there is a window period during which a person may be infected but during which the body has not yet responded to the virus with detectable antibody response. This time period can range from 3 to 12 weeks after infection, although reports of 6 months or more have been made. The screening test used is the ELISA, or enzyme-linked immunosorbent assay. If a specimen has a positive result, a repeat ELISA is generally performed. A persistent positive result is confirmed by a Western blot test. Although both the ELISA and the Western blot test for antibody, the Western blot is considered a more sensitive assay. Therefore persons testing negative on the ELISA are considered seronegative (at least for that point in time), and persons with a positive test confirmed by a Western blot are considered seropositive. For those in whom the results are indeterminate, the tests are repeated.

The Food and Drug Administration (FDA) approved the first antigen test kit in 1996 for use in screening blood donations.[9] Although it may take up to 3 months or more to detect antibodies to HIV, antigens, the virus's own protein, may be detected on an average of 6 days earlier. Transfusion-related HIV infection is low. Current tests fail to detect only 1 in 450,000 to 660,000 HIV-positive donations. This represents about 18 to 27 donations per year. Use of antigen testing will prevent 5 to 10 cases (about 25% of current cases of transfusion-associated HIV) per year. Antigen testing is approved only for blood screening and not as a diagnostic tool.

In 1996 the FDA licensed the first home test for HIV antibody.[10] There is some controversy surrounding this test because in a majority of states and under the professional recommendations testing should not occur without appropriate counseling before and after the test. This first approved test is an over-the-counter specimen collection kit where the user mails a dried blood sample to a laboratory for analysis, with results available after 1 week by telephone. The reported sensitivity is 99.9% and the specificity close to 100%. Therefore 1 in 1000 false-positive results and almost no false-negative results would be expected. Also licensed by the FDA in 1996 is the first saliva-based HIV test. The accuracy of this test is close to that of those using blood samples. The FDA has also approved tests that measure the concentration of HIV in the blood, a more appropriate predictor of the progression of disease then previously available tests such as those that measured CD4 counts. Studies on these viral load tests have shown that individuals with levels below 10,000 viral units per milliliter of serum were more likely to survive the 6-year study period than were those with higher levels of virus.

As of December 1996, more than 581,429 cases of AIDS and 343,000 deaths have been reported to the CDC,[11] and the estimate of those infected with HIV (HIV seropositive without signs and symptoms of AIDS) is about 1.5 million in the United States. It took 9 years for the first 100,000 cases to be reported but less than 2 years for the second 100,000. By the end of 1992, 100,000 people had died of AIDS, and now there is an AIDS death every 15 minutes. Although the HIV epidemic still affects homosexual and bisexual men more than other groups, the spread of the disease into the heterosexual population is becoming more evident. Women accounted for about 22% of new cases reported in 1995, and their cumulative total is about 15% of reported AIDS cases. In 1992 the number of women infected through heterosexual contact exceeded the number infected through IV drug use. In addition, AIDS is the leading cause of death in American males between the ages of 25 and 44 years. It is currently the fourth leading cause in women, but this is expected to rise.[12]

Epidemiologic studies have shown an increase in infection rates among IV drug users and disproportionate rates among minority groups. In *Living with AIDS*,[13] the National Commission on AIDS reported, "As of June 1991, women accounted for 10% of all AIDS cases . . . cases among women are growing faster than AIDS cases among men." Children are becoming infected as well. Nearly 70% of all pediatric AIDS cases are related to the mother's exposure to the disease. Clinical trials reported in 1994 demonstrated that the use of zidovudine (AZT) can reduce by two thirds the risk of HIV transmission from women to their unborn children. The perinatal transmission rate for women taking AZT was 8.3% compared with 25.5% for those taking a placebo. Estimates in 1994 were that between 6000 and 7000 women infected with HIV gave birth in the United States each year, and that 1500 to 2000 of the infants were infected. An FDA advisory panel has recommended that AZT be given to all HIV-infected women during specified prenatal and postnatal periods.[14] This could also have implications for postexposure management in those dental health care workers (DHCW) who are pregnant, although no recommendations have been proposed.

Guidelines and regulations regarding transmissible diseases

What does all this mean for dentistry? Several salient concepts emerge from the data provided by prevalence studies using the HIV antibody tests. First, the concept of "risk groups" is of diminishing usefulness for evaluating who may be at risk. Second, the majority of persons with serologic evidence of infection have no symptoms of infection. Third, 9 of 10 infected persons are unaware that they are infected. Thus, while risk groups become less distinct, the asymptomatic population continues to grow and increasingly consists of individuals unaware of their status. It follows that dentists are treating many unknown HIV-seropositive patients. With this knowledge, it becomes obligatory that all patients be treated as potentially infectious for HIV. There is simply no scientific rationale (nor legal precedent) for selecting certain patients or groups of patients to be subject to particular infection-control procedures. These arguments provide the basis for the use of universal rather than selective precautions in infection control.

Universal precautions have the added advantage of being effective against other viruses transmitted by blood and saliva during the course of oral health treatment. Infectious diseases are not a new threat in dentistry. Although HIV disease carries with it stigmas and fears that are a new phenomenon, hepatitis B (HBV) has always been an occupational hazard. Hepatitis C virus is also recognized as a potential occupational hazard. State, federal, and local regulatory and advisory agencies have caused DHCWs to change the way they practice and to alter the environment in which they place themselves, their staffs, and their patients.

In 1970 Congress passed the Occupational Safety and Health Act, creating, within the Department of Labor, the Occupational Safety and Health Administration (OSHA).[15] The charge to the OSHA was to protect workers and ensure healthful working conditions for every worker in the United States. This act required all employers to provide to all employees "a workplace that is free from recognized hazards that are causing or likely to cause death or serious physical harm." Before finalizing the blood-borne pathogens rule on December 6, 1991, the OSHA relied on this general duty clause to enforce the use of recommended guidelines to control the spread of blood-borne disease among health care workers.[16] OSHA is a regulatory agency with enforcement authority and an ability to make citations and impose fines or penalties for failure to comply with established standards, especially when this failure results in illness, injury, or death.

The CDC is an advisory agency with an intent to protect and promote the health of the public. The CDC has no regulatory authority, and the guidelines issued are for the most part voluntary, although over time these guidelines become standards of practice and, in some cases, the basis for regulation by agencies such as OSHA. Once the CDC published its first infection control guidelines in 1982,[17] standards of care evolved for the dental profession. The early guidelines did not specifically address dental care but outlined suggested precautions to be used when dealing with patients with AIDS, such as the use of gloves, refraining from bending or recapping needles, the use of gowns, and the use of extraordinary care to prevent injury. In general, early in the epidemic the CDC, reasoning by analogy, recommended use of procedures already known to be appropriate for persons infected with HBV. The first actual recommendations for DHCWs in 1983 stated the following:

1. Personnel should wear gloves, masks, and protective eyewear when performing dental or oral surgical procedures.
2. Instruments used in the mouths of patients should be sterilized after use.[18]

State-of-the-art infection control guidelines for dentistry did not emerge until April 18, 1986, when the CDC published "Recommended Infection Control Practices for Dentistry."[19] These recommendations were based on the use of a common set of infection-control strategies to be used routinely in the care of all patients in dental practices. This represented a shift to universal precautions from selective precautions. Of special interest is the editorial note that "All DHCWs (dental health care workers) must be made aware of sources and methods of transmission of infectious diseases."[19] It was emphasized that disease transmission in either direction (patient to DHCW or DHCW to patient) could be minimized by following the infection-control guidelines. In addition, vaccination for HBV was strongly recommended for dental personnel as a supplement to, not a replacement for, strict adherence to universal precautions.

The guidelines for dentistry, updated and released in July 1993, represent a logical progression of knowledge in the emerging science of infection control and exposure management.[20] The new recommendations emphasize behavior-driven components of exposure control and issues of patient safety, including providing a clear understanding of disease transmission mechanisms and associated risk. The overall premise is the same as in 1986, that "Dental patients and DHCWs may be exposed to a variety of microorganisms via blood or oral respiratory secretions. . . . Infection via any of these routes requires that all three of the fol-

lowing conditions be present: a susceptible host; a pathogen with sufficient infectivity and numbers to cause infection; and a portal through which the pathogen may enter the host. Effective infection control strategies are intended to break one or more of these links in the chain, thereby preventing infection."* In addition, there is a shift from the earlier emphasis on bloodborne disease transmission to now include airborne disease concerns, such as *Mycobacterium tuberculosis* and other upper respiratory illnesses. These new recommendations are intended to provide direction where there is no current regulation from OSHA.

Other major guidelines for infection control were released in 1987[21] and 1988[22] from the CDC and referred, in part, to all health care workers but also, in part, specifically to DHCWs. The CDC now made note of the fact, cited previously, that the antibody status of most patients would not be known; therefore these recommendations were to apply to all patients and all health care workers who performed or assisted in invasive procedures. The 1987 guidelines were the first to introduce the concept of universal precautions. All previous recommendations were selective precautions. The recommendations included the wearing of gloves and other personal protective barriers such as masks and eyewear, the handling of needles and other sharp instruments in such a manner as to prevent injury, and the management of specific exposure incidents with a potential for disease transmission. In the recommendations specific to dentistry it was emphasized that gloves were to be regarded as single-use items. Handwashing, the use of masks, protective eyewear, gowns where indicated, disinfection of environmental surfaces, and sterilization of instruments were more fully defined. The precautions recommended for dentistry began to recognize that blood,

*See *MMWR Morb Mortal Wkly Rep* 42 (No.RR-8), 1993.

saliva, and gingival fluid should be considered infective. Handpiece sterilization and infection control procedures for dental laboratory cases emerged as important issues for dentistry. All these recommendations became the basis for the OSHA blood-borne pathogens standard.

Risk to dental health care workers

The first case of occupationally acquired HIV infection, by a needlestick, was reported in Africa in 1984. It also became apparent during this period (1988 to 1990) that DHCWs were themselves susceptible to becoming infected.[23] Indeed, two dentists were reported to have most likely seroconverted as a result of occupational exposure.

As of December 31, 1996, 52 health care workers had been reported to the CDC as having a documented occupational transmission of HIV, through a special study set up to monitor health care workers.[12] *Documented* means that seroconversion occurred after an occupational exposure to blood known to be infected with HIV. This exposed DHCW must also have had a baseline HIV test that was negative at the time of exposure, and seroconversion must have occurred 3 to 6 months later. Among the documented cases, 45 reported percutaneous exposures; 5 reported blood splashes to the eyes, nose, or mouth; 1 reported percutaneous and mucotaneous exposure; and 1 an unknown route. Forty-seven were exposed to blood of an HIV-infected person, 1 to visibly blood-contaminated bodily fluid, 1 to an unspecified fluid, and 3 to concentrated virus in a laboratory. Subsequently, AIDS has developed in 24 of these HCWs.

This report may not represent the total number of exposed and infected health care workers because it may not include those not reporting an occupational exposure or infection. No DHCWs have been reported through this surveillance system as a documented occupa-

tional infection. Reporting occupational incidents to agencies is important in tracking not just seroconversion but the routes and circumstances of the injury as well. The CDC has two programs for voluntary reporting. For incidents related to known HIV-infected source individuals the report is to the National Center for Infectious Disease's Hospital Infections Program. To report documented HIV seroconversion, contact the local or state health department, which reports to the CDC. In addition, reports of medical device failures that may have facilitated the injury should go to the FDA Medwatch program. This program is designed for health care workers to report adverse events and product problems.

One hundred eleven health care workers have been reported to the CDC as a "possible occupational transmission" and among these are seven dental workers. These health care workers have been investigated and are "without identifiable behavioral or transfusion risks; each reported percutaneous or mucotaneous occupational exposures to blood or body fluids, or lab solutions, but HIV seroconversion specifically resulting from an occupational exposure was not determined."[12] Occupational exposure control is a serious issue. In February 1995, OSHA issued a guide to dental employer obligations as a follow-up to the blood-borne pathogens standard in regard to occupational exposure.[24] These detail, in a step-by-step guide to compliance, the recommendations and regulations regarding management of exposure incidents in oral health facilities (Fig. 17-1). The employer is obligated to provide, not perform, a confidential medical evaluation and follow-up by a licensed health care professional at no cost to the employee.

Among the medical services that the employee must be offered are counseling, collection and testing of the employee's blood, postexposure prophylaxis (in accordance with U.S. Public Health Service recommendations) and evaluation of reported illnesses. The employer

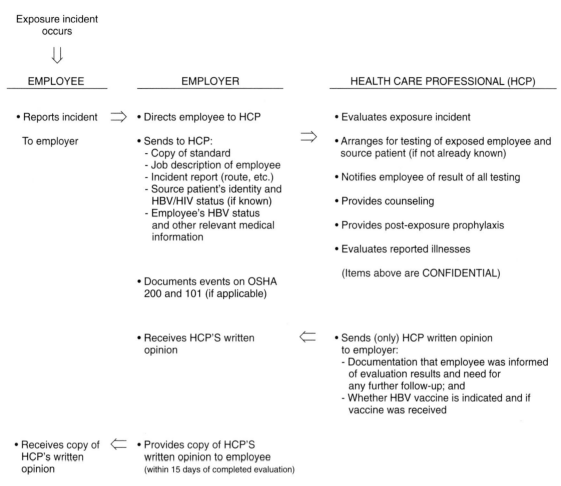

Exposure incident
occurs

⇓

| EMPLOYEE | EMPLOYER | HEALTH CARE PROFESSIONAL (HCP) |

• Reports incident ⇒ • Directs employee to HCP

To employer

• Sends to HCP: ⇒
  - Copy of standard
  - Job description of employee
  - Incident report (route, etc.)
  - Source patient's identity and
    HBV/HIV status (if known)
  - Employee's HBV status
    and other relevant medical
    information

• Documents events on OSHA
200 and 101 (if applicable)

• Receives HCP'S written ⇐ • Sends (only) HCP written opinion
opinion   to employer:
            - Documentation that employee was informed
              of evaluation results and need for
              any further follow-up; and
            - Whether HBV vaccine is indicated and if
              vaccine was received

• Evaluates exposure incident

• Arranges for testing of exposed employee and
  source patient (if not already known)

• Notifies employee of result of all testing

• Provides counseling

• Provides post-exposure prophylaxis

• Evaluates reported illnesses

(Items above are CONFIDENTIAL)

• Receives copy of ⇐ • Provides copy of HCP'S
HCP's written   written opinion to employee
opinion   (within 15 days of completed evaluation)

Fig. 17-1. *Postexposure evaluation and follow-up requirements under OSHA's Standard for occupational exposure to bloodborne pathogens: a guide to dental employer obligations,* Washington, 1995, Department of Labor, Occupational Safety Health Administration.

is only obligated to pay for the cost of treating the incident and not the cost of the subsequent disease should seroconversion occur. All exposure incidents are recordable for purposes of OSHA's recordkeeping requirements. Testing of source patients is in accordance with state laws and with consent of the patient. The U.S. Public Health Service did not officially recommend zidovudine (ZDV) for HIV postexposure prophylaxis until recently. OSHA therefore did

not require the employer to pay for it.[25] It would be prudent to assume that OSHA would expect the employer to now pay for the antiviral regimen since there have been changes in the U.S. Public Health Service recommendations. Previously the U.S. Public Health Service neither recommended nor advised against the use of ZDV for postexposure prophylaxis. However, the agency did recommend offering it to an exposed health care worker. Findings released by the CDC in December 1995 associate the use of ZDV with a lower risk for HIV transmission after studying its use in health care workers who sustained percutaneous injuries to blood known to be infected with HIV.[26] The data suggest that "use of ZDV postexposure may be protective for healthcare workers." The study investigated factors associated with HIV transmission, such as exposure to a large quantity of blood, a deep injury, a visibly contaminated device and terminal illness in the source patient. "Risk for HIV infection among healthcare workers who used ZDV was reduced approximately 79 percent" with other factors controlled. These results prompted the U.S. Public Health Service to evaluate the data and to propose revisions for postexposure management (PEM) on the basis of the severity of an injury and the HIV status of the source patient. Newly released recommendations for PEM of individuals exposed to blood known to be infected with HIV include the use of antiretrovirals either as monotherapy or in combination as determined by source individual and injury information.[27] The current U.S. Public Health Service recommendation is that health care workers who are exposed to HIV on the job should, in many cases, take zidovudine and other antiretroviral drugs after exposure to reduce their risk of becoming infected.

Injury data on DHCWs has been derived from observational, retrospective, and prospective studies (including self-reported data). In 1987 dentists reported about 1 injury in a month, 12 per year. By 1991 dentists reported 0.3 per month, about 3 to 4 per year. More recent data from the CDC indicate a further decline to about 0.18 per month, 2 to 3 per year. This supports the assumption that most injuries are preventable with appropriate administrative, engineering, and work practice controls. Most percutaneous injuries occurred outside the patients' mouth, most on the hands of the dentist. Burs were the most common

source (37%), followed by syringe needles (30%), sharp instruments (21%), and orthodontic wires (6%). The CDC stated that "the rate of percutaneous exposures among dental workers . . . is probably less than among general surgical personnel. Most injuries are outside the mouth, involve the fingers and hands and are self-inflicted."[28]

Of a total population of more than 213,357 professionally active dentists and dental hygienists, the current estimate of dentists and dental hygienists with AIDS is only 424, of which about 332 have died.[11] There are possibly more than 2000 DHCWs with HIV. The best estimates of risk to health care workers is 0.3% for HIV transmission from percutaneous exposures and 0.09% for mucous membrane exposures (even less for skin contacts), 3% to 10% for hepatitis C and 30% for HBV transmission after percutaneous injury from an infected patient.[29] From the data available, it appears that the risk of HIV infection to DHCWs is extremely low. Health care workers represent about 5% of the general population and about 5% of reported AIDS cases, indicating that they are not overrepresented.

Risk to patients

DHCWs had already recognized the potential to transmit disease in either direction. HBV transmission had been well documented from dentists to patients, as well as herpes transmission from dental hygienists to patients. Indeed, health care workers, primarily physicians and dentists, have a threefold to fivefold higher prevalence of HBV than the general population does. However, transmission from HIV-infected health care workers to patients had not yet been reported. Since the early 1970s, when serologic testing became available for HBV, the CDC had reported on 20 clusters of HBV transmission to more than 300 patients from infected health care workers. In 12 of the clusters the health care worker did not routinely use gloves, and some reported skin lesions that could have promoted the transmission. Nine of these clusters were linked to dentists or oral surgeons. Many of the transmissions could have been prevented by strict adherence to current universal precautions. Most of the reports were before the acceptance of universal precautions. The CDC[30] suggested, "The limited number of reports of HBV transmission from HCWs [health care workers] to patients in recent years may reflect the adoption of universal precautions and increased use of HBV vaccine."

Previous experience with HBV transmission suggested that the performance of invasive procedures was more likely to contribute to disease transmission, that the use of universal precautions was likely to reduce the risk of transmission, and that this transmission would be expected to "occur only very rarely."[21] Therefore routine testing of health care workers was not recommended. Recent reports of HBV transmission from a health care worker to patients during performance of invasive, exposure-prone procedures are not among dentists, but refer to a surgeon who is HBeAg(+) and had not been vaccinated against HBV. About 1% of surgeons are infected with HBV and transmission is thought to be rare.[31] In 1992 a female patient was diagnosed with HBV and transmission was associated with cardiac surgery. No deficiencies in infection control were detected and no specific events could be identified. HBV was transmitted to at least 19 patients studied and epidemiologic and laboratory evidence "support the surgeon as the source of infection." Factors of transmission were more likely related to irritations on the surgeons' fingers, and virus, which may have escaped through tiny holes in the gloves, was found in the glove washings. Health care workers who are positive for HBeAg are more infectious, and reports of transmission of HBV since the early 1970s have been associated with this state.

Hepatitis C virus (HCV) transmission in health care facilities has also been documented.

In a study conducted from 1992 to 1994, five patients of a cardiac surgeon were identified in whom infection may have been transmitted by the surgeon. All were infected with the same HCV genotype. The surgeon reported one serious percutaneous exposure from a patient with HBV and was treated for this exposure. Overall, the surgeon reported a rate of about 20 percutaneous injuries per 100 procedures, most of which went unnoticed until after the procedure.[32] This resembles reports of HBV transmission in surgical and dental settings as a cluster of cases. There is also a report of simultaneous transmission of HIV and HCV to a health care worker who sustained a deep needlestick injury from an HIV/HCV-infected source patient in 1990. Use of ZDV was declined. This is the first report of simultaneous transmission.[33]

When the inevitable became the actual with the first report of transmission of HIV from an infected health care worker to a patient during an invasive procedure,[34] it was indeed in dentistry. The first report of a "possible" transmission to "patient A" came in the July 1990 issue of the CDC's *Morbidity and Mortality Weekly Report*.[35] By January 1991 the transmission was no longer considered merely possible, and the report then read, "Update: Transmission of HIV Infection During an Invasive Dental Procedure."[36] The concept of transmission from health care worker to patient had progressed from highly improbable to possible to probable in less than a year, and the involvement had increased from one to six patients.[37] These events, leading up to the death of patient A, Kimberly Bergalis, left an indelible imprint on dentistry.

Guidelines for HIV/HBV–infected dental health care workers

The public outcry over the first real victim of AIDS was deafening. Conservative congressmen called for stiff measures, from jailing infected health care workers who continued to practice to mandatory testing of all health care workers. One of the most serious possible consequences of this event for the health care field in general could be the loss of the professional control over the future of health care workers. At a minimum, proposals ranged from reviewing the health status of infected health care workers (HIV and HBV) by expert review panels to mandatory testing and patient notification. By an act of Congress in October 1991 states were given 1 year in which to adopt the CDC "recommendations for preventing transmission of human immunodeficiency virus and hepatitis B virus to patients during exposure-prone invasive procedures" or else to come up with their equivalent and have it approved by the CDC; all states have complied.[38] In essence, the CDC recommendations cited by Congress are based on a series of assumptions as to the likelihood of transmitting disease from infected providers to patients:

1. Infected health care workers who adhere to universal precautions and who do not perform invasive procedures pose no risk for transmitting HIV or HBV to patients.
2. Infected health care workers who adhere to universal precautions and who perform certain exposure-prone procedures pose a small risk for transmitting HBV to patients.
3. HIV is transmitted much less readily than HBV.

The key phrase is "exposure-prone procedures," and the problem is how to define them and how and when to restrict their practice by infected health care workers. The task may have seemed simple at first, with the plan being to have the professions determine a list of exposure-prone procedures. It proved, however, to be far from a simple matter, and professional organizations either refused to produce a list, were unable to come up with lists, or felt that it was not in their best interest to list these procedures. Data from the CDC were challenged during public testimony by, for ex-

ample, the American Dental Association and the University of Texas Health Science Center at San Antonio, which presented testimony offering that the rates of injury were lower than those estimated by the CDC and that therefore their assumption that 13 to 128 patients were infected with HIV and 406 to 4057 with HBV by surgeons and DHCWs during an invasive procedure was incorrect (*The Nation's Health*, April 1991). A more accurate measure of provider-to-patient transmission potential is not possible until a much larger sample of patients on whom exposure-prone invasive procedures were performed can be studied. Looking back at more than 22,032 patients of 63 HIV-infected providers (including 33 dentists or dental students), no other case of transmission of HIV has been discovered.[39] In 15 years only one cluster of cases has been linked to provider transmission. The CDC cites the risk from an infected health care worker, more specifically, a dentist, to transmit HIV to a patient is between 1 in 263,100 to 1 in 2,631,000 dental procedures. There have been more than two billion dental procedures performed in the United States since the beginning of the AIDS epidemic and not a single documented case of occupationally acquired HIV infection among DHCWs.

Whatever plan a state adopts, it must be in compliance with statutes and court actions on discrimination and disability such as Section 504 of the Rehabilitation Act of 1973, the Americans with Disabilities Act of 1990, and any pertinent state laws. All states have submitted plans to the CDC or verified that they will comply with existing CDC guidelines. The literature suggests that a majority of states rejected mandatory testing in favor of voluntary testing, rejected patient notification, recommended the use of expert review panels, and emphasized the importance of education, training, and the use of universal precautions. Preliminary findings from a research project by a dental intern from Harvard University

School of Dental Medicine in conjunction with the Boston Public Health Commission, HIV Dental Ombudsperson Program, indicate that of states validated as in compliance with CDC guidelines 100% rejected mandatory testing, 96% rejected patient notification, 71% recommended the use of expert review panels for HIV-positive DHCWs and 63% for HBV-negative DHCWs, 90% emphasized the importance of education and training, and 98% recommended the use of universal precautions. Furthermore, 86% stated that currently available data provide no basis for recommendations to restrict HIV- or HBV-positive DHCWs who perform invasive procedures.[30]

OSHA regulations

It is important to note that the recommendations of the CDC are not regulatory, only advisory. Although they may set professional standards, they do not have full legal force behind them. However, these recommendations became, for OSHA, the basis for the final rule on occupational exposure to blood-borne pathogens, issued on December 6, 1991. As an OSHA administrator remarked, "We are providing full legal force to universal precautions—employers and employees must treat blood and certain body fluids as if infectious. Meeting these requirements is not optional. It's essential to prevent illness, chronic infection and even death."[16] The U.S. Department of Labor expects this standard to protect more than 5.6 million workers and prevent more than 200 deaths and 9200 blood-borne infections each year.

The purpose of the OSHA standard is to minimize occupational exposure to blood or other potentially infectious body fluids or materials that pose a risk of transmission of blood-borne disease in a health care setting. It covers any employee exposed, or potentially exposed, during the performance of his or her duties, to blood, body fluids, or potentially infectious materials. Health and safety are recognized as one

aspect of practice administration. Although the OSHA obligates the employer to provide for the employee, free of charge, a series of hazard abatement measures to diminish the risk of exposure, they are in the best interest of each DHCW and will pay for themselves by ensuring a safe dental practice. Some costs are one-time improvements (e.g., an eyewash station) and preventive measures (HBV vaccination), whereas others, such as gloves and masks, are recurring costs. The OSHA estimates that the annual cost per dental establishment, of which there are 100,174, to be about $873. The highest-cost area is personal protective equipment, followed by vaccination and postexposure follow-up. Some costs may vary, depending on the length of employment, turnover, and actual office experience with injuries.

The hazard abatement measures include mandating the use of universal precautions, emphasizing engineering and work practice controls, providing and requiring employees to use personal protective equipment, making available the hepatitis B vaccination (and associated tests and boosters) at no cost to the employee, making available specific procedures for employees who sustain an occupational exposure (including confidential medical evaluation and follow-up), and the communication of hazards to employees by warning signs and labels. The OSHA further mandates that the training provided relate specifically to information about the standard itself, the particular office exposure control plan contemplated, and information about the transmission of blood-borne disease. There are requirements on identifying at-risk employees and their tasks within the context of a written exposure control plan. This plan must be specific as to how the office will comply with the standard. Employers have recordkeeping requirements, including written schedules for housekeeping, plans for waste management, and exposure management.

Some states have their own occupational safety and health plans that may differ from the federal standard. DHCWs should become familiar with their state plan or the federal standard, as appropriate. It will also be necessary to review individual state and local regulations on infectious and hazardous waste management and disposal because there is no federal standard on dental waste as yet. The Environmental Protection Agency did have a pilot medical waste tracking act and will consider whether to make it national in scope.

The OSHA blood-borne standard is not the only regulation from the Department of Labor of concern to dentistry. In 1987, the OSHA extended the hazard communication standard to the health care industry.[40] The standard became final for the health care industry in 1989. The intent of this standard is to protect health care workers from hazards associated with the use of chemical agents during the course of employment. The standard is based on the simple concept that employees have a need and a right to know the hazards and identities of the chemicals to which they are exposed. Employers are obligated to identify and list hazardous chemicals in their workplaces, obtain material data safety sheets (MDSSs) for these chemicals, develop and implement a written hazard communication program, and communicate hazard information to their employees through labels, MDSSs, and formal training programs. Employees must understand what personal protective equipment is necessary to prevent illness or injury and how to manage an exposure incident or an emergency. Unlike the blood-borne standard, training in hazard communication must occur before an initial assignment. Training in both blood-borne exposure and chemical hazard exposure must be renewed whenever the hazard changes. Training is required to be specific to the agents used by an employee.

Transmissible diseases

The oral cavity harbors microorganisms with potential to transmit a wide spectrum of infectious agents. Dental professionals are therefore at risk for any orally transmissible disease from the blood or saliva of the patients they treat. In addition, the trauma of some dental procedures and the mixing of blood and saliva enhance the risk of blood-borne disease transmission. Any patient's blood or saliva is potentially infectious and puts the DHCW at risk.

Before the HIV epidemic there was concern over the transmission of disease in dental settings, and HBV drove the model for infection control. Although HBV is still the basis of infection control procedures, HIV drives many of the evolving regulations and guidelines. The transmissible diseases currently of greatest concern to the dental professional are HBV, HIV, HCV, and *Mycobacterium* tuberculosis, although the list of transmissible diseases is more widely encompassing. Each of these diseases will be discussed in terms of etiology, tests available for diagnosis, risk of transmission, and recommendations for prevention in the professional context.

HEPATITIS B

The disease is produced by a virus known as the Dane particle. This intact virus consists of an inner core antigen (HB_cAg) and an outer coat surface antigen (HB_sAg) and is highly infective. As little as 0.00000001 ml of blood can transmit the disease. Initial symptoms may include the following: vague abdominal discomfort, myalgia, diarrhea, jaundice (30% of cases), lack of appetite, and low-grade fever. However, approximately 80% of individuals infected with the virus are asymptomatic and unaware that they are infected. People who are infected with the virus can transmit HBV whether or not they manifest clinical signs and symptoms. HBV is one of the most common reportable diseases in the United States and is "primarily a disease of young adults, with about 75% of cases occurring in persons aged 15 to 39."[41] Cases reported underestimate the rate of true infection because of the subclinical state. Health care providers also underreport cases despite laws that mandate reporting. The CDC estimates, after correcting for underreporting, that "approximately 300,000 HBV infections occur in the United States each year." The most serious consequence is not acute infection but chronic carrier states that occur in about 6% to 10% of adults, more in children. These carriers also represent a population at risk of spreading infection.

"HBV infection is the major infectious occupational hazard to health care workers."[41] Healthcare workers represent about 2% to 6% of reported cases and this recognition and the availability of the HBV vaccine was the driving force behind the development of the OSHA blood-borne pathogens standard.

Fortunately for dental professionals, a vaccine has been developed to immunize recipients against HBV. Three doses are given to confer immunity: an initial dose, followed by a second dose at 1 month, and then a third dose 6 months after the first. Given dental personnel's high risk of contracting HBV, it is strongly recommended that all dental professionals be immunized. Indeed, there is great emphasis on vaccination in the OSHA blood-borne pathogens standard where the employer is obligated to provide the vaccination free of charge to potentially exposed employees with a specific waiver to be signed by an employee who declines the vaccine. The risks associated with HBV include not only the morbidity of the acute phase of the disease but also the possible sequelae of the chronic carrier state, including cirrhosis of the liver or primary hepatocellular carcinoma. There are no current recommendations for a booster dose of the vaccine, although some have suggested titer testing to determine if an immune response is evident. Although the vaccine is successful in more than 90% of individuals, some do not initially respond, do not develop HB_sAg and therefore are not protected; however, in a majority of these cases an additional dose is effective. There is a very small percent who never respond and in whom immunity cannot be assured.

Approximately 86% of DHCWs have been vaccinated.[42] Before the vaccine, about 250 health care workers died per year as a result of complications from HBV. After compliance with the vaccination recommendations, the estimate dropped to about 100 per year. Vaccination should be received before exposure occurs or it will be of no benefit.

Serologic testing is available to determine the presence in the blood of HBV antigens and antibodies to those antigens. The presence of hepatitis B core antigen (HB_cAg) is associated with active viral infection and infectivity. The hepatitis B surface antigen (HB_sAg) appears before acute illness and usually disappears quickly. Antihepatitis B core antibody (anti-HB_cAb) is not protective, appears early in the illness, and decreases in titer in those who become immune. Persistent high titer indicates ongoing infectivity. HB_sAb does not appear for several months and then rises to a high titer in those who become immune. The e antigen (HB_eAg) is associated with higher risk of chronic liver disease and higher risk of infectivity. Also of concern is delta hepatitis (HDV), a single-stranded circular RNA virus. Often referred to as the "delta agent," this is a defective virus that relies on HBV for its pathogenicity. It is a piggyback virus that cannot infect on its own but depends on the presence of HBV for infectivity. The combination results in a "supervirus" and a more fulminant course of disease. Vaccination against HBV will prevent HDV coinfection, as long as the person has not already become an unknown HBV carrier. For an estimated 1% of health care workers who are HBV carriers, prevention of HDV would be difficult. Essentially, prevention relies on strict compliance with universal precautions and practicing in such a manner as to avoid injury or exposure. Research is being conducted on the use of interferon alpha or other antiviral agents.

HEPATITIS C

Hepatitis viruses that were not A and not B became known as NANB, non-A, non-B in the early 1970s. Diagnosis was not based on identification of an agent but by mode of transmission, for example, whether it was serologic or enteric. In 1989 one of the NANB viruses was identified as hepatitis C (HCV), a single-stranded RNA virus that appears to have cytopathic activity. HCV is implicated in viral hepatitis and is of concern to DHCWs. Transmission is similar to HBV in the parenteral routes identified and mostly is associated with intravenous drug use or administration of blood products, less with sexual or vertical transmission. HCV has been found in saliva. As with HBV, acute infection is usually asymptomatic and may go undetected.[43] Studies indicate that HCV may be responsible for 90% of the posttransfusion hepatitis and about 60% to 70% of sporadic NANB hepatitis. The community prevalence of anti-HCV has ranged from 1% to 3% in the United States. About 170,000 people become infected each year and mortality is estimated at 8000 to 10,000 per year. The clinical course of the disease is similar to HBV. At least 50% will, however, have chronic hepatitis, and 20% of these chronic carriers will have cirrhosis or even hepatocellular carcinoma.

Blood transfusions are thought to be the most efficient route of transmission. A screening test for HCV antibody was developed in 1990; however, the test fails to detect all infections and has a low predictive value in populations with low prevalence. A supplemental or confirmatory test comparable to that available for HBV is needed to eliminate false-positive and identify true-positive results. However, this was not available with first-generation tests and only by specific physician request with second-generation tests. Third-generation tests are being released and more data are needed to determine their efficacy. These tests also fail to differentiate between active HCV infection, immunity to HCV, or a carrier state.[43] Screening of blood donors has reduced the risk of transmission associated with transfusions by about 80% in studies conducted in the early

1990s. Fewer than 5% of cases now reported to the CDC are related to transfusions. There is no consistently effective antiviral treatment nor is there a vaccine or postexposure prophylaxis available, so therefore prevention is paramount. Compared with HBV, HCV is less transmissible after a single exposure. The average risk of infection after a needlestick injury has "ranged from 2 to 3 percent."[31] This range falls between risk estimates of HBV and HIV transmission. In terms of acute infections annually, HBV is most prevalent and HCV next; however, higher rates of chronic infection and death are reported with HCV.[28] HCV seroconversions are more likely to occur where there are breaches of infection control. The CDC stresses that, "Bloodborne pathogens, wherever they are and whatever the titer, can be transmitted in either direction." The most important steps a DHCW can take is the appropriate use of recommended hazard abatement procedures to prevent exposure.

It does not appear that health care workers (including dentists) have a disproportionate rate of HCV infection. Results of a voluntary study suggest that the rate of infection of health care workers may even be less than found in voluntary blood donors.[44] As expected, the risk is more evident in health care workers frequently exposed to large quantities of blood. In one study the highest infection rate was among maintenance workers.[43] Among health care workers in the early 1970s, as detection became available, HBV rates were as high as 17%, whereas HCV rates are significantly lower. This low risk estimate is validated by at least one needlestick study wherein HCV developed in only 4% after injury from blood known to be HCV positive, and in only three health care workers was seroconversion demonstrated. Other studies have shown anywhere from 0% to 1.3% seroprevalence of anti-HCV in health care workers. There appear to be significant differences between HBV and HCV in terms of transmission risk to health care workers. However, there are very few studies of DHCWs.

TUBERCULOSIS

Although the major infectious diseases of greatest concern to dentistry are HBV, HCV, and HIV/AIDS, other diseases pose a risk to the health care worker. Of emerging concern is tuberculosis (TB), which made a comeback in direct proportion to AIDS cases.

"Tuberculosis is a recognized risk in health-care settings."[45] A 1990 report by the CDC was prompted by outbreaks of TB over recent years, including some multidrug-resistant strains. Transmission is most likely from patients without recognized disease, not from those receiving anti-TB therapy. Environmental factors, such as inadequate ventilation and contact with patients in "small, enclosed areas," can play a part in transmission. Estimates are that for every active TB case there are 15 asymptomatic yet infected people. The risk of disease progression after infection may be heightened in persons with HIV disease.

In April 1994 OSHA issued a notice of proposed rule making for a standard to regulate indoor air quality, which is currently in a comment and review period. The standard is designed for nonindustrial workplaces; the effect on dental facilities is undetermined, but it may consider the effects of aerosolized dental unit water. Also, in 1992 OSHA was petitioned, much in the same fashion as with the Bloodborne Pathogens Standard, for a national compliance directive on occupational exposure to TB. When no action was taken, the Secretary of Labor was petitioned in August 1993 to initiate rule making to promulgate a national standard on TB. As a result, on October 20, 1993, OSHA issued "Enforcement Guidance in the Face of Increased Exposure to Tuberculosis," which is based on guidelines issued by the CDC in 1990 for preventing the transmission of tuberculosis in health care settings. In October 1994, CDC issued the final version of "Guidelines for Pre-

venting the Transmission of *Mycobacterium tuberculosis* in Health-Care Facilities." The intent is to emphasize the importance of a hierarchy of control measures to reduce the risk of exposure. The fundamentals of TB infection control are not based on universal precautions but require the application of a selective hierarchy of controls to identify, isolate, and treat TB. The three levels of control include administrative measures, engineering controls, and personal respiratory equipment. Measures recommended are based on community and facility risk of exposure to TB. Most oral health care facilities fall into the minimal or very low risk determinations. The CDC provides specific guidance for dental facilities depending on the setting. At a minimum, a risk assessment must be done annually; there must be a written TB infection control plan; protocols should be in place for identifying and managing patients who have active TB; DHCWs must be educated, trained, and screened; and a method of evaluating problems must be established. With specific regard to oral health care facilities, the CDC states, "In general, the symptoms for which patients seek treatment in a dental care setting are not likely to be caused by infectious TB. Unless a patient requiring dental care coincidentally has TB, it is unlikely that infectious TB will be encountered in the dental setting. Furthermore, it has not been demonstrated that oral health care procedures generate TB droplet nuclei. Therefore, the risk for transmission of *M. tuberculosis* in most dental settings is probably quite low." More specifically, the CDC recommends that patient medical histories include questions on TB and that those with suggestive symptoms be referred for medical evaluation. Such patients should not remain in the dental care facility any longer than required for a referral and should wear masks and be instructed to cover their mouths and noses when coughing or sneezing. Elective dental treatment should be deferred until a physician confirms that the patient does not have infectious TB. If urgent care is required, such care should be rendered in a facility that can provide TB isolation. DHCWs providing care in these circumstances should use respiratory protection. DHCWs symptomatic for TB should be evaluated and not return to the workplace until a diagnosis of TB has been excluded or until the DHCW is on therapy and determined to be noninfectious.

Prevention: infection control

Because treatment of HBV, HCV, HIV/AIDS, and other transmissible diseases is symptomatic at best, prevention is the most important aspect in the discussion of these diseases. Even if a cure were available, protection from the untoward effects and discomfort of each disease would be desirable. Because many diseases can go undetected for long periods of time, the focus must be on preventing disease transmission from providers to patients, from patients to providers, and between patients and families. Again, it is important to emphasize that one of the most important personnel barriers is the HBV vaccine, and as a result the CDC has recommended its inclusion in the childhood vaccination series.[41]

In 1993 the CDC updated all previously published recommendations relative to infection control in dental facilities.[20] The following recommendations should be used routinely in the care of *all* patients in dental practice to control the spread of infection.

Medical history

Always obtain a complete medical history. Include specific questions about lymphadenopathy, recent weight loss, and infections. Follow up on all positive responses. Remember that an individual may not be aware of an infectious state, so diagnostic acumen may be required.

Vaccinations

Vaccines for vaccine-preventable diseases are indicated for all DHCWs. OSHA recommends that all health care workers with potential for exposure be offered the HBV vaccination at no charge.

Protective attire and barrier techniques

Protective attire and barrier techniques should be used wherever there is the potential for contacting blood, blood-contaminated saliva, or mucous membranes. This includes, but is not limited to, the use of appropriate personal protective equipment such as gloves, masks, chin-length face shields, and protective eyewear when involved in procedures likely to generate splashing or splattering of blood or other potentially infectious materials, as is the case in most dental procedures. These should be changed when visibly contaminated or compromised and between patients. They should be removed when leaving the patient area. Protective clothing is indicated when contamination is likely. Appropriate maintenance and disposal should be in accordance with OSHA and CDC recommendations. Environmental barriers are indicated for surfaces that are difficult to clean and disinfect and that may become contaminated during oral health care procedures. These should be removed and replaced between patients in accordance with state and federal recommendations. Use of rubber dams, high-velocity evacuation, and proper patient positioning will minimize aerosolization.

Handwashing and care of hands

Handwashing is indicated before and after patient care, at any time hands become contaminated (even if gloved), and after touching surfaces likely to be contaminated. Handwashing with plain soap is adequate for examinations and nonsurgical procedures. Antimicrobial surgical hand scrubbing is necessary with surgical procedures. Gloves compromised by a puncture or tear should be removed as soon as patient safety permits, hands should be thoroughly washed, and new gloves used when continuing patient care. NOTE: The CDC recommends that "DHCWs who have exudative lesions or weeping dermatitis, particularly on the hands, should refrain from all direct patient care and from handling dental patient-care equipment until the condition resolves."

Use and care of sharp instruments and needles

Any sharp instrument, contaminated or not, should be considered potentially infectious and handled in a manner such as to prevent injuries. Needles should not be recapped or otherwise manipulated with both hands nor should a technique that involves directing the point of a needle toward any part of the body (the operator's or someone else's) be used. A one-handed technique or a mechanical device designed to isolate a needlestick hazard should be used. Disposal of all sharp instruments, including needles, scalpel blades, and other items or instruments, should be in puncture-resistant containers located as close as practical to their area of use. Removal of needles from nondisposable syringes should not be attempted if uncapped, and recapping only by approved methods with one hand should be used.

Sterilization or disinfection of instruments

Reprocessing of instruments used in dental practices should follow the classifications of critical (used to penetrate soft-tissue or bone and require sterilization), semicritical (do not penetrate, but have contact with oral tissues and should be sterilized if capable of withstanding the process or at least high-level disinfection), and noncritical (contact skin and require intermediate or low-level disinfection). Appropriate cleaning and use of appropriate personal protective equipment during reprocessing is necessary. CDC guidelines should be reviewed for reprocessing. Critical and semicritical heat-stable instruments should be routinely sterilized by autoclave, dry heat, or chemical vapor, with appropriate packaging and in biologically monitored units. Use of high-level disinfection should be according to

manufacturers' directions with Environmental Protection Agency–registered agents. CDC guidelines should be reviewed.

Cleaning and disinfection of dental unit and environmental surfaces

All surfaces that become contaminated should be appropriately maintained according to schedules recommended in the guidelines with Environmental Protection Agency–registered tuberculocidal hospital disinfectants.[11] General housekeeping in keeping with the guidelines may be accomplished through the use of low-level Environmental Protection Agency–registered chemical agents. These agents are not recommended for critical or semicritical instruments.

Disinfection in the dental laboratory

Manufacturers' guidelines should be reviewed for appropriate cleaning and disinfection of materials before they are manipulated in the laboratory, after handling, and before placement in the patient's mouth. At least an intermediate-level disinfectant is recommended. The dental facility and laboratory should review the guidelines and establish communication.

Use and care of handpieces, antiretraction valves, and other intraoral dental devices attached to air and water lines of dental units

All high-speed dental handpieces, low-speed components used intraorally, and reusable prophy angles should be sterilized between patients by a heating process capable of sterilization. Manufacturers' directions should be reviewed. Surface disinfection is not acceptable. Retraction valves should be used to prevent fluid aspiration and reduce the potential of transmitting infectious material. Routine maintenance is required. Flushing of water lines and discharging water and air from high-speed handpieces is indicated. The guidelines should be consulted for details.

Single-use disposable instruments

Single-use disposable instruments are not designed or intended for reuse and should be appropriately handled and disposed of properly.

Use of extracted teeth in dental education settings

Extracted teeth should be considered infective and be handled with universal precautions in the same manner as a biopsy specimen. Workers in contact with extracted teeth should be vaccinated against HBV. Guidelines should be reviewed for cleaning and disinfection. Extracted teeth given to a patient are not considered regulated waste.

Disposal of waste materials

State, local, and federal guidelines should be reviewed and waste disposed of according to the requirements and published recommendations.

Other recommendations

Written protocols and training should be in place in all dental facilities. In addition, research into factors that may contribute to the risk of transmission of blood-borne pathogens and other infectious agents is necessary to assess risk and offer suggestions to reduce risk.

These guidelines are meant to provide the reader with an awareness of the precautions that should become a routine part of the daily practice of dentistry. Variations on these basic precepts may exist within certain school, clinic, or hospital settings. However, common sense and good judgment will help each professional determine the best preventive techniques for each environment. Because the art and science of infection control is continually evolving, practitioners must make every effort to remain up-to-date through continuing education and by reviewing journals and other resources.

AIDS and HIV disease have generated a new set of professional standards for infection control, a series of federal obligations to meet these standards, and other federal regulations to deal with the chemicals we use in controlling infection. However, HIV disease has also presented dentistry with the insidious issue of discrimination. In their 1990 report on AIDS discrimination, the American Civil Liberties Union noted that the most frequent complaints were against dentists and nursing homes.[46] "Dentists turn AIDS patients away," noted Mitchell Karp, a supervising attorney for the New York City AIDS Discrimination Unit. A recent analysis of dental discrimination identified three major factors associated with negative attitudes of dentists toward persons with HIV: (1) fear of infection, (2) concerns about the competence to treat patients with HIV safely or effectively, and (3) business-based concerns about the effect of treating patients with HIV on other patients and staff.[47] The first two factors are reduced by education and experience, but business-based concerns remain significant. There are many other reasons given for refusal to treat: low reimbursement rates by Medicaid, a lack of understanding about the disease, fear of transmission, fear of becoming known as an "AIDS dentist," prejudice, and more.

LEGISLATION AND LITIGATION

Refusals to treat people with HIV/AIDS by dentists and other health care professionals may well be the most common and blatant form of discrimination against people with HIV today.

In a survey of U.S. dentists in 1995, only 50% of male dentists and 38% of female dentists believed that a private dental office was an acceptable location in which to treat people with HIV.[48] During the first 3 years, 1990 to 1993, of the HIV Dental Ombudsperson Program (a Ryan White CARE Act program in Boston) 12% of all callers indicated that they had experienced discrimination by a dentist. About 20% of callers throughout the duration of the program indicated that they were uncomfortable seeking dental care out of a concern over discrimination.[49]

STATE AND FEDERAL DISABILITY DISCRIMINATION LAWS

People with HIV (or other disabilities) are protected under state and federal disability discrimination laws, the Americans with Disabilities Act (AwDA) and the Rehabilitation Act of 1973. Most state statutes and both federal statutes define disability as having the following:

1. A physical or mental impairment that substantially limits one or more of the major life activities of such individual
2. A record of such impairment
3. Being regarded as having such impairment

Courts have uniformly found that people with HIV are protected by disability discrimination laws. The legislative history of the AwDA and interpretive guidelines written by the United States Department of Justice specifically provide that people with asymptomatic HIV are substantially limited in numerous major life activities, including procreation and intimate sexual relations, and are therefore covered by the AwDA. In addition, these individuals are covered by the "regarded as" prong of the definition even if they are not limited in any major life activity.

When Congress passed the Rehabilitation Act of 1973, it was an effort to provide some national protection against discrimination on the basis of a "handicap." The Civil Rights Restoration Act of 1987 added a clarifying position to section 504, "which implicitly acknowledged this act's coverage of HIV infection" (including asymptomatic HIV).[50] Section 504 prohibits discrimination against people with disabilities from agencies or programs who receive federal funds, including private dental or medical offices and hospitals that accept Medicare or Medicaid.

In 1990 Congress passed the AwDA, which extended disability discrimination protection to private places of public accommodation. A place of public accommodation is any place that is open to and accepts the general public, including the professional offices of dentists and physicians. Section 504 was limited in its scope of application to those receiving federal assistance.

Most states also have laws that prohibit discrimination in places of public accommodation that do not receive federal assistance. Many states have similar civil rights laws, which vary in their scope of protection. In addition, most states have regulatory boards that license and discipline DHCWs and can pursue complaints of discrimination. Although each state law is different, the AwDA is the most specific and comprehensive disability discrimination law affecting dental offices.

The AwDA of July 26, 1990, "is perhaps the most sweeping civil rights legislation passed since the enactment of the Civil Rights Act of 1964 nearly 30 years before."[51] The AwDA is "to provide a clear and comprehensive national mandate for the elimination of discrimination against individuals with disabilities" and picks up where Section 504 left off, that is, to extend coverage to those not receiving federal assistance. Titles I and III of the AwDA hold the most significance for dental offices. Title I prohibits employment discrimination and Title III prohibits discrimination by a "place of public accommodation," which explicitly includes the "professional office of a health care provider."

TITLE III OF THE AWDA

Title III is specific in the type of discriminatory conduct that is prohibited. As applied to the delivery of oral health services, it is illegal to do the following:

1. Deny an HIV-positive patient the "full and equal enjoyment" of dental services or to deny an HIV-positive patient the "opportunity to benefit" from dental services in the same manner as other patients
2. Establish for the privilege of receiving dental services "eligibility criteria" that

tend to screen out patients who have tested positive for HIV

3. Provide "different or separate" services to patients who are HIV positive or fail to provide services to patients in the most "integrated setting"

4. Deny equal services to a person who is known to have a "relationship" or "association" with a person with HIV, such as a spouse, partner, child, or friend

Although the act has specific prohibitions against discrimination by places of public accommodation, it does permit the denial of services to an individual where there is a "direct threat to the health and safety of others." The AwDA defines the term "direct threat" as a "significant risk to the health and safety of others that cannot be eliminated by a modification of policies, practices, or procedures." The assessment of whether an individual poses a direct threat is made on the basis of reasonable judgment that relies on current medical knowledge or on the best available objective evidence to ascertain (1) the nature, duration, and severity of the risk; (2) the probability that the potential injury will occur; and (3) whether reasonable modifications to policies, practices, and procedures will mitigate the risk.

Abbott v Bragdon, 912 F. Supp. 580 (D. Me. 1995), a case litigated in federal district court in Bangor, Maine, involved a dentist who had a written policy stating that he did not treat any patient with an active infectious disease, including HIV, in his office. The dentist argued that the performance of invasive dental procedures on a patient with HIV was such a "direct threat" because of the potential for blood-to-blood contact. The plaintiff presented evidence that it is safe to provide routine dental care to persons with HIV. The CDC testified through Donald Wayne Marianos, DDS, MPH, Director of the Oral Health Division, that people with HIV may be safely treated in a private dental office with use of standard universal precautions for all patients. This testimony is of particular importance because the U.S. Supreme Court has specifically ruled that courts addressing the issue whether discrimination against a person with a contagious disease is justified by a health or safety risk "should normally defer to the reasonable medical judgments of public health officials" unless those judgments are "medically unsupportable."[52] The court deferred to the judgment of the CDC in deciding that it is safe to treat patients with HIV and ruled that Dr. Bragdon had not been able to counter that judgment with any admissible evidence about the significance of the risk. Of all facts considered, the court gave the most weight to the "probability" of HIV transmission in dentistry, stating that "[N]either the duration or severity [of HIV infection] outweigh the evidence as to how the disease is transmitted and the slight probability of transmission."[53]

The U.S. Court of Appeals for the First Circuit upheld the trial court's ruling on March 5, 1997. Like the trial court, the appeals court ruled that each of Dr. Bragdon's claims about a "significant risk" of HIV transmission from patient-to-dentist was "too speculative or too tangential" to establish a "direct threat" under the AwDA.[54] The court relied on guidelines from the CDC and the American Dental Association to conclude that it is safe for a dentist to provide routine dental care in a private dental office to a patient with HIV. The court concluded that Dr. Bragdon violated the AwDA by refusing to provide routine dental care in his office to a patient with HIV. Several state public health departments and national public health associations submitted a friend of the court brief indicating that not only is it safe to provide routine dental care to patients with HIV but that a decision for Dr. Bragdon would result in a public health disaster.[55] The American Dental Association filed a brief in support of the dentist arguing, in spite of its policy that a dentist ethically must treat patients with HIV, that people with asymptomatic HIV should not be covered by disability discrimination laws. To date, every court has ruled that it is illegal for a dentist to refuse to treat a patient on the basis of HIV status. It is important to remember, however, that HIV instills fear and discomfort in judges who are ruling on these cases.

ILLEGAL REFERRALS

Another common form of discrimination by dentists is automatic referral of patients with HIV on the assumption that routine dental treatment of an HIV-positive patient requires a specialist. The U.S. Department of Justice has issued regulations that provide that a health care worker may refer a patient with a disability such as HIV in the following cases:

1. The treatment being sought is outside the referring provider's area of specialization.
2. If in the normal course of operations, the referring provider would make a similar referral for an individual without HIV who seeks or requires the same treatment.[56]

In the *United States v Morvant*,[57] a 1995 federal court decision, the court rejected the notion that dental treatment of patients with HIV requires specialization. The court agreed with the extensive testimony that no special training or expertise is necessary to provide such care and that there is no medical or scientific basis to refer all patients with HIV. Of particular importance is that the court rejected the dentist's argument that he had not kept up with the literature and training necessary to understand HIV. The court specifically noted the extensive educational materials available to dentists and said that Dr. Morvant "chose to ignore the information and in doing so ran afoul of the law as it now stands."[57]

IN OTHER DECISIONS

Under Title III of the AwDA the Department of Justice recently settled a complaint against a dentist in East Hartford, Connecticut, for al-legedly refusing to treat a patient with AIDS. The dentists agreed to implement a policy that would not discriminate on the basis of HIV/AIDS. In addition, they paid the estate of the complainant $20,000 in compensatory damages and $9000 in civil penalties.[58]

In Houston a large chain of dental offices agreed under a consent decree to pay $80,000 in compensatory damages for refusal to treat an HIV-positive patient. In addition, the owner of Castle Dental and its management company each agreed to pay $10,000 in civil penalties to the federal government. The agreement includes staff training on nondiscrimination and requirements to provide "equal services" to persons with HIV/AIDS and "send periodic reports to the DOJ [Department of Justice] so that compliance can be monitored."[58]

Also under the AwDA, a federal court in New Jersey ruled that a dentist violated the AwDA and New Jersey state law by refusing to treat a patient with HIV and referring him to a "special clinic for HIV . . . better suited to take care of [his] needs." The court ruled the referral "a pretext for discrimination because no specialized skills are required to treat patients who are HIV positive."[57] In addition to paying compensatory damages of $25,000 and punitive damages of $25,000, the defendants were ordered to institute and maintain a policy of nondiscrimination on the basis of HIV status and to post this policy prominently in the waiting room.

THE FUTURE

Even after 16 years into the epidemic and more than 10 years of promoting universal precautions as procedures to minimize the risk of disease transmission from DHCW to patient, patient to DHCW, or patient to patient, confusion and questions still persist. During the 1996 World Congress of the American Dental Association, members who questioned the efficacy of universal precautions were soundly defeated by the scientific community reaffirming the effectiveness of universal precautions. Policies on professional judgment and designated centers to treat persons with HIV/AIDS were also debated. Courts have decided that it is safe to provide oral health services to persons with HIV/AIDS, but appeals to these decisions will determine the future role of the profession, the protection of the HIV infected (both patient and provider), and the safety of providing oral health care services.

REFERENCES

1. As AIDS epidemic approaches second decade, report examines what has been learned, *JAMA* 264:431, 1990.
2. Pneumocystis pneumonia—Los Angeles, *MMWR Morb Mortal Wkly Rep* 30:250, 1981.
3. Kaposi's sarcoma and pneumocystis pneumonia among homosexual men: New York City and California, *MMWR Morb Mortal Wkly Rep* 30:305, 1981.
4. Follow-up on Kaposi's sarcoma and pneumocystis pneumonia, *MMWR Morb Mortal Wkly Rep* 30:40, 1981.
5. The HIV/AIDS epidemic: the first 10 years, *MMWR Morb Mortal Wkly Rep* 40:22, 1991.
6. A cluster of Kaposi's sarcoma and pneumocystis carinii pneumonia among homosexual male residents of Los Angeles and Orange Counties, California, *MMWR Morb Mortal Wkly Rep* 31, 1982.
7. Centers for Disease Control and Prevention *AIDS case definition change*, Atlanta, 1993, Centers for Disease Control and Prevention.
8. *Diagnostic tests for evidence of HIV infection (supplement on testing). PI Perspective: A Publication of Project Inform*, San Francisco, October 11, 1988.
9. US Department of Health and Human Services, *FDA approves first test for HIV antigen screening of blood donors*, press release, March 14, 1996.
10. US Department of Health and Human Services, *FDA approves first home kit to test for HIV*, press release, May 14, 1996.
11. AIDS information hotline, personal communications, Centers for Disease Control and Prevention, March 14, 1997.
12. HIV/AIDS surveillance report: Year-end edition, vol 8, No. 2, June 1997, U.S. Public Health Service, Centers for Disease Control and Prevention.
13. National Commission on Acquired Immune Deficiency Syndrome: *Living with AIDS*, Washington, 1991, US Government Printing Office, Superintendent of Documents.
14. Bednarsh H, Eklund K: AZT reduces perinatal HIV transmission, *Access* 8(7): 1994.
15. Washington, 1970, Department of Labor.
16. *Occupational exposure to bloodborne pathogens, final rule*, Washington, 1991, Department of Labor, OSHA, Part II, 29 CFR Part 1910.1030.
17. Acquired immunodeficiency syndrome (AIDS): precautions for clinical and laboratory staffs, *MMWR Morb Mortal Wkly Rep* 31, 1982.
18. Acquired immunodeficiency syndrome (AIDS): precautions for health care workers and allied professionals, *MMWR Morb Mortal Wkly Rep* 32, 1983.
19. Recommended infection control practices for dentistry, *MMWR Morb Mortal Wkly Rep* 35:15, 1986.
20. Recommended infection control practices for dentistry, 1993, *MMWR Morb Mortal Wkly Rep* 42:RR-8, 1993.
21. Recommendations for prevention of HIV transmission in health-care settings, *MMWR Morb Mortal Wkly Rep* 36:2S, 1987.
22. Update: universal precautions for prevention of transmission of HIV, HBV, and other bloodborne pathogens in health care settings, *MMWR Morb Mortal Wkly Rep* 37:24, 1988.
23. Klein RS et al: Low occupational risk of human immunodeficiency virus infection among dental professionals, *N Engl J Med* 318:86, 1988.
24. *Post-exposure evaluation and follow-up requirements under OSHA's standard for occupational exposure to bloodborne pathogens: a guide to dental employer obligations*, Washington, 1995, Occupational Safety Health Administration, Department of Labor.
25. Bednarsh H, Eklund K: Prevention and management of bloodborne occupational exposure incidents—it's not as easy as 1,2,3 . . ., *Access* 8(9): 1994.
26. Case control study of HIV seroconversion in health care workers after percutaneous exposure to HIV-infected blood—France, United Kingdom, and United States, January 1988—August 1994, *MMWR Morb Mortal Wkly Rep* 44(50), 1995.
27. Update: provisional public health service recommendations for chemoprophylaxis after occupational exposure to HIV, *MMWR Morb Mortal Wkly Rep* 45:22, 1996.
28. Centers for Disease Control and Prevention, ACGIH: *Frontline healthcare workers*. National Conference on Prevention of Sharps Injuries and Bloodborne Exposures, August 14-16, 1995, Atlanta.
29. *Estimates of the risk of endemic transmission of HBV and HIV to patients by the percutaneous route during invasive surgical and dental procedures*, Draft, January 30, 1991, Centers for Disease Control and Prevention.

30. Recommendations for preventing transmission of HIV and HBV to patients during exposure prone invasive procedures, *MMWR Morb Mortal Wkly Rep* 40:RR-8, 1991.

31. Harpaz R et al: Transmission of hepatitis B virus to multiple patients from a surgeon without evidence of inadequate infection control, *N Engl J Med* 334(9):549-54, 1996.

32. Estebon J et al: Transmission of hepatitis C virus by a cardiac surgeon, *N Engl J Med* 334(9):555-60, 1996.

33. Ridzon K et al: *Simultaneous transmission of both human immunodeficiency virus (HIV) and hepatitis C virus (HCV) with delayed seroconversion in a healthcare worker (HCW)*, (abstract) Proceedings of the Thirty-Fifth Interscience Conference on Antimicrobial Agents and Chemotherapy, American Society for Microbiology.

34. Gerbert B et al: Possible health care professional to patient HIV transmission: dentists' reactions to a Centers for Disease Control and Prevention report, *JAMA* 265:1845, 1991.

35. Possible transmission of human immunodefiency virus to a patient during an invasive dental procedure, *MMWR Morb Mortal Wkly Rep* 39:489, 1990.

36. Update: Transmission of HIV infection during an invasive dental procedure—Florida, *MMWR Morb Mortal Wkly Rep* 40:21, 1991.

37. Update: investigations of persons treated by HIV-infected health-care workers—United States, *MMWR Morb Mortal Wkly Rep* 42:17, 1993.

38. Davenport R, Bednarsh H: Unpublished data on an analysis of state plans regarding HBV and HIV infected health care workers, 1996.

39. Robert LM et al: Investigations of patients of health-care workers infected with HIV. the Centers for Disease Control and Prevention database, *Ann Intern Med* 122:653, 1995.

40. *OSHA hazard communications, final rule, standards only*, Department of Labor, OSHA, 29, CFR, August 24, 1987.

41. Kane M et al.: Hepatitis B infection in the United States, *Am J Med* 87(suppl 3A):3A-11S, 1989.

42. Cleveland J: Division of Oral Health, Centers for Disease Control and Prevention, August 1996, personal communication.

43. Molinari J: Hepatitis C virus infection, *Dent Clin North Am* 40(2):309, 1996.

44. Cooper B et al.: Seroprevalence of antibodies to hepatitis C virus in high-risk hospital personnel, *Infect Control Hosp Epidemiol*, 13(2):82, 1992.

45. Guidelines for preventing the transmission of tuberculosis in health care settings with special focus on HIV related issues, *MMWR Morb Mortal Wkly Rep* 39:RR-17, 1990.

46. *Epidemic of fear.* American Civil Liberties Union, 1990.

47. Burris S: Dental discrimination against the HIV-infected: Empirical data, law and public policy, *Yale J Regul* 13(1), 1, 1996.

48. Kunzel C, Sadowsky D: Assessing HIV related attitudes and orientations of male and female dentists, *J Am Dent Assoc* 126, 1995.

49. Boston Public Health Commission: *Ryan White CARE Act, Title I.*

50. Public Law No. 100-259, 56 U.S.L.W. 46 (Apr. 5, 1988); 134 Cong. Rec. H587-8 (daily ed. Mar. 2, 1988).

51. US Department of Justice, Office of Justice Programs, National Institute of Justice: *The Americans with Disabilities Act and Criminal Justice: an Overview*, Sept. 1993.

52. *School Board of Nassau County v Arline*, 480 U.S. 273 (1987).

53. *Abbott v Bragdon*, 912 F. Supp. 580 (D. Me. 1995).

54. *Abbott v Bragdon*, No. 96-1643, U.S. Court of Appeals for First Circuit (March 5, 1997), Slip Opinion at 31.

55. *Abbott v Bragdon*, No. 96-1643, U.S. Court of Appeals for First Circuit. Brief of *Amici Curiae* Rhode Island Dept. P.H., Dept. P.H. Commonwealth of Mass., Bureau of Health, Maine Dept. Human Services, APHA, ASTDD, ASTHO.

56. Bednarsh H, Eklund K, Klein B: Courts strike down HIV discrimination in dental offices, *Access* 10(3) 1996.

57. *United States v Morvant*, 898 F. Supp. 1157 (E.D. LA. 1995).

58. US Department of Justice: *Enforcement highlights: fighting discrimination against persons with HIV/AIDS*, Washington DC, Civil Rights Division.

CHAPTER 18

Risk management in dental practice

Burton R. Pollack

Licensed health providers occupy a special place in society. The license granted them by the community enables them to pursue their profession in a virtual monopoly. Only those who are specially trained and who meet rigid qualifications and standards may hold themselves out to the community as providers of care and engage in practice defined by law. However, once having accepted the license, licensees are subjected to life-long regulation by society as a whole and by individual patients whom they treat. The risks in practice are many. This chapter examines the risks in dental practice and presents methods that enable practitioners to reduce and control them. The process is called *risk management.*

After the crisis in medical and hospital malpractice in the early 1970s, risk management concepts borrowed from industry were adapted to the health field—particularly to hospitals. Lately risk management principles have been applied to individual practice settings. These principles are designed primarily to protect the financial resources of an industry (e.g., hospital, private practitioner) from losses resulting from legal action. An effective risk management program includes the following:

1. Loss identification (exposure to legal claims)
2. Loss analysis (evaluation of loss experience)
3. Loss avoidance or reduction
4. Loss financing (financing claims exposure)

The following three activities are associated with risk management:

1. Identifying areas of legal vulnerability
2. Instituting corrective or preventive measures
3. Purchasing liability insurance

This chapter provides information related to the first two of these activities. It is based on a thorough review of cases brought against dentists and opinions of courts deciding medical and dental malpractice suits. The text summarizes the areas of legal vulnerability associated with the practice of dentistry. The italicized risk management rules (i.e., recommendations, suggestions) represent corrective or preventive measures associated with the subject matter of the text. The amount of liability insurance purchased (the third listed activity) is a personal matter; practitioners must consider cost, scope of coverage, and amount of indemnification of losses that are desired on the basis of their ability to afford premium costs.

Risk management principles are applied to professional and general liability. General liability relates to negligence associated with injuries that result from the physical structures within the office. Professional liability relates to injuries that result from the treatment of patients. For example, if a patient falls in the waiting room as a result of tripping over an electric cord, the incident comes under the general liability category. If the patient's tongue is lacerated during a crown preparation, the incident becomes one of professional liability. This chapter deals solely with professional liability. An effective risk management program does much to control the cost of malpractice insurance and to protect the reputation and resources of the practitioner.

This chapter also provides dentists, hygienists, dental assistants, and other office personnel with information about the legal risks of practice and methods designed to eliminate or reduce them. The goal is to enable the health practitioner to practice in a worry- and claims-free environment. Because so much of risk management relates to law and the legal system, it is necessary to describe how the system works in the regulation of the health professions to fully understand both the risks in practice and the methods recommended to reduce or eliminate them.

Courts and legal precedents

What courts do is important to matters relating to the practice of dentistry, public health, and to the lives of all who reside in the United States, whether citizens of the country, simply residents, or for that matter, those just passing through. The foundation of the laws of the land is what we took from the English when the 13 colonies declared their independence. Thus English common law became the cornerstone of the making of the laws of the United States. The English model still serves us. The law in the United States springs from two distinct

sources that in some cases overlap: case law and black letter law. Further, the organization of the courts plays an important role in establishing just what is the law.

COURTS

Courts may be classified in many ways: as to their organization, whether upper or lower; their geographic jurisdiction, based on where they sit; their subject matter jurisdiction, criminal or civil; trial or appellate; etc. For purposes of this chapter, upper and lower, trial and appellate are of concern. The issue is how legal precedent is set and how it affects the health professions in general and dental practice in particular.

Lower courts, also known as *trial courts,* are the courts of original jurisdiction. These courts are the first to hear and decide a case. Those lower courts that decide suits in which one party alleges that he or she suffered an injury due to the negligence (malpractice) of another are heard in a lower court assigned that jurisdiction by the state, either by its constitution or through its court rules. The default setup is a jury trial with a judge and jury, although each side may affirmatively waive having a jury and have the judge sit alone (bench trial). Decisions made in the lower courts may be appealed to a higher (appellate) court should either party feel that (1) the procedure in the lower court violated procedure as established by appellate courts or court rules or (2) the judge in the instructions to the jury applied the wrong law to guide the jury in arriving at a decision in the case. Juries decide the facts, the judge applies the law.

Upper courts are courts in which appeals are heard from decisions made in the lower courts; they are appellate courts—in different states with different names. The highest appellate court in the land is the U.S. Supreme Court. Cases taken to appeal are heard by judges, without juries—this fact is of major importance because the lower court decides the facts and its decision about the facts is dependent on testimony of witnesses. Appellate courts do not receive testimony of witnesses; therefore they accept the facts as determined by the jury or judge in a bench trial. (There are some few exceptions to this general rule, but they have no bearing on the subject of this chapter.) These courts, in reviewing the appeal, decide whether the wrong law was applied by the lower court, or if an error was made during the trial. The appeal court may (1) affirm the decision of the lower court, (2) declare that a procedural error was made in the lower court and thus vacate the decision and remand the case for retrial, (3) reverse the decision on the basis of the fact that the wrong law was used in the lower court's decision, or (4) modify the decision as it relates to damages, etc.

When an appellate court decides a case, *precedent law* is established. All lower courts within the geographic jurisdiction of the appellate court are required to follow the precedent established by the appellate court. If the court does not and the case is appealed, the decision of the lower court will be reversed. If the case is not appealed, the decision of the lower court is final, notwithstanding the fact that in arriving at the decision precedent law was ignored. It is important to remember that only appellate courts establish precedent, and that no one, not even the most experienced attorney, can ever predict with any degree of certainty how a judge, or jury, will decide a case. Fifty percent of all lawyers representing clients end up on the losing side and are proved wrong by either a judge or jury or by an appellate court.

CASE LAW

Case law, also known as court law, is that law established through decisions made by the courts. All appellate decisions are officially published and made available to all law libraries and included in electronic databases of legal publishing companies. Only the appellate courts make precedent law. The precedents they establish are known as case law. Except for cases decided in federal courts, case law is state specific. Only the jurisdiction in which the appellate court sits is affected by its case law. The decisions and opinions of the appellate courts are available within hours throughout the country. Case law may change with every decision reached by an appellate court. Attorneys must remain current on changes in case law that affect their fields of practice. It is not a simple task. Although appellate decisions are officially published, decisions of the lower courts are not. These are recorded in the court in which they are heard. There are thousands of trial courts scattered throughout the country. The result is that there is no simple way to collect national data on what takes place at the trial court level. For this reason it is not possible to obtain reliable data on what is taking place in the field of malpractice litigation. Only the insurance companies know, and they do not share information unless it suits them.

Black letter law

Black letter law (BLL) is law written in black ink on white paper. These are laws that come from several sources: from elected officials serving in some form of formal organization (e.g., Congress, a state legislature, a city council, etc.) and from administrative agencies established by the elected body. Those laws adopted by Congress, a legislature, or any other elected body are called by different names: by Congress, acts of Congress; by a state legislature, statutes; and by lower jurisdictions, a variety of names (i.e., codes, ordinances, etc.). State BLL is state specific; therefore the BLL regulating the practice of dentistry in Vermont has no impact on dental practice in Ohio.

Caveats in risk management and the law

There are 51 jurisdictions in the United States: 50 states and the federal government. Each of the 50 states has exercised its right to regulate the health professions, including dentistry. In addition, Puerto Rico, the Virgin Islands, and the District of Columbia regulate health practices. The federal government also regulates some elements of health practice. Therefore 54 separate jurisdictions regulate the practice of dentistry. Except for federal regulations that apply to practitioners in all states, each jurisdiction has independent regulations. Except for some federal laws, there is no generic law in the United States. There are, however, legal principles that apply nationwide. For example, the legal principle of the statute of limitations is the same in all jurisdictions, but the statute may operate at different times and for different lengths of time in each individual jurisdiction.

The caveat is that for practitioners to know the specifics of the regulation of dental practice they must know local law. The same act may be legal in one state and illegal in another. As an example, in New York it is legal for a dental laboratory to select a shade for a crown. In Massachusetts it is illegal for a dentist to refer a patient to a laboratory for the purpose of selecting a shade. Therefore a dentist in New York who sends a patient to a dental laboratory for the selection of a shade is not in violation of the law, nor is the laboratory in violation of the state law. The same act performed by a dentist in Massachusetts would be in violation of the law.

Except for the purpose of presenting examples, this chapter describes generic legal principles. Local attorneys, or government agencies, should be of assistance in determining the specific laws of the jurisdiction in which you conduct your practice.

LEVELS OF LEGAL RISK

This artificial legal concept of "levels of legal risk" relates to the degree to which a dentist is willing to take a risk in the performance of a professional act. Clearly, refusing to treat a patient who does not follow the advice of a dentist presents the lowest level of legal risk to the dentist. However, if the dentist agrees to treat the patient although the patient did not comply with the dentist's advice, the risk is great. A good example of the concept relates to a dentist's advice that the patient have a thorough radiographic examination before treatment is begun. If the patient refuses and the dentist proceeds with the care, there is a risk that, because radiographs were not taken, an important pathologic condition was not discovered and as a result the patient suffered an injury. The dentist may lose a suit should the patient allege that the dentist was negligent in not discovering the condition. The dentist's defense is that the patient refused to have radiographs taken. Given the uncertainty of the outcome of jury trials, the dentist may lose the case. Therefore the lowest level of legal risk is to refuse to treat the patient. The highest level of legal risk is to treat a patient who refuses to follow advice. Under some circumstances, the dentist may be willing to take the risk after assessing the benefits of continuing to treat the patient.

While you review the risk management rules, you should keep the concept of levels of legal risk in mind. Prudent dentists make certain that they are aware of the risks attached to any professional decision before acting. That is what this chapter is all about: describing the risks.

LOSS WITHOUT FAULT

Another artificial legal concept is "loss without fault." It evolved from a study I conducted in the early 1980s during the crisis in dental malpractice litigation. Four hundred cases in which a dentist was accused of malpractice were tracked from the initial service of suit papers to the closing of the case. The results were that in 80% of 400 cases brought against dentists the insurance company, on the advice of a panel of dental experts and an attorney experienced in dental malpractice litigation, sought settlement before trial because it was apparent that the case could not successfully be defended. In only 20% of the cases the panel felt that the dentist was guilty of malpractice. In

60% of the cases where settlement was sought the dental experts were of the opinion that no negligence was present. The 60% represents "loss without fault"—no malpractice, but little or no chance of successfully defending the suit. Looking at the data from another perspective, of 400 cases alleging malpractice brought against dentists, in 80% there was no evidence of malpractice, but according to the expert panel in only 20% could the suit be successfully defended. Loss without fault is the foundation of much of risk management. More on that issue will be described later in the chapter.

Although there is no hard evidence that malpractice suits against dentists are on the decline (there is some speculation that such is the case), there is no doubt that dollar awards and settlements are on a dramatic increase.

Regulation of dental practice

As stated previously, each of the jurisdictions has exercised its right to regulate dental practice. Except for federal regulation, the mechanism for regulation is similar. The elected body, the legislature, enacts legislation designed to regulate dental practice. Because the members of the electorate have neither the time nor the expertise to exercise control over the daily activities of the profession and the details of practice, they enact additional legislation (enabling legislation or statutory authority) establishing an administrative agency to further regulate the profession and grant to that agency the power to adopt administrative laws (rules and regulations) to carry out its mission.

Each state may vary the name of the administrative body and adopt any organizational structure to accomplish the goal of regulating the health profession, but the general regulatory structure is the same. In New York, for example, two administrative agencies regulate dentists and other health professionals: the state education department and the Board of

Regents. The commissioner of education is empowered by legislative act to adopt regulations, the Board of Regents, to adopt rules. In New York the state Board for Dentistry is not authorized to adopt rules or regulations for the purpose of regulating dental practice. It serves as an examining body, recommends licensure, and advises the commissioner, the Board of Regents, and the legislature on dental matters. Also, it serves as an administrative body to hear alleged violations of the rules and regulations and to recommend actions to be taken against the dentist to the state education department. In Massachusetts one administrative agency regulates the practice of dentistry: the Massachusetts Board of Registration in Dentistry. It combines all the functions assigned to the three agencies in New York. Most other states, like Massachusetts, have only one administrative agency.

A combination of the statutes and the rules and regulations make up the body of dental BLL, commonly referred to as the Dental Practice Act. However, in all jurisdictions there are many other laws that affect the practice of dentistry. These may be found in the public health law, the sanitary code, the education law, and others. The practitioner should be aware that the laws regulating dental practice are spread throughout the statutes and administrative laws of the state. In addition, a multitude of federal laws exercise control over dental practice. The old adage that ignorance of the law is no excuse should not be ignored.

The risk management principle is: *Learn the laws of the jurisdiction in which you practice and the federal laws that apply to the practice of dentistry, and remain current on changes in the laws. Although it is difficult, much can be learned by attending continuing education courses, reading journals and texts on the subject, and attending seminars. Also, annually request of the local licensing agency a copy of the current Dental Practice Act. If you are in doubt about a provision, consult the licensing agency or a local attorney.*

Legal vulnerability in dental practice

Legal vulnerability in dental practice may be divided into two broad categories: criminal and civil. Each broad category has subcategories, as shown in Fig. 18-1. The intentional torts listed on the chart are those most frequently associated with dental practice. False imprisonment, abuse of process, trespass to real property, conversion, interference with performance of a contract, and others are recognized in law but have little relevance in dental practice.

Criminal and quasicriminal vulnerability

Violations of statutory law are termed *crimes*. They constitute acts that are deemed by the government to be against the public interest. They may be defined as misdemeanors or felonies. Violations of that part of the Dental Practice Act that is statutory, enacted by the legislature, are classified as crimes and may include penalties such as loss or suspension of license, mandatory psychiatric counseling, drug rehabilitation, mandatory continuing education, fines, or even jail. If the legislature declares the violation a misdemeanor, the jail sentence may be less than if it classifies the violation a felony. In New York, for instance, aiding or abetting an unlicensed person to perform a service that requires a license is classified a class E felony, punishable by up to 3 years in jail. In other jurisdictions it is classified as a misdemeanor.

Violations of administrative laws (rules or regulations of administrative agencies, e.g., the state board, the state education department, the board of regents), are termed *quasicrimes*. Penalties may include all actions that are possible under crimes, except loss of personal freedom (jail). Because members of administrative boards and agencies are appointed rather than

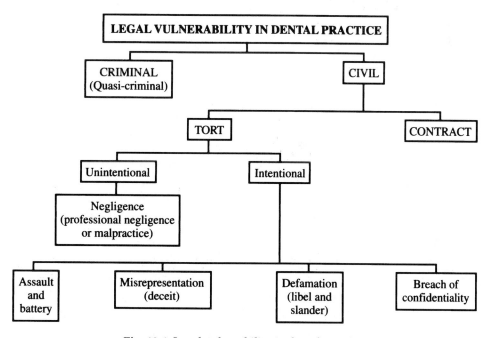

Fig. 18-1. Legal vulnerability in dental practice.

elected, the framers of the constitution felt that appointed individuals should not be granted the power to deprive anyone of liberty.

One of the major differences between a violation of a statute and that of an administrative law is the degree of evidence necessary to convict. In allegations of criminal behavior the state must prove "beyond a reasonable doubt" that the law was violated. For violations of administrative law the proof necessary is considerably less. (In civil actions the burden on the plaintiff is to prove by a "fair preponderance of the evidence" [more than 50%] that the defendant is guilty.)

In all dental practice acts there is authority granted to an administrative agency to impose punitive sanctions against a dentist who is found guilty of a violation. Therefore a dentist who is found guilty of violating the law regulating the prescription or the administration of controlled substances may have an additional action taken by the dental board, or if the violation occurs in New York, by the Board of Regents, against the license of the offender.

Professional liability insurance does not provide protection against either criminal or quasicriminal allegations as it does in civil actions (those brought by a patient). However, if there is an allegation of negligence attached to a violation of the law, either criminal or quasicriminal, the defense of a civil suit based on an injury resulting from the alleged illegal act becomes more difficult because of trial practice procedures.

The risk management admonition is: *Don't break the law!*

Doctor-patient contract
WHEN THE DOCTOR-PATIENT RELATIONSHIP BEGINS

The legal foundation of the doctor-patient relationship is contract law. At the moment a dentist expresses a professional opinion to an individual who has reason to rely on the opinion, the doctor-patient relationship begins, and the doctor is burdened with implied warranties (duties). The fact that no fee is involved does not affect the relationship that attaches to the contract or the duties.

The example best demonstrating the moment the relationship begins and the duties that attach is a situation where a dentist gives a fellow party-goer dental advice at a social gathering. If the advice results in an injury, the dentist may be held liable for negligence. It is not a valid defense that no fee was charged or expected. The dentist would be held to the standard that patients should not be given dental advice unless an examination and a history are completed.

The risk management principle is: *In social settings, never provide anyone, unless that person is a bona fide patient, with advice regarding dental problems.*

Must you accept anyone who comes to you for care? The answer is a qualified *no.* You may refuse to treat a patient for any reason except race, creed, color, or national origin. With the effective date of the federal Americans with Disabilities Act of 1990, refusal to accept a patient on the basis of a disability may be in violation of the law. Patients with acquired immunodeficiency syndrome (AIDS), who test positive for human immunodeficiency virus (HIV), or who have any infectious disease, fall into the category of disabled persons and may not be refused care if the refusal is based solely on the presence of AIDS or the HIV-positive status. The law declares that all health providers' offices are "places of public accommodation" and therefore subject to antidiscrimination laws. Local jurisdictions have followed the same course as Congress. Therefore in many jurisdictions a dentist's office is subject to the jurisdiction of the local Human Rights Commission and the antidiscrimination policies that it enforces. For more on the care of patients who have AIDS or are HIV positive, see the section on histories (p. 347).

As long as the person is not a patient of record, you may even refuse to provide emergency care, subject to the limitations stated previously. It may be unethical, but it is not illegal and cannot form the basis of a criminal or civil suit. However, remember that just as soon as you express a professional judgment or perform a professional act the doctor-patient relationship begins, and duties begin to attach.

WHEN THE DOCTOR-PATIENT RELATIONSHIP ENDS

The relationship ends when any of the following takes place:

1. Both parties agree to end it.
2. Either the patient or the dentist dies.
3. The patient ends it by act or statement.
4. The patient is cured.
5. The dentist unilaterally decides to terminate the care.

The dentist's unilaterally terminating the relationship may support an abandonment claim by the patient unless the dentist follows a procedure acceptable to the courts. Abandoning a patient before the agreed treatment is completed is unethical, and in some jurisdictions it is a violation of the law. In all jurisdictions abandonment may lead to a civil suit.

The major causes that contribute to a decision to terminate treatment before it is complete are (1) the patient has not fulfilled the payment agreement, (2) the patient has not cooperated in keeping appointments, (3) the patient has not complied with home care instructions, and (4) there has been a breakdown in interpersonal relationships. Any of these is ample justification for the dentist to terminate treatment.

A risk management rule is: *Discontinue treatment of patients who do not cooperate in care, become antagonistic, or exhibit a litigious attitude.*

The procedure recommended to discontinue care without running the risk of a finding of abandonment by a court follows. It begins with a discussion of the problem with the patient as follows. (1) Advise the patient that it is in his or her best interest to seek care elsewhere. (2) Assure the patient that you will cooperate by making copies of the records available should the patient make the request in writing. (3) Let the patient know that you will be available to provide emergency care for a reasonable period of time. Note the conversation on the patient's record. Follow up the conversation with a certified letter, signed receipt requested, stating the above facts.

A risk management caveat is: *Do not discontinue treatment at a time when the patient's health may be compromised. (This decision is professional rather than legal.) It is best not to suggest any dentist the patient should see. Have the patient select the substitute practitioner.*

Express terms

An *express term* is one in which both parties are in agreement. Putting the term in writing is not required to make it enforceable, although to prevent misunderstandings a written agreement is always preferred. Usually, the express terms define items such as the fee, the treatment, and the manner in which payments are to be made. The risk management principle is when in doubt, write it out. It may be done on separate forms or entered into the record of the patient. It is best done on a separate form because the treatment record should contain only treatment notes and patient reactions to treatment.

Guarantees

Guarantees made by the dentist or an employee constitute an express term in the agreement. In some jurisdictions guarantees attached to health care are illegal. They are also in violation of the Principle of Ethics and Code of Professional Conduct of the American Dental Association (ADA). You may be held to a guarantee even if the treatment meets acceptable standards of care. A statement made by a dentist to the patient that the patient will be satisfied with the treatment is a guarantee. If the patient is not satisfied, the dentist has breached the contract despite the excellent quality of the service.

Therapeutic reassurances—statements whose purpose is to induce patients to accept care that is clearly in their best interest—are rare in dentistry, except in unusual situations and usually when related to oral surgery. Courts generally do not consider therapeutic reassurances guarantees.

Risk management rule: *Never guarantee a result.*

Implied warranties (duties) owed by the doctor

Attached to the doctor-patient relationship are additional duties that are implied, unless the express terms serve to void or modify them. They are enforceable although not written or stated. Over the years the courts have identified many of these implied duties. Some of the more important ones are included in the list that follows.

In accepting a patient for care the dentist warrants that he or she will do the following:

1. Use reasonable care in the provision of services as measured against acceptable standards set by other practitioners with similar training in a similar community.
2. Be properly licensed and registered and meet all other legal requirements to engage in the practice of dentistry.
3. Employ competent personnel and provide for their proper supervision.
4. Maintain a level of knowledge in keeping with current advances in the profession.
5. Use methods that are acceptable to at least a respectable minority of similar practitioners in the community.
6. Not use experimental procedures.
7. Obtain informed consent from the patient before instituting an examination or treatment.
8. Not abandon the patient.
9. Ensure that care is available in emergency situations.
10. Charge a reasonable fee for services based on community standards.
11. Not exceed the scope of practice authorized by the license or permit any person acting under direction to engage in unlawful acts.
12. Keep the patient informed of progress.
13. Not undertake any procedure for which the practitioner is not qualified.
14. Complete the care in a timely manner.
15. Keep accurate records of the treatment rendered to the patient.
16. Maintain confidentiality of information.
17. Inform the patient of any untoward occurrences in the course of treatment.
18. Make appropriate referrals and request necessary consultations.
19. Comply with all laws regulating the practice of dentistry.
20. Practice in a manner consistent with the code of ethics of the profession.

The list generates a host of risk management rules. They are all important as principles of good risk management.

Implied duties owed by the patient

Patients, as well as doctors, are expected to comply with some rules of behavior relative to their care, without the rules being stated. In accepting care the patient warrants the following:

1. Home care instructions will be followed.
2. Appointments will be kept.
3. Bills for services will be paid in a reasonable time.
4. The patient will cooperate in the care.
5. The patient will notify the dentist or office of a change in health status.

Depending on the treatment, there may be additional warranties.

It is best to make the last duty part of the express written terms of the agreement. This can be done by placing the statement at the end of the history form and reminding the patient of the need to notify the office of a change in health status. If the patient breaches any of these duties, notes to that effect should be made in the patient's record.

For purposes of risk management: *If any of the warranties should be broken by the patient, this should be noted on the patient's record, and consideration should be given to discontinue the care of the noncompliant patient.*

Risk reduction in the transmission of blood-borne infectious diseases
USE OF BARRIER TECHNIQUES

The legal issue of the dentist's right to refuse to treat patients in groups that engage in high-risk behaviors for AIDS or those patients who have AIDS or are HIV-infected, whether symptomatic or asymptomatic, has not been decided by any court to give positive direction to practitioners. However, as stated previously, with the passage of the Americans with Disabilities Act of 1990, Congress has imposed its will on the courts, and by its declaration of a health provider's office a "place of public accommodation" a dentist who refuses to treat a patient who has AIDS or is HIV positive is in violation of the law and subject to excessive and severe penalties. Not all patients are aware of their HIV status or know they have other blood-borne contagious diseases; therefore the use of barrier techniques in the treatment of all patients becomes increasingly important. In addition, many high-risk patients who are in need of dental care may decide not to disclose any information on their health history form relating to the presence of AIDS or HIV infection or their presence in groups that engage in high-risk behaviors for fear of being refused care. The result is that all patients must be treated as high-risk patients. It is clear that the provider of care is at greater risk of contracting AIDS from an infected patient than the healthy patient is of contracting AIDS from an infected health care worker.

The fact that the risk of contracting and transmitting AIDS in the dental office is low does not change the responsibility of the dentist to use appropriate barrier techniques. Hepatitis B represents a greater risk in dental practice, and, to ensure protection from transmission in the treatment of patients with hepatitis, barrier techniques must be employed.

As a further complication, it is virtually impossible for the dentist to identify, with any high degree of accuracy, patients who may engage in high-risk behaviors for either AIDS or HIV infection or patients with hepatitis. Therefore appropriate measures should be taken in the treatment of all patients to prevent the transmission of a blood-borne disease to other patients, to the staff in the office, or to the dentist and his or her family. As these measures relate to the use of barrier techniques, the legal issue is to what standard the dentist will be held. During the past several years the standard has seen dramatic changes.

Currently, dentists must use six basic infection control procedures to meet an acceptable standard of office practice:

1. All office personnel involved in the treatment of patients must wear protective eye shields.
2. All office personnel involved in the treatment of patients must wear surgical gloves.
3. All office personnel involved in the treatment of patients must wear surgical masks, and splash shields when aerosol sprays are used or blood or saliva may splatter.
4. All instruments used in or near the oral cavity in the treatment of patients must be sterilized in a heat or heat-pressure sterilizer.

5. All touch or splash surfaces must be disinfected with an Environmental Protection Agency–registered hospital-grade disinfectant.

6. All contaminated, hazardous, and medical wastes must be disposed of in a manner consistent with local law.

In addition, some states have mandated the use of these and other barrier techniques in the treatment of all patients. Some have addressed the issue of hepatitis B carrier testing and regular monitoring of sterilization equipment.

Dentists should remain current with the latest Centers for Disease Control and Prevention (CDC) recommendations, Occupational Safety and Health Administration (OSHA) standards, ADA recommendations, and local law to determine what measures must be taken to prevent transmission of blood-borne diseases. Failure to meet the standards exposes the dentist to legal risk of action by a government agency for violation of the law and civil action by an individual (i.e., patient, staff) who contracted a blood-borne disease traced to the dentist's office.

Following are contact agencies from which information and their rules may be obtained:

ADA: Council of Dental Therapeutics, 211 E. Chicago Ave., Chicago, IL 60611; telephone 800-621-8099, ext. 2522.

CDC: Centers for Disease Control and Prevention, 1644 Freeway Park, Atlanta, GA 30333; telephone 404-639-1830.

Local law: Either the state dental board, the department of health, or a local attorney.

OSHA (by regional office):

Region I (CT,* MA, ME, NH, RI, VT*). 16-18 North St., 1 Dock Square Building, 4th Floor, Boston, MA 02109; telephone 617-565-1161.

Region II (NJ, NY,* PR*). 201 Varick St., 6th Floor, New York, NY 10014; Telephone 212-337-2325.

Region III (DC, DE, MD,* PA, VA,* WV). Gateway Building, Suite 2100, 3535 Market St., Philadelphia, PA 19104; telephone 215-596-1201.

Region IV (AL, FL, GA, KY,* MS, NC,* SC,* TN*). 1375 Peachtree St., N.E., Suite 587, Atlanta, GA 30367; telephone 404-347-3573.

Region V (IL, IN,* MI,* MN,* OH, WI). 230 S. Dearborn St., 32nd Floor, Room 3244, Chicago, IL 60604; telephone 312-353-2200.

Region VI (AR, LA, NM,* OK, TX). 525 Griffin St., Room 602, Dallas, TX 75202; telephone 214-767-3731.

Region VII (IA,* KS, MO, NE). 911 Walnut St., Room 406, Kansas City, MO 64106; telephone 816-374-5861.

Region VIII (CO, MT, ND, SD, UT,* WY*). Federal Building, Room 1576, 1961 Stout St., Denver, CO 80294; telephone 303-844-3061.

Region IX (AZ,* CA,* HI,* NV*). 71 Stevenson St., 4th Floor, San Francisco, CA 94105; telephone 415-995-5672.

Region X (AK,* ID, OR,* WA*). Federal Office Building, Room 6003, 909 First Ave., Seattle, WA 98174; telephone 206-442-5930.

Torts

A *tort* is a civil wrong or injury, independent of a contract, that results from a breach of a duty. The tort may be unintentional or intentional. An unintentional tort is one in which harm was not intended, as is the case in the tort of negligence. As the name implies, the intentional torts contain the element of intended harm.

Negligence is an unintentional tort. If the negligence involves an act that is performed in a professional capacity, it is termed *professional negligence,* or *malpractice.* Thus if a dentist is accused of negligence in the performance of dental treatment, the allegation is one of malpractice.

The intentional torts of major concern to the dentist include *trespass to the person* (commonly known as *assault and battery), defama-*

*These states and territories operate their own OSHA-approved job safety and health programs (except Connecticut and New York, whose plans cover public employees only).

tion, breach of confidentiality, and *misrepresentation (deceit).*

MALPRACTICE (PROFESSIONAL NEGLIGENCE) AND THE STANDARD OF CARE

Only malpractice related to dentistry is presented here. The New York courts have provided the most comprehensive definition of malpractice as it relates to physicians and dentists. Included are some editorial changes and updating; important risk management concerns are italicized.[1]

A doctor's responsibilities are the same whether or not he/she is paid for the services. By undertaking to perform a medical (dental) service, he/she does not—nor does the law require him/her to—guarantee a good result. He/she is liable only for negligence.

A doctor who renders a medical (dental) service is obligated to have that reasonable degree of knowledge and ability expected of doctors (or specialists) who do that particular (operation, examination) treatment in the community where he/she practices, or a similar community. (The trend in some jurisdictions, the most recent being New York for some of its appellate jurisdictions, is to apply a national standard. See the section called A National Standard Of Care?).

The law recognizes that there are differences in the abilities of doctors, just as there are differences in the abilities of people engaged in other activities. To practice his/her profession a doctor is not required to be possessed of the extraordinary knowledge and ability that belongs to a few people of rare endowments, but *he/she is required to keep abreast of the times and to practice in accordance with the approved methods and means of treatment in general use.* The standard to which he/she is held is measured by the degree of knowledge and ability of the average doctor (or specialist) in good standing in the community where he/she practices (or in a similar community).

In the performance of medical (dental) services the doctor is obligated to use his/her best judgment and to use reasonable care in the exercise of his/her knowledge and ability. The rule requiring him/her to use his/her best judgment does not make him/her liable for a mere error in judgment, provided he/she does what he/she thinks is best after careful exami-

nation. The rule of reasonable care does not require the exercise of the highest possible degree of care; it requires only that he/she exercise that degree of care that a reasonably prudent doctor (or specialist) would exercise under the same circumstances.

If a patient should sustain an injury while undergoing medical (dental) care and that injury results from the doctor's lack of knowledge or ability, or from his/her failure to exercise reasonable care or to use his/her best judgment, then he/she is responsible for the injuries that are the result of his/her acts.

Courts do not require that all dentists use the same modality of treatment. The standard can be met if a "respectable minority" of practitioners use the same treatment method. Therefore the Sargenti method in endodontic treatment and the Keyes technique in periodontal therapy may be acceptable to the courts as meeting the standard of reasonable care. It should be noted that the standard to which a dentist is held is the standard set by other dentists, not what a text, article, or a guideline from a professional organization recommends. These are hearsay, not available for cross-examination, and therefore may not be directly entered into evidence.

Additional risk management principles applied to malpractice prevention are the following:

1. *Do not undertake treatment beyond your ability and training, even if the patient insists that you provide the care.*
2. *If, in your professional judgment, you believe that specialty care is required before the care you intend, do not undertake your treatment unless the patient follows your recommendation to obtain specialty care. This is of importance when the patient needs to receive periodontal therapy before the fabrication of crowns or fixed bridges.*
3. *If you recommend to the patient that specialty care is necessary and the patient refuses to follow your recommendation, the legal risk is increased if you undertake the care that, by your own admission, should have been provided by a specialist.*

4. *If you believe that certain tests or diagnostic procedures should be completed before you undertake treatment and the patient refuses, as in the case of the need for radiographs, the legal risk is markedly increased if you treat the patient without the diagnostic aid you recommend.*

In the last three items above, the dentist has established a standard of acceptable care. By acceding to the patient's refusal to follow recommendations and treating the patient, even at the patient's request, the dentist has departed from the standard. This action presents a situation that is difficult to defend. Having the patient sign a statement to the effect that he or she is aware of the risk of noncompliance somewhat reduces the risk but does not eliminate it. A court might declare the statement exculpatory and void as against public policy. An exculpatory statement excuses an individual from liability for negligence. Agreements entered into by patients that relieve health practitioners from responsibility for negligent acts have not been enforced by the courts. When having to address the issue, courts have declared exculpatory clauses in doctor-patient agreements against public policy and therefore void.

A NATIONAL STANDARD OF CARE?

Establishing a standard of care to which a defendant dentist is held directly relates to who the court will permit to present testimony (the expert), as to the standard to which the defendant dentist is to be held. If the court limits the experts to those who practice in the community, be it local or even statewide, the standard would be "local," not "national." There is now a trend among the courts to apply a national standard of care. The trend is most evident when practitioners are certified by a specialty board. Under these circumstances a board-certified specialist from California may be permitted to present testimony as to the standard of care to which a board-certified specialist in the same speciality would be held in New York.

Another somewhat disturbing effect of the trend is that there are two standards of care in those jurisdictions that accept a different standard of care for specialists than for generalists. The result is that a board-certified specialist would not be permitted to testify as to the standard of care of a generalist or non-board-certified specialist. Thus, there are two standards of care in the community—one for generalists and another for board-certified specialists. A court in New York, in applying a national standard of care for board-certified Radiologists, by permitting a board-certified radiologist from California who never practiced in New York to testify against a board-certified radiologist in New York, noted that the result is that a two-tiered level of care has been accepted.[2] The trend in the courts to apply a national standard to generalists is taking place but is progressing at a steady but slower rate.

TRESPASS TO THE PERSON (ASSAULT AND BATTERY)

The civil counterpart of the criminal act of assault and battery is trespass to the person. It constitutes a threat to harm (assault) and unauthorized touching (battery). Traditionally, lack of informed consent to care was treated as assault and battery. Recent decisions classify lack of informed consent as negligence. The change resulted in part from the recognition by the courts that, except in the most unusual cases, doctors do not intend to harm their patients, although the touching was not authorized by the patients. In some jurisdictions if the consent is present but faulty, the rules of malpractice will apply. If there is a total absence of consent, the case may be treated as trespass to the person.

Assault and battery cases not associated with lack of consent have occurred in dentistry. The use of force or unnecessary physical restraints in the treatment of uncooperative children has led to allegations of criminal assault and battery and civil trespass to the person. Dentists should be aware that if the allegation is criminal professional liability insurance will not provide coverage. In some older professional liability policies, civil actions of assault and battery were covered. However, recent professional liability policies limit coverage to professional negligence.

The risk management principle applied to trespass to the person is: *Avoid the use of physical force or unnecessary restraints in the treatment of children. If you feel that such measures are necessary, discuss the matter with the parents and have them present in the operatory.*

Risk management as it applies to consent is discussed later in the chapter.

MISREPRESENTATION (DECEIT)

Patients must be kept informed of their treatment status. This is one of the implied duties that the courts have attached to the doctor-patient relationship. If information is withheld that places a patient's health in jeopardy or deprives the patient of the legal right to bring suit against the practitioner, a legal action in deceit or fraudulent concealment may result. In the civil action of deceit and fraudulent concealment, the statute of limitations may be extended, and professional liability insurance may not provide coverage. In addition, a criminal action of fraud may also be alleged. The problems in dentistry most frequently associated with deceit and fraudulent concealment include the failure to inform the patient when an instrument breaks off in a root canal, when a root is fractured and the tip remains in the jaw, and when the dentist is aware that the success of the treatment will be compromised because of lack of cooperation by the patient. Informing the patient of an untoward event at the time it occurs defeats any future attempt by the patient to extend or toll (delay the beginning of) the statute of limitations. A note on the patient's record of the event and of the fact that the patient was informed should be made; if possible, the patient should be asked to initial or sign the entry.

The risk management rules are: *Never lie to patients about their treatments and keep them informed about their health status while in your care.*

Third-party payment coverage has led to many allegations of fraud and deceit. It is usually associated with passing off one metal for another in the fabrication of prosthetic appliances by substituting nonprecious for precious metals, with not collecting copayment fees from the patient, or with substituting an approved-for-payment treatment for one that is not covered by the third party. Actions in criminal fraud also may result. Insurance companies are alert to such activities and are relentless in their pursuit of suspected dentists. The patient may also institute an action for the same act against the errant practitioner. Actions in fraudulent misrepresentation overlap actions in breach of contract. The choice is left to the plaintiff's attorney, and the one most damaging to the dentist's interests or most favorable to the success of the lawsuit will be selected.

The risk management rule is worth repeating: *Never lie to or deceive a patient or an insurance company.*

DEFAMATION

The intentional tort of defamation is not of major concern in dentistry because most dentists are aware of the problem and its consequences.

The risk management admonition is: *Keep your opinions about your patients to yourself unless the opinions are essential to successful treatment. Expressions about the mental health of a patient are particularly risky.*

BREACH OF CONFIDENTIALITY

Breach of confidentiality was not known as a tort under English common law. It is a product of recent case law (law as stated by courts in deciding cases) and BLL (including statutes enacted by elected officials and administrative laws, rules, and regulations adopted by administrative agencies).

Information obtained from the patient in the course of diagnosis or treatment must remain confidential. Unless the patient waives confidentiality, a breach may lead to a suit. Patients may waive confidentiality by their actions or words. It may also be waived by action of law, as in the case of the requirement to report certain communicable diseases to government health agencies. When a patient visits a specialist or another health practitioner at the dentist's request, the dentist is expected to inform that practitioner of the health status of the patient. In going to the specialist the patient, by his or her action, has waived confidentiality. A patient who seeks care from a group practice and is aware that the practitioners practice as associates has waived confidentiality. There are many other situations in which confidentiality is waived. However, there are many situations that a practitioner should be aware of when a specific waiver is required. Recently the matter of whether a health practitioner is permitted to inform another health practitioner who is to provide care to a patient who has AIDS or is HIV positive, that the patient has these conditions has been settled in many jurisdictions. In those that have addressed the issue, it can be done. However, it is best for the dentist faced with this problem to determine the local ruling. Under federal law it is permitted.

The risk management rule is: *Never reveal any information about a patient to anyone without first obtaining permission from the patient—preferably in writing.* (See the following section on patient records.)

In some jurisdictions information related to sexual activity obtained from a minor must not be revealed to the parent without the minor's consent. Both criminal and civil actions may result from this specific form of breach of confidentiality.

PATIENT RECORDS

Treatment records serve as documentation of the care the patients have received. They are essential to the defense of a practitioner accused of negligence.

One of the legal authorities in the field of medical malpractice and editor of a major text on the subject had the following to say about dental records: "Dentists seem to be among the worst record keepers. It is not unusual for the complete dental records to consist mainly or solely of a billing chart. Such scant records should be considered malpractice in and of themselves."[3]

The patient's dental record is considered by the courts as a legal document and must be treated as such. It serves many purposes in the judicial process. It contains information about the patient's complaint, health history, and basis for the diagnosis, and it reports all treatment rendered, the patient's reaction to treatment, and the results of the treatment. Case law requires that health practitioners keep accurate records of the diagnosis and treatment of their patients. These records constitute an essential part of patient care. Treating a patient without maintaining accurate records represents a serious departure from an acceptable level of care as defined by the courts. Some jurisdictions require that accurate records be kept as part of the rules and regulations of administrative health or licensing agencies.

The outcome of many suits against dentists is decided on the content and quality of patient records. For the treating doctor the record is the only documentation of the course of treatment of the patient and the patient's reactions to the treatment. Memory alone is often viewed as self-serving and, as stated in one court decision, "the shortest written word lasts longer than the longest memory." In cases in which the doctor and patient disagree on what took place and there is no written documentation of the event, the question of how much weight will be given to the oral statements may be determined in court by who makes the most credible witness. It can become a risky situation for the doctor.

In summary, failure to keep accurate records may constitute negligence and, in some jurisdictions, a violation of law. In addition, failure to keep accurate records markedly increases the chance of losing a malpractice suit.

The risk management rule is: *Accurate and complete records must be maintained for each patient you treat or examine.*

Record ownership

The right to ownership of the patient's treatment record has undergone considerable change during the past several decades. Courts have separated the physical record from the right of the patient to its contents. At one time doctors had the exclusive right to the possession of the record and its contents. Today, after many suits, the law has evolved so that the doctor is considered the custodian of the record and the patient has a property right in its contents. Some jurisdictions have codified court decisions.

If the patient demands in writing to be sent a copy of the treatment record or demands that a copy be sent to another practitioner or to any other person or agency, the practitioner should comply with the request (in some jurisdictions, *must* comply with the request), but, in either case, supply only copies. The term *record* includes the treatment record, radiographs, casts, results of tests, and consultation reports.

If the dentist believes that the patient, when demand is made for the record, intends litigation, the dentist should report the request to the insurance carrier after complying with the request. If there is no local law that the dentist must comply with the request for copies of the record, the dentist should not comply unless the carrier approves in writing. If an attorney demands the record, the dentist should not comply without first informing the carrier. However, if the dentist does decide to comply, the attorney's demand should also include a written release from the patient. Should another dentist ask for a copy of the record, the original dentist should make certain that the request includes a written release from the patient.

Remember, in no case should the original records or radiographs be sent. The one exception is if the request is made by a court.

The risk management rules that are generated by the new view of the courts about the patients' rights to record ownership are: *On the patients' written request for their records, comply but supply only copies. If you believe a patient intends to sue, before you comply, contact your insurance carrier for advice.*

The risk management rule that the dentist retain the original of all patient records is underscored by what a California court said about a doctor's not producing the originals: "The inability of the physician to produce the original of the clinical record concerning his treatment of the plaintiff creates a strong inference of consciousness of guilt."[4]

Form and content

The changing law on ownership of patient records has had a profound effect on the form and content of the record. Keeping in mind that what is written on the record may be seen by the patient will serve as a guide to what should be entered on the record.

Financial information has no place on the treatment record. Separate records should be kept to record charges and payments.

The treatment record should be written in black ink or black ballpoint pen. It should be neat, well organized, and easily read. A sloppy record implies a sloppy dentist and has a negative effect on the jury and judge. Patient records, as all legal documents, should be legible and complete. There should be no blank spaces where information is supposed to be inserted. A decision by a New York court stated: "[A] patient record so sparse as to be accurate and meaningful only to the recording physician fails to meet the intent of the requirement to maintain records which accurately reflect the evaluation and treatment of the patient."[5] A later section of this chapter provides suggestions on the form and content of record keeping.

How long should patient records be retained? In many jurisdictions, laws specify the minimum time period for retention of patient treatment records. Failure to comply brings with it risk of allegations by a state agency of a violation of the law. On the civil side, practitioners are advised to keep the original treatment records for as long as possible. Although the statute of limitations runs for a specific period, the exceptions suggest that the records be kept for a period considerably longer than the statute. For example, in New York, an occurrence state (where the statute of limitations begins to run from the time of the occurrence of the negligent incident), if you are accused of withholding information from a patient about a mishap in treatment, the courts may extend the statute on the basis of your fraudulent concealment. In Massachusetts, a discovery state (where the statute does not begin to run until the patient discovered, or should have discovered, the act that produced the injury), the suit may begin many years after the patient completed treatment. Two thirds of the states have the discovery rule. The rest have the time-of-injury rule. But even in those states there are exceptions, which may include fraudulent concealment (noted previously), foreign body exception, and an exception for continuous treatment. In the case of minors, in many jurisdictions the statute on retention of records does not begin to run until the minor reaches majority. Therefore the records of minors must be kept for an extended period of time.

The appointment log, or book, is an integral and essential part of office records. It records appointments made for patients, either for consultation or treatment. It may serve the dentist well should the log accurately record not only the scheduled appointments but, in addition, late arrivals, canceled appointments, and no-shows. All entries on the log should be made in ink or ballpoint pen. Like the patient's treat-

ment records, there should be no erasures obliterating original entries. Like the patient's treatment records, the appointment log should be kept for as long as possible—not discarded at the end of each year.

Without records, it is virtually impossible to succeed in defending a suit.

The risk management rule is: *Retain original patient treatment records, including radiographs, the appointment log, and all other documents related to the diagnosis and treatment of the patient, for as long as possible.*

Record keeping rules

1. Entries should be legible, written in black ink or ballpoint pen. In one case decided by a court, the court stated that the physician's records were not "accurate" as required by the law because they were illegible and contained nonstandard abbreviations. The physician's license was suspended.

2. In offices where more than one person is making entries, the entries should be signed or initialed. A sample of the initials and signatures of all persons who make entries on records should be maintained.

3. Entries that are in error should not be blocked out so that they cannot be read. Instead, a single line should be drawn through the entry and a note made above it stating "error in entry, see correction below." The correction should be dated at the time it is made.

4. Entries should be uniformly spaced on the form. There should be no unusual or irregular blank spaces. Always write between the lines and never in the margins.

5. On health information forms there should be no blank spaces in the answers to health questions. If the question is inappropriate, draw a single line through the question, or record "not applicable" (NA) in the box. If the response is normal, write "within normal limits" (WNL).

6. Record all cancellations, late arrivals, and changes of appointments.
7. Document consents, including all risks and alternative treatments presented to the patient. Include any remarks made by the patient. Enter telephone conversations that relate to the care of the patient.
8. It is important to inform the patient of any adverse occurrences or untoward events that take place during the course of treatment and to note on the record that the patient was informed. If possible, have the patient initial or sign the entry.
9. Record all requests for consultations and their reports.
10. Document all conversations held with other health practitioners relating to the care of the patient.
11. All patient records should be retained for as long as possible.
12. If the practice is terminated, local law should be checked to determine the requirements on how, where, and in what form the records must be retained.
13. Guard confidentiality of information contained on the record.
14. *Never* surrender the original record to *anyone,* except by order of a court or to your own attorney.
15. *Never* tamper with a record once there is some indication that legal action is contemplated by the patient.
16. Keep patient records in a safe place, fireproof, etc.

What not to put on the treatment record

1. Financial information should not be kept on the treatment record. Use a separate financial form.
2. Do not record subjective evaluations, such as your opinion about the patient's mental health, on the treatment record unless you are qualified and licensed to make such evaluation. Record such observations on a separate sheet marked "Confidential—Per-

sonal notes." In most jurisdictions such notes are not discoverable, and the practitioner is not required to deliver them when a request is made for the records.
3. Do not record any correspondence with your professional liability insurance company, your attorney, or the attorney representing a patient on the treatment record. Record all such notes and any conversations with the above on a separate sheet marked "Confidential—Personal notes."

HISTORIES
Medical history

An area of growing concern for dentists in malpractice liability relates to the health history. There have been major financial and professional losses caused by the dentist's failure to discover information about the patient's medical history. The primary cause of the problem is the design of the typical self-administered health history form and the manner in which the dentist deals with the completed form. The form used by most dentists has led to considerable difficulties. The most common has two columns in which patients may indicate whether they have a particular health problem. They are asked to place a checkmark in a "yes" or "no" box or to circle a "yes" or "no" word. In many cases there have been disputes at trial about who placed the checkmark or circle, notwithstanding the fact that the patient signed the form. Facts in dispute lead to problems for the defense attorney in the trial of a case. Questions have been raised as to whether a question on the health history form can be asked about if the patient has AIDS or is HIV positive. Currently there appears to be no problem related to asking the question provided it is asked of all patients and the answer is not used to refuse care to the patient. If the refusal to treat is based on other medical or dental considerations there would be no violation of any antidiscrimination laws.

The risk management rule is: *If you use a self-administered health history form in which patients are to respond by marking a box, have them initial the appropriate box rather than using a checkmark.*

Other problems have arisen with the self-administered health history form. Did the patient understand the questions? Did the patient know the answer at the time the form was completed? Was the patient aware of the importance of the question to care? If the answer to any of these questions is no, the patient may leave a blank in place of an answer or may provide an answer that is not accurate. Blanks left on a completed history form may lead to difficulties: was the question ignored or was the answer negative?

If a self-administered health form is used, there should be four columns instead of two, to avoid a possibility of blanks. The column headings should be "Yes," "No," "Don't Know," and "Don't Understand the Question."

Another problem is related to the manner in which the dentist follows up the self-administered health history. It is usual for the dentist to question the patient further but limiting the questioning to the positive answers on the form. Most forms are designed to alert the dentist solely to the positive answers. This process may lead to major errors. The patient may have misinterpreted or not understood the question and incorrectly answered in the negative. This has resulted in large malpractice losses. Several cases have been reported where the dentist, using a "Yes-No" form, failed to discover that the patient had a history of rheumatic fever and thus took no precautions in treatment. Do not leave it to patients to decide whether the answers to the questions on the health history are important to the success and safety of their care.

The risk management rule is: *If you use a self-administered health history form and the choices to the patient are two—"yes" or "no"—follow up on the "no" answers as well as the "yes" answers to make certain the patient understood the questions, their importance in treatment, and the reason the questions were being asked.*

The best policy for the use of a self-administered health history form is not to use it. It leaves too much to chance in discovering medical problems that may compromise the successful and safe treatment of the patient. There is much more at stake than legal liability. When a history of rheumatic fever is not discovered, no matter who is at fault, the consequences to the patient and the dentist may be disastrous.

A more effective way to determine medical history is to have the history taken by someone who has been trained in the procedure and who has the background to interpret the responses—preferably, the treating dentist. If the history is elicited by someone other than the treating dentist, the dentist should review the history with the patient before treatment.

Another type of history-taking form is simple to design. Use a blank sheet of paper with a reminder list of the questions to be asked in the left margin. It is better to spend the extra time this takes than to have a patient, because of your negligence, suffer permanent injury as a result of the use of an inadequately designed form.

Updating the medical history

Good dental practice requires that the patient's health history be updated at regular intervals. The frequency at which it should be done is a professional, not a legal, decision. The process is simple and effective: allow the patient to review the documented health history that was obtained at the last history-taking visit and ask if there are any changes. Make notes of the procedure and the patient's responses in the patient's record. An abbreviated history update form is simple to design. For example, the form may state the following: "I have reviewed the health history form completed on ____, and I report the following: ____." If there has been no change, the patient writes, "No change." If there is a change, the patient so indicates on the form. At times, depending on the nature of the change, the dentist may ask the patient to complete another full health history form.

The risk management rule is: *Update the health history at appropriate intervals and document the process and responses.*

If you continue to use a self-administered health history form, place the following statement before the space for the patient's signature: "I understand and agree that in the event there is any change in my health status, I will notify your office at the earliest possible time." As an express term in the doctor-patient contract it places some of the burden on the patient but will not relieve the doctor of the responsibility for updating the health status of the patient. Follow up on positive findings.

It is essential to good patient care and to risk management concerns that positive findings in the medical history be followed up by consulting the patient's physician or another appropriate health provider or health facility. It is best to have consultant reports in writing. If this is inconvenient, information received by telephone should be noted on the patient's record.

The risk management rule is: *Document all conversations with other health practitioners and health facilities that are or were involved in the treatment of your patient and from whom you received information. If you receive a written report, it should be placed in the patient's treatment folder.*

The dental history

The dental history presents fewer problems to the dentist than does the general health history. However, one issue not as yet addressed by the courts deserves attention. Dental disease is chronic and almost everyone suffers from it. It does not begin when the patient comes to the dentist. Most patients change dentists several times throughout their lives. To have a complete picture of the etiology of the patient's current dental problem and the history of the treatment, it is essential that, in addition to the dental history obtained from the patient, the treating dentist should make every effort to obtain the records of the previous dentist(s). It is possible that the previous dentist's notes may assist in the treatment of the patient in areas such as an abnormal reaction to the administration of a drug, the level of patient cooperation, breaking of appointments, and delinquencies in the payment of fees. Not obtaining information that is available and may be essential in the treatment of the patient may constitute malpractice.

A good risk management practice is: *Obtain the records and radiographs of prior dentists and other health care providers who have treated your patient. Determine whether there is some law in the state that enables patients to secure copies of their records and radiographs and, if such a law is present, use it to obtain the records rather than making a direct request. If you decide to make a direct request, make it in writing and include an authorization signed by the patient to release the records.*

EXAMINING THE PATIENT AND COMPLETING A TREATMENT PLAN

"Failure to diagnose" represents a growing area of legal vulnerability. A thorough clinical examination and radiographic review should be completed on each patient. The results should be recorded on the patient's record.

It is difficult to defend a case successfully when many of the questions on the form used to record the dental examination have been left blank. It is impossible to determine whether the blank indicates that the question was mistakenly omitted in the examination or if the result was within normal limits. If the form you use has questions that are not germane to your practice habits or are seldom answered, design your own form or purchase one that is more suited to your particular needs and habits of practice.

Many recent cases involve failure to diagnose periodontal disease. Periodontal issues present a major problem if there is no evidence that the patient was examined to determine periodontal needs, for example, pocket depth, plaque scores, bleeding points, mobility, or oral hygiene index. The answers to the following questions may become important if a suit alleging periodontal neglect is brought against the dentist: If periodontal disease was diagnosed, was the patient informed? Was the need for periodontal care neglected? Was a recommendation made for the patient to seek the services of a periodontist? In summary, was there failure to diagnose, failure to inform, failure to make a timely referral, or failure to treat? If the answer to any part of the question is positive, the dentist is at risk of an allegation of malpractice and is likely to lose the suit.

Issues related to the temporomandibular joint (TMJ) and surrounding tissues have become a target of litigation. The same questions raised about periodontal neglect apply equally to the joint, and the same risks in practice apply. The area of the joint should be examined and monitored during treatment. Problems may arise during orthodontic care, after the extraction of lower molars, and after procedures that require the jaws to remain open for long periods of time, such as the use of a rubber dam for an extended period of time during endodontic procedures. In a recent appellate court decision the court stated that all reversible and conservative forms of therapy to correct problems related to the TMJ should be ruled out as ineffective before surgery is performed. In that case, after multiple surgeries the patient, a 26-year-old woman, committed suicide.[6]

Acceptable dental practice includes completing both a recommended treatment plan and a reasonable alternative. Either have the patient sign or initial the accepted plan or make a note of the patient's acceptance in the record.

Good risk management practice includes completing a thorough dental examination and treatment plan before treatment is begun. The results should be accurately recorded, and all questions on the dental examination form should be answered. There should be documentation that the treatment plan was accepted by the patient.

CONSENT

Legal problems related to lack of informed consent to dental care began to surface as a result of the explosion in medical malpractice in the early 1970s. The general principle that a doctor who treats a patient without the patient's express consent is guilty of an unauthorized touching, for which the doctor can be held liable to the patient in damages, began early in the century. The fact that the patient needed the treatment and benefited as a result of the treatment did not relieve the doctor of liability. In the early years the civil claim was that the doctor was guilty of trespass to the person, or assault and battery. Today the courts feel that the legal action of malpractice is more appropriate, given the lack of intent to harm by the doctor. The legal procedure is quite different if the action is brought in trespass compared with actions brought in malpractice. In addition, many courts opined that the failure to obtain the consent of the patient before initiating treatment was a breach of the doctor-patient contract. Actions in contract law differ in procedure from both trespass actions and malpractice actions. The modern view is that if *no* consent was obtained the action may be in contract. However, if the consent was obtained but was faulty, as most of them are, the action in malpractice is more appropriate. The defendant dentist benefits if the action is in malpractice rather than in trespass or contract. In trespass and contract actions the patient-plaintiff is not required to produce an expert witness relating to the standard of professional care and whether the dentist-defendant departed from the standard. In malpractice actions an expert testifying on behalf of the patient-plaintiff is required.

Content of consent: what and how much to tell

Having discussed the legal form of action, we now turn our attention to the content of the consent. As the years progressed since the first major case dealing with the consent to medical care, the courts turned their attention to the issue of whether the consent was informed: Was the patient given enough information on which to make an intelligent decision? The modern view is that the patient must be informed of all the following:

1. A description of the proposed treatment
2. The material or foreseeable risks
3. The benefits and prognosis of the proposed treatment
4. All reasonable alternatives to the proposed treatment
5. The risks, benefits, and prognosis of the alternative treatments

All these factors must be described to the patient in language the patient understands, and the patient must be given an opportunity to ask questions about the treatment and alternatives and to have the questions answered.

What of the description of the risks?

How much of the risk must be told to the patient for consent to meet the test of being informed? There is no agreement among state courts on which to present a bottom-line rule. In most states the patient must be given enough information about the risks to make an intelligent decision about whether to proceed with the proposed treatment. It is called *the subjective prudent person rule.* Another standard is whether a reasonable person in the patient's situation was given enough information to make an intelligent decision. It is called *the objective reasonable person rule.* In both rules the risks are called *material* because they are material either to the patient or to the reasonable person. The third standard is the *professional community standard;* that is, what do other practitioners tell their patients about the risks when the same condition exists? These risks are termed *foreseeable.* As an example, in a state that follows the *professional community standard,* a dentist would not have to explain the risk of breaking an instrument in a canal during an endodontic procedure if it can be shown that few, if any, dentists in the community warn

their patients of the possibility. In a *reasonable-person* state, whether objective or subjective, a dentist may not be required to inform an 80-year-old retiree of the possibility of permanent paresthesia after the extraction of an impacted lower third molar because the risk is not material to the patient or to any reasonable person in the same situation as the patient; the risk is not material. However, if the same dental situation is present where the patient is a trial lawyer, the risk becomes *material* and should be told to the patient before treatment is begun.

In *material-risk* states the patient-plaintiff is not required to present the evidence of an expert dentist. In *foreseeable-risk* states the patient-plaintiff is required to produce an expert witness for the judge or jury to determine the standard of disclosure of the professional community. Thus the burden on the patient-plaintiff in *professional-community (foreseeable risk)* states is greater than that in *reasonable-person (material-risk)* states.

Many states have adopted statutes, administrative rules, or court procedural rules, superimposed on court decisions, that may have modified their courts' decisions. However, all fall in with the standards described previously.

The prudent dentist will tell each patient both the *foreseeable* and the *material* risks. This approach will satisfy all court-imposed and BLL (i.e., statutes, administrative rules and regulations) standards. Thus the dentist is advised to inform each patient faced with the extraction of an impacted lower third molar the risk of permanent paresthesia regardless of who the patient is, the educational level, age, occupation, or whatever, no matter what the dentist believes other dentists tell their patients.

Another issue relating to what the patient should be told is the "common knowledge" doctrine. There are certain risks of which the patient should be aware, by common knowledge, without having to be told by the dentist. All reasonable adults are expected to know that after the extraction of a tooth they will have some bleeding and, when the anesthetic wears off, some pain. By contrast, no reasonable person would expect to have permanent loss of sensation of the lower lip after the extraction of an impacted lower wisdom tooth. However, the admonition is not to rely on common knowledge in describing the risks of the proposed procedure.

The risk management rules are: *Tell the patient everything about what you recommend and the reasonable alternatives. Use language the patient understands. Give the patient an opportunity to ask questions, and provide answers. Document the entire process.*

Form of consent: written or oral?

Consent to health care, like all agreements between parties, may be written or oral, and further it may be expressed or implied. An expressed consent is one in which both parties agree, either orally or in written form. An implied consent is present either by the action of the parties or by law. Expressed and implied consents will be discussed in the next section. Here we will examine written and oral consents.

As long as there is no dispute between the parties as to the details of the agreement, an oral agreement is effective and enforceable. Only when the parties disagree as to the details of the agreement does a written document become important. In general, laws that require agreements (contracts) to be written do not directly affect dental care. These include agreements relating to real property, contracts of sale over a specified amount, and contracts that cannot be completed within a year. They fall into a legal category called the "statute of frauds" and must be written to be enforceable.

In a few situations the law requires that consent to health care be in writing and signed by the patient. Health facilities such as hospitals may require that the consent to treatment be written and signed by each patient. If you work in such a facility, you should comply with the rules and obtain the written and signed consent of each patient you treat in the facility. Failure to do so may compromise your legal position, and that of the institution, if a patient claims that you proceeded with treatment without valid consent. Other than institutional rules, few regulations require written consent to health care. Most refer to abortions, donation of human organs, in New York to acupuncture, in some jurisdictions to HIV testing, and in others to surgical procedures. You should check the local law to determine whether any require that for the treatment you propose consent must be written and signed. Also, you should check to see whether local law requires that you include specific information in informing the patient about the treatment you propose.

As a general rule, despite the absence of any law requiring that consent be written, you should have documentation that a valid consent was obtained for a procedure that has high risks or is invasive. The best documentation is to have a written and signed consent to care that contains all the elements required for it to be valid. The problem is that without a written document there may be conflicting testimony as to exactly what the dentist informed the patient about the procedure and its attendant risks and exactly to what the patient agreed. In nonemergency situations it is best to allow patients to take consent forms home before signing, to allow time to discuss the matter with family or friends. Your records should indicate that this was done and that the consent was discussed before treatment was begun.

Form of consent: implied or expressed?

In some dental practice situations implied consent may serve as an effective defense for the dentist. In simple, common, noninvasive procedures implied consent is likely to be supported by the courts. A routine dental examination is a good example of one in which the dentist does not have to rely on a written signed consent. Another situation is one in which the patient understands what is being done and makes no attempt to interrupt the procedure. In both situations consent is implied by the action of the party. However, as stated before, if the procedure is invasive or the risks are great and likely to occur, written consent may prepare the patient for the possible consequences and serve to defuse a lawsuit.

In an emergency situation in which care must be rendered at once and consent of the patient could not be obtained, consent is implied by law, as compared with the previous situation in which consent is implied by the action of the party. Courts have applied the following test to support consent implied by law in an emergency situation: (1) consent would have been granted had the patient been able to do so, (2) a reasonable person in the patient's condition would have granted consent, and (3) an emergency was present where treatment was necessary and time was of the essence to preserve the life or health of the victim. This legal theory is present in Good Samaritan situations; consent is implied by law.

Who should obtain consent?

As a general rule the health provider is the person charged with obtaining consent to care. However, in practice, others associated with the office or institution in which the care is provided are assigned the responsibility to obtain consent. Two recent court cases, one in Pennsylvania[7] and the other in New York[8], stated that anyone designated and trained by the provider may obtain a valid consent to care. Despite the rulings, the dentist is advised to review the consent document with the patient; offer to answer any questions concerning the procedure, its risks, benefits, and alternatives; and note on the patient's record that this was done.

Who may grant consent?

As a general rule, only the recipient of care may grant a valid consent. As with all general rules, there are exceptions. The most obvious

is that minors cannot grant valid consent for their health care. Only a minor's parent or legal guardian can grant a valid consent for the care of the minor—not the minor's adult sibling, not a neighbor, not even a grandparent who supports and pays for the care of the grandchild, and not the child's schoolteacher. However, the parent may grant to any of these people authority to consent to health care for the minor child. The authorization should be written and signed by the parent for the dentist to rely on the authorization.

The obvious question is: When does a minor become an adult? Most states set the majority age at 18 years. There are exceptions. The age at which a minor may grant a valid consent to health care may be established by state statute. It may be as low as 14 years. In addition, many states have defined an "emancipated minor" in contract law and extended it to include consent to health care. In general, an emancipated minor is one no longer dependent on parents for support. In addition, pregnant minors are emancipated, as are married minors. The net result is that emancipated minors may grant a valid consent to health care independent of parental consent. Who pays for the service has no effect on the consent to care. Payment for it is a separate issue; the parent may consent to the payment, but the emancipated minor must consent to the care.

In the case of divorced or separated parents, either may consent to the care of the child, unless there is a modification of the custody agreement. Again, payment is a separate issue but it may be part of the custody agreement.

Keeping in mind that only the patient can grant a valid consent to health care, a husband cannot grant a valid consent to the care of his wife despite her inability to do so, nor can an adult for an aged parent. In either case the spouse or adult child of the aged parent must be appointed the legal guardian of the patient.

In the case of a mentally impaired adult, in some states consent granted by the parent may not be valid unless the parent is designated by the court as the patient's legal guardian. In others, a mentally impaired adult may be considered a minor and the rules of consent to the health care of minors apply. You are advised to check the local law of the state in which you practice.

Telephone consent

Telephone consent, properly executed, is acceptable to the courts. It must, however, contain all the elements that constitute a valid consent. In addition, it must be properly documented. In the case of a minor, the parent or guardian should be contacted by phone and told that a third party is listening on an extension. The parent should be told of the situation and the need for treatment, including all the facts that would be required to meet a valid consent. After the consent is obtained, appropriate notes should be made on the patient's chart, signed by the one who obtained the consent, and countersigned by the third party.

Summary

For a summary of consent as it relates to risk management, see Box 18-1.

Box 18-1

CONSENT: A RISK MANAGEMENT GUIDE

1. In general, the more invasive the procedure or the greater the risk, the more the requirements of a valid consent must be met; documentation that consent was obtained becomes important. For example, to obtain consent for an examination in which no invasive procedure is to be performed, it might be that implied consent by the actions of the patient is sufficient with little or no documentation on the patient's record. By contrast, in a situation where an invasive procedure is to be performed, all the requirements of a valid consent should be met, and documentation in the patient's record is essential.

2. The better the documentation, the less the legal risk. Written forms may be used, provided that the delivery of the form is linked to the patient's awareness by sufficient notes made on the patient's record, such as "Patient given handout number __ to read, the proposed treatment and alternatives were discussed, and all the patient's questions were answered."

3. Make certain that the one from whom consent is obtained has legal standing to grant consent.

4. When consent for the treatment of a minor is obtained by telephone, it is best to follow up on the telephone conversation by sending a written consent in the mail to be signed by the parent or guardian and then returned to the office.

5. Check the local law to determine if written consent is required in situations related to specific treatment.

6. If you delegate to anyone in your office the responsibility to obtain consent from a patient, document that the person was trained in obtaining consent and that you reviewed the consent, discussed it with the patient, and answered all the patient's questions about the procedure.

7. Make certain that in obtaining the consent all elements to make the consent valid are included: a description of the procedure, why it is necessary, an estimate of the anticipated success, the prognosis if the procedure is not done, the foreseeable and material risks in having it done, and alternatives to the recommended procedure, including their risks, benefits, and prognoses. Present this in language the patient understands (use lay terms), and give the patient an opportunity to discuss all these topics with you. By describing the material risks and the foreseeable risks all bases are covered to satisfy any local law or court decision.

8. When the treatment includes an invasive procedure, it is best to allow the patient to take the consent form home before signing it.

INFORMED REFUSAL

A new legal concept appears to be developing in the arena of malpractice litigation as an outgrowth of informed consent: informed refusal. In a medical malpractice case a woman was advised to undergo a Papanicolaou (PAP) smear. She refused. Later cervical cancer developed and the woman died. The physician was sued for failing to sufficiently inform the patient of the consequences of her refusal. Several members of the court agreed that the patient must be told of the possible consequences of refusal to make an intelligent decision in refusing a recommended course of treatment.[9] Thus the concept of informed refusal is gradually emerging.

If a practitioner recommends to a patient that surgery is the best course of treatment, the patient must be informed of the consequences of refusal. If the patient refuses the care and later has an injury because of not having the surgery performed, the practitioner may be liable to the patient in damages because the patient was not informed of the consequences of the refusal. Having now been informed of this modification to the informed consent concept, it must be incorporated into practice documentation that the patient has been told of the risks of refusal.

The risk management rule relating to the refusal of a patient to follow professional advice: *Document that the patient was informed about the best course of action to take to preserve or improve his or her oral health and about the likely consequences if the advice is not followed.*

EMERGENCIES AND THE GOOD SAMARITAN LAW

The Good Samaritan law, enacted in all states, provides immunity from suit for specified health practitioners who render emergency aid to victims of accidents. Generally the statutes require that the aid is provided with no expectation of financial remuneration. Should an injury result from negligence, the victim is precluded by law from instituting a suit, provided there was no evidence of gross negligence. *Gross negligence* is defined as a wanton disregard for another's safety or the failure to exercise slight care. Immunity does not extend to acts performed in the office or in any health facility.

The standard to which the Good Samaritan is held is based on education and experience. Therefore an act performed by an oral and maxillofacial surgeon may constitute gross negligence, whereas the same act performed by a general practitioner may not be considered negligence at all.

Not all states include dentists in the Good Samaritan law.

The risk management rule is: *Determine whether the jurisdiction in which you practice includes dentists in the Good Samaritan law. Be guided by the answer in rendering emergency aid at the scene of an accident, but keep in mind there are ethical responsibilities that attach to your role as a health professional.*

An *emergency* is defined as any situation when care must be provided at once to preserve the life or health of the patient. Because the interpretation is broad in most states, dental care may fall within the definition. In cases where a dental emergency exists and consent cannot be obtained because of a time constraint, consent to care is implied by operation of law.

The risk management rule in dealing with emergencies in which a minor is involved and brought to the office by someone other than a parent is: *Efforts should be made to obtain the consent of the parent before treatment is begun. These efforts should accurately be recorded on the record. If consent was obtained by telephone, the third listening party should sign the record following the note.*

One of the duties owed by the dentist to patients of record, by case law, and in some jurisdictions by BLL is to make care available to patients in emergency situations. Generally the patient determines what constitutes an emergency.

The risk management rule in emergency situations for patients of record is: *The availability of care is a 24-hour-a-day, 7-day-a-week responsibility. If you are on vacation or otherwise unavailable, someone must cover for you, and that information be made available to your patients—the most effective way to do this is with a message left on your answering machine or with a member of your staff who is available.*

Miscellaneous issues
PACKAGE INSERTS

Inserts in drug packaging have been accepted into evidence in malpractice cases. Dentists and physicians have been found guilty of negligence for not following the warnings contained on the package inserts. Statements contained in the *Physicians' Desk Reference* (PDR) have also been admitted into evidence.

The risk management rule is: *Read all drug package inserts and the PDR before administering or prescribing a drug. Because inserts and the PDR are updated frequently, they should be consulted regularly.*

WHAT TO DO WHEN DOCTORS DISAGREE

Situations may arise when the treating dentist and the patient's physician disagree on what prophylactic measures should be taken with a cardiac-compromised patient. The physician may recommend that no preventive measures be taken or that measures be taken that are not consistent with those the dentist feels are appropriate. If the physician's advice is followed and an injury results, it is difficult for the dentist to claim immunity on the basis of the physician's recommendation. The patient is a patient of the dentist, and the dentist operates on his or her own license. Dentists are not employees of physicians or required to carry out a physician's orders if they believe the orders are not consistent with the patient's needs. Whatever care is rendered by a dentist to the patient is interpreted as what the dentist, in her or his best judgment, thinks should be done.

If the dentist does not follow the advice of the physician and an injury occurs, the dentist will be judged on what other dentists in the community would do under similar circumstances and not on what the physician recommended. If the dentist's care meets acceptable community standards, there may be no liability.

If the patient demands that the physician's advice be followed by the dentist and the dentist feels that the advice is not in the best interests of the patient's health, the best course for the dentist to follow is to refuse to treat the patient—the principle is one of Level of Legal Risk.

The risk management rule is: *Exercise your own judgment when deciding on the dental care of the patient. Use advice by others, including physicians, as recommendations that you may either accept or reject. The final decision as to what is done is yours and the patient's.*

ASSOCIATES AND EMPLOYEES

There are several important legal issues involved with associates and employees of the dentist. Those with an impact on legal vulnerability are discussed in this section. It is important for dentists to be aware that the more complex the arrangements of practice, the more exposure there is to legal entanglements.

Associations in practice may take many forms, some of which increase legal risk. The employer-employee relationship between dentists makes the employer-dentist individually or jointly liable for the negligent acts of the employee dentist. The legal doctrine for this transfer of liability to the employer, an innocent party, is known as *respondeat superior* (the person in the superior position, the employer, must answer for the acts of the one in the inferior position, the employee, to injured third parties). It is a form of vicarious liability (the substitution of an innocent party for a guilty one in the matter of liability to third parties). However, the employer may sue the employee for indemnification of the employer's losses. If both are insured by the same professional liability insurance company, complications may be avoided.

The same principle of respondeat superior applies to all employees of the dentist, including hygienists, dental assistants, receptionists, and others. The employer-dentist is held liable for all acts performed by an employee in the course of conducting the business of the employer-dentist, even if the acts are specifically prohibited or illegal.

Another form of associate practice among dentists is the partnership. All partners are individually liable for the negligent acts of one partner. The choice of whom to sue is exercised by the plaintiff or the plaintiff's attorney. If a generalist, who is at low risk, has a partner who practices oral and maxillofacial surgery, which is of high risk, the generalist may be held liable for the negligent acts of the surgeon. It is not unusual for all partners to be joined in the suit. Vicarious liability is supported by the legal theory that all partners are united in interest (each benefits from the acts of others). To avoid serious complications, all should be covered by the same professional liability insurance company. From the standpoint of legal liability for negligent acts, practicing in a partnership agreement brings with it serious risks. In several cases, courts have stated that if the patient considers the practice to be a partnership, the courts will treat it as such; even if the agreement among a group of dentists is to practice as solo and independent practitioners. If they engage in sharing to the extent that the arrangement appears to be a partnership, they may take on the liability risks of a partnership.

The third form of association is the professional corporation. This relationship represents the lowest level of the transfer or sharing of legal risk. Except in unusual circumstances, innocent shareholders are not liable for the negligent acts of other shareholders. Only the guilty practitioner and the corporation are liable. However, all shareholders and the corporation should be insured by the same professional liability insurance company.

Recently all states have enacted legislation to enable businesses to enter into a new form of legal entity, the limited liability company, designated as the LLC or the L.L.C. It has all the advantages of the traditional corporation as it relates to liability, or lack of shared liability of "innocent parties." Dentists may form an LLC, known as a professional limited liability company, or PLLC. Currently two states permit a single dentist to form a PLLC: Texas and New York. In the future other states may permit solo practitioners to form a PLLC. The advantage of an LLC over a corporation is that it is considerably less costly to form and maintain.

The independent contractor (IC) is the final form of association to be considered. With this arrangement, the principal hopes to avoid liability for the negligent acts of the IC. The courts examine, in detail, the arrangement between the parties before determining whether the principal is free from liability for the negligent acts of the IC. The matter of control of the ICs, who sets the hours for the IC, whose patients they are, who hires and pays auxiliary personnel, and who provides the equipment and supplies used by the IC are all questions that determine whether the IC is truly an IC or simply an employee in determining the liability of the principal (employee). Having the same professional liability insurance company prevents many complications. Recent court decisions have examined whether a dentist working with another under the cloak of an IC for the principal to avoid withholding a portion of the IC's earnings and the payment of unemployment and worker's compensation taxes was consistent with the law. The decisions reached clearly point out that such an arrangement is employer-employee. The rules to qualify as an IC are many and complex. The principal is at risk and will be penalized, not the bogus IC.

The lowest level of legal risk in associateship practice is to practice as a professional corporation or as a professional limited liability company and in any form of joint practice for all parties to be insured by the same professional liability insurance carrier. Before you agree to join another dentist or group as an IC, check the law.

The acts or statements made by nondentist employees present forms of legal risks to the employer-dentist other than those described previously. Employees of a dentist are treated by the courts as agents of the dentist when they are serving in the capacity for which they were employed. Thus if a receptionist, hygienist, or assistant assures a patient that after treatment the patient will be satisfied with the result or makes other such statements related to the services provided by the employer-dentist, an express guarantee has been made to which the dentist will likely be held.

The risk management advice is: *Educate your employees to the precise role they are to play in communicating and dealing with patients. Supervise them carefully and monitor their activities at regular intervals. Remain current on changes in the law that affect dental auxiliaries.*

INTERPERSONAL RELATIONSHIPS

A deterioration in good interpersonal relations between patient and dentist or between patient and staff still ranks as one of the leading causes of malpractice allegations. When a patient becomes angry, upset, or frustrated, instituting a lawsuit is one of the methods available for retaliation against the dentist or the dentist's staff. The resulting annoyance to the dentist may be reason enough to sue, regardless of the merits of the claim. For the patient, it works. For the dentist, it becomes a real problem involving time, effort, emotional distress, and at times dollars. Too often, efforts of the auxiliary staff made in the interest of shielding the dentist from complaints of difficult patients or patients with annoying problems result in a patient seeking redress through the courts. Most of these situations can be defused by an understanding and compassionate staff. The dentist must be accessible to patients, particularly to those with perceived problems. The judgment of the staff as to what is important to the patient should not be substituted for the patient's judgment of what is important.

The risk management advice is: *Monitor the staff in their interpersonal relationships with patients. Listen to your patients. Make certain that patients with problems have access to you. Do not hide from your patients. Arrange for substitute care when you are absent for extended periods. If all efforts fail to restore a cordial relationship with a difficult patient, the safest course to follow is to discontinue treatment.*

RETURN OF A FEE AND SUING TO COLLECT ONE

At one time, courts viewed the return of a fee by a doctor as an admission of wrongdoing. Today, it is viewed as an expression of good faith and interest in the welfare of the patient. If the return of a fee, or part of it, will appease a hostile patient and defuse a difficult situation, it is best to do so. With a patient who threatens to sue unless the fee is returned, and the dentist decides to return the fee, it is best to have the patient execute a release-from-liability form with acceptance of the returned fee. You should weigh the refusal to return the fee with the trauma and loss of time in defending a claim of malpractice; you might even lose the case.

At one time the return of a fee, no matter what the amount, by a health practitioner to a patient had to be reported to the National Practitioners Data Bank. On interpretation of the law by an administrative law judge, the reporting requirement was declared not to include private practitioners. Thus a dentist who returns a fee to a patient is not required to report it to the National Practitioners Data Bank.

One of the major causes of malpractice allegations is a response to an attempt by a doctor to collect a fee. Patients who are delinquent or refuse to pay are inclined to claim poor quality of care as the reason. Should the doctor press to collect, especially through the courts, the patient is likely to countersue for malpractice. Weighing the risk of a countersuit in malpractice should be a guide before suing to collect the fee.

If the dentist uses a collection agency to act on his or her behalf for fee collection, all correspondence sent to a patient should be reviewed. Usually there is more at stake for the practitioner than the fee.

The risk management advice is: *Think of what might be prevented if a fee is returned and of the possible consequences if a suit is instituted to collect a fee. Do not let pride and principle interfere with making a practical decision. If you return a fee, insist that the patient execute a release-from-liability form.*

CURRENT TARGETS IN MALPRACTICE LITIGATION

The traditional problems leading to allegations of malpractice are still with us· ill-fitting dentures and extraction of wrong teeth. The ill-fitting denture problem is often linked with statements made by the dentist that constitute guarantees of satisfaction or serviceability (see the previous section, Guarantees). Most wrong-tooth extraction cases are the result of poor office practices and, in situations that involve oral and maxillofacial surgeons, with inadequate communication with the referring dentist.

Over the past several years new grounds of vulnerability have been discovered by patients and their attorneys. In addition, risks have increased because of the introduction of new and more sophisticated techniques into dental practice. New fertile grounds of litigation include the following:

1. Failures in treating problems related to the TMJ
2. Failures associated with implants
3. Failure to diagnose, monitor, treat, refer (particularly, periodontal disease and TMJ dysfunctions)
4. Failure to obtain the informed consent of the patient by not informing the patient of the risk of failure and its consequences (particularly endodontics and orthodontics)
5. Failure to take necessary precautions (rubber dam, use of assistants, etc.) to prevent mechanical injuries to the patient, such as aspiration of foreign bodies (crowns and instruments) and lacerated soft tissues
6. Continuing to treat when the dentist is aware that the result will not be satisfactory, for example, in orthodontics when the patient is not cooperating in home care
7. Failure to identify a patient with a compromised medical history, such as rheumatic fever, heart murmur, or allergies
8. Failure to take precautions to protect a patient having a compromised medical condition, for example, to prevent subacute bacterial endocarditis
9. Performing a service at the insistence of the patient that is not in the best interest of the patient and will not produce acceptable results, such as treating periodontal disease that should be treated by a specialist; the same holds true in oral surgical cases
10. Not performing a service, at the insistence of the patient, that should be performed before certain treatment is undertaken, for example, radiographs before any treatment and periodontal care by a specialist before fabrication of fixed prostheses
11. Failure to inform the patient about the risk of paresthesia after surgical procedures

12. Failure to provide follow-up care after surgery, for example, abandonment
13. Failure to consult the patient's physician when the patient's health is compromised.

The risks are significantly increased for failure to maintain adequate records or remain current with new advances in the profession. Deteriorating interpersonal relationships between patient and dentist or patient and office staff and attempts by the dentist to collect the fee may be causes of the patient seeking redress in the courts.

WHAT TO DO AND WHAT NOT TO DO IF YOU ARE SUED

If a patient threatens you in writing with a suit, if you receive a letter threatening suit from an attorney representing a patient, or if you receive a summons, the following precautionary measures apply.

Things to do

1. At the earliest time after receiving the letter or summons, report it to your insurance carrier by telephone.
2. Make a copy of the papers and send the originals to your carrier; use certified mail, signed receipt requested. Include a copy of any envelope that contained the papers.
3. Write a summary of the treatment of the patient using the treatment record to refresh your memory. Include all you recall, even if it is not on the record. Sign and date the summary.
4. Make a copy of the records, including radiographs, reports, and the summary. Lock the originals in a safe place.
5. Tell your staff about the suit and instruct them not to talk, without obtaining your permission, to anyone asking questions about the case.
6. Cooperate with your insurance carrier and the attorney assigned by it to your case.

Things not to do

1. Do not tell the patient or the patient's representative that you are insured.
2. Do not agree to or offer a settlement.
3. Do not agree to or offer to pay for a specialist's services without first consulting with your carrier or the attorney assigned to your case.
4. Do not alter your records in any way.
5. Do not lose or misplace any of your records.
6. Do not discuss the case, or the treatment of the patient, with anyone except representatives of your insurance company or the attorney assigned to your case.
7. Do not admit fault or guilt to anyone.
8. Do not contact any other practitioner about the case, even if the practitioner has written a report.
9. Do not agree to treat or treat the patient-plaintiff during the course of the action.

ON BEING A WITNESS

In a case alleging malpractice a dentist may be a fact witness, an expert witness, or a defendant. However, there are some general rules that apply to all who appear as a witness at trial: (1) dress properly, (2) do not be professionally arrogant, (3) face the jury when answering a question, (4) answer questions directly with either "yes," "no," "I don't know," or "I don't understand the question; please repeat it," (5) don't elaborate unless asked for a narrative, (6) don't be baited into an argument with either the lawyers or the judge, (7) wait before answering to give you time to think about the question and your answer and to give your lawyer time to object to the question, and, finally, (8) always tell the truth. A fact witness is at trial to recite the facts as the witness found them, not to render an opinion as to the standard to which the defendant dentist is held or to whether the defendant dentist departed from the standard. An expert witness is anyone who possesses special knowledge related to the issue at trial. Thus any dentist who is aware of the professional issues to be decided by the jury may qualify as an expert witness. The question becomes: How much weight will be given by the jury to the testimony of the expert? This in turn depends on the credibility of the expert. An experienced practitioner in the field, who has contributed to texts and journals, has more credibility than one who recently graduated from dental school, so the jury is likely to give more weight to the opinion of the former than the latter. Cases often end up as a battle of the experts.

The defendant dentist as a witness has a greater burden at trial than either the fact witness or the expert. For the defendant dentist much depends on the dentist's credibility before the jury. To be believed is the major issue. Not all that transpires between a dentist and a patient is recorded. Many facts in almost all cases are in dispute. Who the jury believes depends solely on who is more credible: the dentist or the patient. The credibility of the dentist depends on many factors as stated above in the general rules on how to be a witness. In addition, how the dentist conducts practice as described at the trial, the records kept by the dentist, etc., may influence the jury in accessing the credibility of the dentist. Many cases in which there is a legitimate question as to whether the dentist was guilty of malpractice are decided against the dentist on the basis of a lack of credibility notwithstanding lack of evidence for the jury to find the dentist guilty of malpractice. One major caveat that all dentists named as defendants where malpractice is alleged should be aware of is the following: tell your attorney everthing you know about the case—hold back nothing—and don't distort the facts to make yourself look good. The most damaging thing that can take place at trial is for the attorney to be surprised by some damaging fact that the attorney should have known about and should have been prepared to deal with and then finding out that the dentist knew about it all along.

AN EMERGING RISK IN DENTAL PRACTICE (NOT RELATED TO PATIENT CARE)

Employment practices litigation (allegations of discrimination, sexual harassment, or wrongful termination brought against an employer) is now the fastest growing area of commercial litigation. The Equal Employment Opportunity Commission reported settlements in employment practice–related claims in 1993 of $105 million dollars. It was up from only $35 million in 1991. The expectation is that future year's figures, when fully tabulated, will continue to set new records. Employees are becoming more litigious. Settlement and awards costs are skyrocketing. All employers in business, no matter how small, including dentists, can be the target of an employment practices liability lawsuit. Even an unintentional violation of the laws has the potential of placing the dentist's practice and future in financial jeopardy. Neither general liability, professional liability, nor workers compensation policies will provide coverage for these claims.

Federal laws that relate to employment discrimination include the following:

1. Americans with Disabilities Act of 1992
2. Civil Rights Act of 1991
3. Age Discrimination in Employment Act of 1967
4. Older Workers Benefit Protection Act of 1990
5. Title VII of the Civil Rights Law of 1964
6. Equal Pay Act
7. Rehabilitation Act of 1973
8. Pregnancy Discrimination Act of 1978.

Employment practices liability insurance coverage is available to dentists. Coverage may be provided for liability and defense costs for claims arising out of discrimination, sexual harassment, or wrongful termination brought by an employee, a former employee, or a prospective employee. Such practices may be both criminal in violation of the law or civil in violation of the civil rights of the person. It should be noted that policies of employment practices liability are limited to cover the dentist for cases brought by the employee, not by a government agency protecting the individual from such illegal practices.

Summary statement on risk management

Data obtained over a period of 10 years, 1982 to 1992, in New York relating to malpractice litigation indicate that 56% of the cases were decided in favor of the dentist. If the judge and jury are convinced that the doctor acted in the best interest of the patient, notwithstanding the injury to the patient, they will be likely to decide that the doctor was free of culpability.

The best advice that an attorney can give to health practitioners to enable them to enjoy a professional life free from malpractice litigation brought by patients is to be careful and caring in all they do. It is advice that is simple and short but goes a long way to prevent legal entanglements with patients and courts, should a lawsuit become a reality. Finally, the dentist should keep current on all laws that have an impact on dental practice and not break any of them. If in doubt, the dentist should consult an attorney before acting.

REFERENCES

1. Modified from PJ1 2:150. Malpractice—Physician, *Pattern jury instructions-civil, vol 1,* ed 2, Rochester, NY, Lawyers Co-operative Publishing.
2. *Riley v Weiman,* 528 NYS2d 925.
3. Louisell DW, Williams H: *Medical malpractice.* New York, 1988, Matthew Bender.
4. *Thor v Boska,* 38 Cal App 3rd 558, 11 Cal Rptr 296.
5. *Schwartz v Board of Regents,* 453 NYS 2d 836.
6. *Estate of Sandra Coert v Federal Insurance Company &* _____, DDS, 430 NW 2d 379 (Table).
7. *Bulman v Myers,* 467 A.2d 1353, 321 Pa.Super. 261.
8. *Hoffson v Orentreich,* NYLJ, June 21, 1989, p. 22, col. 5.
9. *Truman v Thomas,* App. 155 Cal. Rptr. 752.

APPENDIX A

Departments of the federal government

Although the department most closely associated with public health–related activities is the Department of Health and Human Services (HHS), there are currently 13 other departments in the executive branch of government. The other 13 are the Departments of Agriculture, Commerce, Defense, Education, Energy, Housing and Urban Development, Interior, Justice, Labor, State, Transportation, Treasury, and Veterans' Affairs. Although HHS is the primary department that addresses issues of public health concern and develops and implements public health related policy programs, virtually all the other departments are also engaged in various levels of public health–related activities.[1]

Department of Defense

The Department of Defense (DOD) is responsible for maintaining the health of members of the armed forces and their dependents.

Department of Veterans' Affairs

The Department of Veterans' Affairs (VA) maintains a large network of facilities that provide health services to eligible veterans. The Veterans Administration was established as an independent agency in 1930 for the purpose of consolidating and coordinating federal agencies created for or concerned with administration of laws providing benefits to veterans. In March 1989 legislation elevated it to cabinet-level status as the Department of Veterans' Affairs.[2]

The difference between the DOD and the VA is that the DOD primarily serves current and retired members of the armed forces, whereas the VA serves those with some service-connected disability who have honorably left the service.[3] The VA provides some dental care to eligible patients through its system of hospitals and absorbed 12% of all public expenditures for dental care in 1977. In 1980 the VA spent $6.2 billion on medical care.[4] In 1990 $12.6 billion was spent on medical care, with $138 million of that amount expended on dental care.[5,6]

Department of Justice

The Department of Justice along with another governmental agency, the Federal Trade Commission, has the responsibility for the enforcement of the federal antitrust laws, which have in more recent years been applied to health care providers. Although not often thought of by the public or even by public health practitioners as public health–related, the impact of the Department of Justice and the Federal Trade Commission on the public's health is significant. The Department of Justice in addition supervises the activities of the Bureau of Prisons. The Bureau's Health Services Division has oversight for all dental, medical, and psychiatric programs as well as for environmental, occupational, and food and nutrition services in federal prisons.

Department of Agriculture

The Department of Agriculture, although not often considered an important public health agency has, with its responsibility for the inspection of various food products, a major role in protecting the public's health.

Department of Transportation

The Department of Transportation is responsible for automobile, highway, and airline safety.

Department of the Treasury

The Department of the Treasury is responsible for the manufacturing and labeling of alcohol and tobacco products and the health of members of the Coast Guard.

Social Security Administration

The Social Security Administration, although not officially a department, administers a national program of contributory social insurance whereby employees, employers, and the self-employed pay contributions that are pooled in special trust funds. When earnings stop or are reduced because of death, retirement, or disablement, monthly cash earnings are paid to partially replace part of the earn-

ings the family has lost. The responsibility for the administration of the Medicare program was transferred from the Social Security Administration to the Health Care Financing Administration (HCFA). Medicare is a health insurance program for the aged, disadvantaged, and physically and mentally challenged. In 1995 the Social Security Administration was transferred from HHS to independent agency status in the executive branch of the federal government. The Administration is headed by a commissioner appointed by the President with the advice and consent of the Senate.[1,7,8]

Department of Health and Human Services

HHS has four major agencies under its jurisdiction. The Administration on Aging, the Administration for Children and Families, the Health Care Financing Administration, and the Public Health Service. The HHS budget is second only to that of the Department of Defense.[3,9]

ADMINISTRATION ON AGING

The Administration on Aging (AOA) is the principal agency designated to carry out the provisions of the Older Americans Act of 1965.

ADMINISTRATION FOR CHILDREN AND FAMILIES

The Administration for Children and Families (ACF) is responsible for federal programs that promote the economic and social well-being of families, children, individuals, and communities and is responsible for the Head Start program, which provides educational, social, medical, dental, nutritional, and mental health services to preschool children from low-income families.

HEALTH CARE FINANCING ADMINISTRATION

The Health Care Financing Administration (HCFA) is responsible for the oversight of the federal portion of the Medicaid program and has full responsibility for the Medicare program and related federal medical care quality control staffs. HCFA also administers the Utilization and Quality Control Peer Review Organization Program, which reviews services provided to Medicare patients to ensure that services are medically necessary, provided in the appropriate settings, and meet professionally recognized standards of quality health care.[1] Currently, HCFA serves 68 million elderly, disabled, and poor Americans through Medicare and Medicaid, approximately one fourth of the U.S. population. The two largest federal health care programs are Medicare and Medicaid, which account for about 80% of annual federal health care expenditures (which totaled $335 billion in fiscal year 1995). The remaining federal health care–related expenditures are divided mostly among the eight PHS agencies (22.4 billion), the VA (17.3 billion), the DOD ($10 billion), and the Environmental Protection Agency ($7.3 billion).[10]

THE PUBLIC HEALTH SERVICE

In 1995 there was a significant reorganization of the Public Health Service (PHS). Until recently, the Assistant Secretary of Health was in charge of the PHS. In the reorganization the Office of the Assistant Secretary (OASH) was significantly downsized and changed to the Office of Public Health and Science.[11] The OASH still reports to the Secretary of HHS but is now responsible for the coordination of interagency activities and no longer has authority over the PHS's eight divisions. Each of the eight divisions now reports directly to the Office of the Secretary. Although the new organizational chart of the Department of HHS does not indicate the existence of the PHS, it still exists in name only.[12]

The result of the reorganization appears to be a weakening of the influence of public health and public health staff within HHS and a strengthening of the influence of the social services staff. It has been suggested that because a good part of the blame for the failure

of health care reform was placed on high level public health staff in the department who had worked for its passage, the downsizing of the OASH and the cutting back of power was in part an act of retribution.

Since the formation of the PHS, which was created in 1789 to provide for "The temporary relief and maintenance of sick or disabled seamen," the federal government's role in regard to the health of its citizens has greatly expanded. From the singular role of responding to the health care needs of the many merchant seamen who arrived ill and unattached in American port cities, cities that had little capacity to take care of them, the PHS has grown to prominence as a federal enterprise dedicated to promoting and protecting the public's health.

There are three different sets of Congressional committees that authorize laws governing federal public health–related activities. These committees establish overall spending ceilings and appropriate moneys annually for program operations. The House Commerce Committee and the Senate Labor and Human Resources Committee establish many overall policies of the eight PHS agencies through the Public Health Service Act. The House and Senate budget committees set overall annual spending ceilings for all government agencies, including the PHS. The House and Senate appropriations committees and their related subcommittees approve annual spending under these ceilings.

Although public health and politics are often better kept separate, the reality is that the political environment in a society has a major impact on the value placed on the public's health and the funding and role of public health agencies within that society. When in 1994, for the first time in more than 40 years, the Republicans gained a majority in both Houses of Congress, one of their clear goals was to downsize government and limit the regulatory powers, activities, and functions of federal agencies. Between 1994 and 1996 the

Republican-controlled Congress with the acquiescence of the Clinton administration had begun to change the PHS and other federal agencies in significant ways. The first true casualty was the Office of Technology (OTA), which was eliminated. The OTA was a small nonpartisan agency created by Congress in 1972 to advise the legislative branch on important issues involving science and technology. In lieu of this agency, Congress will now depend on getting this kind of information from private sources, which may not provide as unbiased a perspective.[10]

The PHS* is charged with the responsibility of promoting health standards, ensuring that the highest level of health care is available for all U.S. citizens, and cooperating with other nations on health projects. It has always been charged with the following:

1. The physical diagnosis of the entire population
2. Setting goals for protecting and improving its health
3. Devising and initiating programs to achieve those goals
4. Measuring whether these goals have been met.[13]

The PHS's eight operating agencies are the Agency of Health Care Policy and Research, the Agency for Toxic Substances and Disease Registry, the Centers for Disease Control and Prevention, the Food and Drug Administration, Health Resources and Services Administration, the Indian Health Service, the National Institutes of Health, and the Substance Abuse and Mental Health Services Administration.[1,14]

1. The *Agency for Health Care Policy and Research (AHCPR)* was established by the Omnibus Budget Reconstruction Act of 1989 as the successor to the National Center for Health Services Research and Health Care Technology

Assessment. The agency is the federal government's focal point for health services research. It develops and disseminates scientific and policy information about the quality, effectiveness, and cost of health care.

2. The *Centers for Disease Control and Prevention (CDC)* is the federal agency charged with protecting the public health of the nation by providing leadership and direction in the prevention and control of diseases and other preventable conditions and responding to public health emergencies. Among its 11 major operating components are the National Center for Prevention Services, the National Center for Chronic Disease Prevention and Health Promotion, the National Center for Infectious Diseases, and the National Center for Health Statistics.

Among CDC's oral activities are dental infection control, community water fluoridation, oral health surveillance, oral pharyngeal cancer and tobacco-related issues, and support for state and oral health programs.[15]

In early 1996 CDC announced a reorganization of its dental program, which was indicative of the continuing diminution of the organizational status of dental public health programs throughout the country at the federal, state, and local levels. In this announced reorganization, what was formerly the Division of Oral Health was to lose its divisional status and become the Oral Health Program (OHP). The OHP would be located in the Division of Cancer Prevention and Control (DCPC), which is located in the National Center for Chronic Disease Prevention and Health Promotion (NCCDPHP). At the announcement of this change the director of NCCDPHP[16] stated that he believed that this transfer would "strengthen current oral health activities," a view that was not held by organized dentistry and most dental public health practitioners, who believed that the administrative demotion of the dental program would be deleterious to the public's dental health.[17]

Shortly after the announcement, the American Dental Association went to Congress, alert-

*The PHS as described here should not be confused with the U.S. Public Health Service Commissioned Corps described in Chapter 1.

ing key members to the shifting emphasis in government health programs at the expense of dental health. At the end of 1996 this effort bore fruit and CDC officials told the association that the OHP would be restored to divisional status in early 1997.[15] In addition, it was announced that CDC had received a half million dollars more and four new staffers to carry out its dental disease prevention activities.[18]

3. The *Agency for Toxic Substances and Disease Registry (ATSDR)* carries out health-related responsibilities in regard to the various laws relating to sites and the substances found at those sites and other forms of uncontrolled releases of toxic substances into the environment. The agency functions to protect the public and workers from exposure or the adverse health effects of hazardous substances.

4. The *Food and Drug Administration (FDA)* is responsible for protecting the health of the nation against impure and unsafe foods, drugs, cosmetics, and other potential hazards.

5. The *Indian Health Service (IHS)* focuses on the goal of raising the health status of Native Americans and Native Alaskans. It provides a comprehensive health services delivery system for both groups.

6. The *National Institutes of Health (NIH)* is the principal biologic research agency of the federal government; its mission is to use science in the pursuit of knowledge to improve health. Among its 19 institutes are the National Cancer Institute; National Heart, Lung and Blood Institute; and the National Institute of Dental Research (NIDR). NIDR supports and conducts clinical and laboratory research designed to understand, treat, and prevent the infections and inherited and acquired craniofacial-oral-dental diseases and disorders that compromise millions of human lives. NIDR staff conduct basic, clinical, and epidemiologic research. The three divisions in NIDR are the Division of Extra-Mural Research, the Intra-Mural Laboratory and Clinic Research Center, and the Division of Epidemiology and Oral Disease Prevention.

7. The *Substance Abuse and Mental Health Services Administrations (SAMHSA)* provides national leadership to ensure that knowledge, based on science and state-of-the-art practice, is effectively used for the prevention and treatment of addictive and mental disorders. SAMHSA includes the Centers for Substance Abuse Prevention, Substance Abuse Treatment and Mental Health Services.

8. The *Health Resources and Services Administration (HRSA)* has leadership responsibility in the PHS for general health services and resource issues relating to access, quality, and cost of care. It supports states and communities in their efforts to plan, organize, and deliver care, especially to underserved area residents, migrant workers, mothers and children, the homeless, and other special need groups.[1] HRSA, at over $3 billion, has the second highest annual budget of any PHS agency.[19]

There are several major components of the HRSA. The Bureau of Primary Health Care serves as a national focus to help ensure the availability and delivery of health care services in health professional shortage areas and to those with special needs. The bureau administers the National Health Service Core Program, which recruits and places health care practitioners for health professional shortage areas and populations.

The Bureau of Health Professions provides national leadership in coordinating, evaluating, and supporting the development and utilization of the nation's health personnel.

The bureau operates the National Practitioner Data Bank and the Vaccine Injury Compensation Program, and it supports through grants health professions and nurse training institutions, among which are grants to support dental public health residencies.

The Bureau of Health Resources Development has four major programs: the Health Facilities Program, the Organ Transplantation Program, the Division of HIV Services, and the Division of Trauma and Emergency Medical Systems.

The Maternal and Child Health Bureau develops, administers, directs, coordinates, monitors, and supports federal policy and programs concerning health and health care–related systems for the nation's mothers and children.[1,16]

Activities related to dental care in the PHS can be found primarily in the (1) Centers for Disease Control and Prevention; (2) Health Resources and Services Administration, Bureau of Health Professions; (3) National Institutes of Health, National Institute of Dental Research (NIDR); which carries out support programs of basic and clinical dental research; and (4) Agency for Health Care Policy and Research.[3,20,21]

Department of Health and Human Services Regional Offices

Ten regional offices of the Department of HHS serve all HHS agencies. The following are the locations and states within the jurisdiction of each region.[1]

No. of region	States in jurisdiction	Location of regional office
1	CT, MA, ME, NH, RI, VT	Boston, MA
2	NJ, NY, Puerto Rico, Virgin Islands	New York, NY
3	DC, DE, MD, PA, VA, WV	Philadelphia, PA
4	AL, FL, GA, KY, MS, NC, SC, TN	Atlanta, GA
5	IL, IN, MI, MN, OH, WI	Chicago, IL
6	AR, LA, NM, OK, TX	Dallas, TX
7	IA, KS, MO, NE	Kansas City, KS
8	CO, MT, ND, SD, UT, WY	Denver, CO
9	AZ, CA, HI, NV, American Samoa, Guam, Territories of the Pacific	San Francisco, CA
10	AK, ID, OR, WA	Seattle, WA

REFERENCES

1. Congressional Quarterly: *Congressional Quarterly's federal regulatory directory*, 7th ed, Washington, DC, 1994, Congressional Quarterly.
2. Office of Inspector General: *Inspector General semiannual report Oct 1, 1989-March 31, 1990*, No RC550-0568, Washington, DC, 1990, Department of Veterans' Affairs.
3. Wilson FA, Neuhauser D: *Health services in the United States*, ed 2, Cambridge, Mass, 1985, Ballinger.
4. Burt BA: *Financing for dental care services.* In Striffler DF, Young WO, Burt BA, editors: *Dentistry, dental practice and the community*, ed 3, Philadelphia, 1983, WB Saunders.
5. Deputy Assistant Secretary for Planning and Management Analysis: *Geographic distribution of VA expenditures fiscal year 1990 state, county, and congressional district.* Washington, DC, 1991, Department of Veterans' Affairs.
6. Floyd D, Director of Dental Policy and Planning, Department of Veterans' Affairs, Washington, DC: Personal communication, July 10, 1991.
7. Office of the Federal Register: *US government manual, 1995/1996*, Washington, DC, July 1, 1995, National Archives and Records Administration.
8. Barrett JK, Hubbard MM, editors: *Government research directory, 9th edition, 1996-7*, Detroit, Mich, 1996, Gale Research.
9. Greene JC: Federal programs and the profession, *J Am Dent Assoc* 92:689, 1976.
10. Inglehart J: "Health Policy Report Politics and Public Health," *N Engl J Med* 334(3):1 203-207, 1996.
11. US Department of Health and Human Services: *Office of Public Health and Science organizational chart*, March 11, 1996.
12. US Department of Health and Human Services: *Organizational chart*, March 13, 1996.
13. Sommer A: Viewpoint on public health's future, *Public Health Rep* 110:657-661, 1995.
14. Brandt E: The federal contribution to public health. In Scutchfield FD, Keck CW, editors: *Principles of public health practice*, Albany, NY, Delmar Publishers.
15. Palmer C: CDC oral health division to return. *ADA News* 17(21):1, 1996.
16. Marks JS: Letter from Director National Center for Chronic Disease Prevention and Health Promotion, Department of Health and Human Services, Feb 28, 1996.
17. Wyatt S: E-mail message, Division of Cancer Prevention and Control, Centers for Disease Control and Prevention, Department of Health and Human Services, Feb 20, 1996.

18. Palmer C. Oral health division comes out stronger: more funding, more people. *ADA News,* 27(21):20, 1996.

19. Sumaya CV: Oral health for all: The HRSA perspective, *J Public Health Dent* 56(1):S35-6, 1996.

20. Agency For Health Care Policy and Research: *AHCPR purpose and programs.* Public Health Service No OM90-0096, Rockville, Md, 1990, US Department of Health and Human Services.

21. Forward plan for health, FY1977-1981, DHEW Pub No (05) 76-50024, Washington, DC, 1975, US Department of Health, Education, and Welfare.

APPENDIX B

National resources hotlines

Alliance of Genetic Support Groups	800-336-GENE
American Academy of Pediatrics	800-433-9016
American Dental Association	800-621-8099
American Dental Hygienists' Association	800-234-ADHA
American Association of Orthodontists	800-STRAIGHT
American Board of Medical Specialties	800-776-CERT
American Cancer Society	800-ACS-2345
American Heart Association	800-AHA-USA1
American Lung Association	800-LUNG-USA
Arthritis Foundation Information Line	800-283-7800
Centers for Disease Control and Prevention National HIV/AIDS HOTLINE	800-342-AIDS
Centers for Disease Control and Prevention Sexually Transmitted Diseases Hotline	800-227-8922
Consumer Product Safety Commission	800-638-2772
Environmental Protection Agency Safe Drinking Water Hotline	800-426-4791
Multiple Sclerosis Association of America	800-833-4672
National Clearinghouse for Drug and Alcohol Information	800-729-6686
National Coalition against Domestic Violence Washington, DC 202-683-6388	202-683-6388
Denver, CO	303-839-1852
National Eating Disorder Organization	614-436-1112
National Headache Foundation	800-843-2256
National Heart, Lung, and Blood Institute's High Blood Pressure Line	800-575-WELL
National Mental Health Association	800-969-6642
National Oral Health Information Clearinghouse	301-402-7364
National Organization of Rare Diseases	800-999-NORD
National Safety Council	800-621-6244

Index

O

OBRA; *see* Omnibus Budget and Reconciliation Act
Observational studies, 122
Occupational exposure to blood-borne pathogens, 55
Occupational Safety and Health Act, 310
Occupational Safety and Health Administration (OSHA), 55, 310, 312-313, 317-318, 321, 340
Odds ratio, 123
OHI-S; *see* Oral Hygiene Index–Simplified
OHL; *see* Oral hairy leukoplakia
OHP; *see* Oral Health Program
Older adult; *see* Geriatric patient
Older Americans Act of 1965, 364
Omnibus Budget and Reconciliation Act (OBRA), 100
One-time visits, dental health education as, 191
On-site dental programs, geriatric oral health and, 100
Open and Closed Plan, 66
Operational phase of health program, 240
Opinion Research Corporation, 187
Oral candidiasis, 135-136, 307
Oral consent, 352
Oral diseases, community prevention programs for; *see* Community prevention programs for oral diseases
Oral epidemiology, 121-143
 of dental caries, 125-129
 of enamel fluorosis, 137-138
 importance of, 121-125
 of oral cancer, 133-135
 of oral manifestations of HIV infection, 135-136
 of periodontal disease, 129-133
 of temporomandibular disorders, 136-137
 of tooth mortality, 133
Oral hairy leukoplakia (OHL), 136
Oral Health 2000, 16-17
Oral Health America, 202, 204
Oral Health Coordinating Committee, 15
Oral Health Program (OHP), 366
Oral Health Status Index (OSHI), 68
Oral Hygiene Index–Simplified (OHI–S), 228
Oral hygiene instructions, 114
Oral injuries, intentional, 165
Oral physician, 26
Oral screening for cancer, 180-181
Oral self-care behaviors, 180
Oral-facial injuries
 sports and, 166, 167
 unintentional, 165-167, 168
Oral-pharyngeal cancers, prevention and early detection of, 167-169, 171
Oregon Health Plan, 293
Oregon Health Program, 19-20
OSHA; *see* Occupational Safety and Health Administration
OSHI; *see* Oral Health Status Index
Outcome measures
 of dental care delivery system, 35
 evaluation of dental plan options and, 65, 70
Outcomes
 measuring, program evaluation in health care and, 241
 program evaluation in health care and, 238

Outcomes assessment, program evaluation in health care and, 246-247

P

P. gingivalis, 133
Pacifiers, 110
Package inserts, risk management and, 356
Pan American Health Organization (PAHO), 11
Papanicolaou (PAP) smear, 355
Parameter, biostatistics and, 254
Parametric tests, biostatistics and, 266
Participation, managed care and, 37-38
Patient
 implied warranties owed by, 338-339
 risk to, from transmissible diseases, 314-315
Patient records, risk management and, 344-347
PDI; *see* Periodontal Disease Index
PDR; *see* Physicians' Desk Reference
PEM; *see* Postexposure management
People v Duben, 59
PEP; *see* Pregnancy, education, and parenting program
Periodontal attachment, loss of, 95, 130
Periodontal disease, 13-14
 epidemiology of, 129-133
 geriatric oral health and, 95
 measurement of, 130-131
 prevention of, 163-164
 tooth loss and, 133
Periodontal Disease Index (PDI), 130
Periodontal Index (PI), 130, 228
Periodontitis, 129-130, 131-133
 adult-onset, 130, 131-132, 133
 early-onset, 130, 132
 generalized juvenile, 132
 geriatric oral health and, 95
 HIV-associated, 136
 juvenile, 132
 prepubertal, 132
 prevention of, 163
 rapidly progressive, 132
 refractory, 132
Personnel; *see* Dental workforce
Personnel for Health Needs of the Elderly Through the Year 2020, 102
Pew Commission report, 26
Pharyngeal cancer, 133-134, 135
Physicians' Desk Reference (PDR), 356
PI; *see* Periodontal Index
Pit and fissure sealants, 114, 160-161, 202
Placebo, 124
Planning
 for community dental programs, 217-236
 alternative strategies for, 232
 definition of, 220-221, 222
 determining priorities in, 229
 development of program goals and objectives for, 229-232
 evaluation of, 232-234, 235
 implementation of, 232-234, 235
 needs assessment for, 221-229